Through a series of major reviews by influential scientists from Britain and elsewhere, this book details the contribution which nutrition research has made and continues to make to the health of man and animals. The volume has been prepared on the Golden Jubilee of the Nutrition Society and celebrates 50 years of nutrition research. Here the reader will find state-of-the-art chapters on energy and the major nutrients including vitamins and trace minerals and their influence on reproduction, lactation, growth and development. Research on malnutrition in the developing world and in Germany in the 1940s, together with the successful feeding of the British people during the Second World War, are discussed. The volume also surveys the impact of diet on human health today and the opportunities for further reducing the risk of major chronic disease.

THE CONTRIBUTION OF NUTRITION TO
HUMAN AND ANIMAL HEALTH

THE CONTRIBUTION OF NUTRITION TO HUMAN AND ANIMAL HEALTH

Edited by

E. M. WIDDOWSON
Formerly on Scientific Staff of Medical Research Council, University of Cambridge

& J. C. MATHERS
Department of Biological and Nutritional Sciences, University of Newcastle upon Tyne

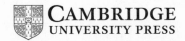

CAMBRIDGE
UNIVERSITY PRESS

Published by the Press Syndicate of the University of Cambridge
The Pitt Building, Trumpington Street, Cambridge CB2 1RP
40 West 20th Street, New York, NY 10011–4211, USA
10 Stamford Road, Oakleigh, Victoria 3166, Australia

First published 1992

Printed in Great Britain at the University Press, Cambridge

A catalogue record for this book is available from the British Library

Library of Congress cataloguing in publication data

The Contribution of nutrition to human and animal health / edited by E. M. Widdowson
& J. C. Mathers.
p. cm.
Includes index.
ISBN 0 521 42064 4 (hardback)
1. Nutrition.   2. Nutrition policy.   3. Health.   I. Widdowson, E. M.
(Elsie May), 1906–   .   II. Mathers, J. C.
[DNLM: 1. Energy Metabolism.   2. Food.   3. Health.   4. Nutrition.
5. Policy Making.   QU 145 C7635]
QP141.C743   1992
612.3′9 – dc20   92-8126 CIP
DNLM/DLC
for Library of Congress

ISBN 0 521 42064 4 hardback

Contents

Contributors

M. Ashwell
British Nutrition Foundation, 15 Belgrave Square, London SW1X 8PS, UK

C. J. Bates
MRC Dunn Nutrition Unit, Downham's Lane, Milton Road, Cambridge CB4 1XJ, UK

D. E. Beever
AFRC Institute of Grassland and Environmental Research, Hurley Research Station, Hurley, Maidenhead, Berkshire SL6 5LR, UK

D. H. Buss
Nutrition Branch, Ministry of Agriculture, Fisheries and Food, London SW1P 3JR, UK

P. J. Buttery
Department of Applied Biochemistry and Food Science, University of Nottingham, Sutton Bonington, Loughborough, LE12 5RD, UK

W. A. Coward
MRC Dunn Nutrition Unit, Downham's Lane, Milton Road, Cambridge CB4 1XJ, UK

J. H. Cummings
Dunn Clinical Nutrition Centre, 100 Tennis Court Road, Cambridge CB2 1QL, UK

J. V. G. A. Durnin
Institute of Physiology, The University, Glasgow G12 8QQ, UK

J. Edelman
55 Black Lion Lane, London W6 9BG, UK

H. N. Englyst
Dunn Clinical Nutrition Centre, 100 Tennis Court Road, Cambridge CB2 1QL, UK

S. J. Fairweather-Tait
AFRC Institute of Food Research, Colney Lane, Norwich NR4 7UA, UK

G. Fine
British Nutrition Foundation, 15 Belgrave Square, London SW1X 8PS, UK

M. I. Fiorotto
Children's Nutrition Research Center, Medical Towers Building, 6608 Fannin, Suite 601, Houston, Tx 77030, USA

J. M. Forbes
Department of Animal Physiology and Nutrition, The University, Leeds LS2 9JT, UK

D. R. Fraser
Department of Animal Husbandry, University of Sydney, NSW 2006, Australia

J. S. Garrow
Department of Human Nutrition, St Bartholomew's Hospital Medical College, Charterhouse Square, London EC1M 6BQ, UK

M. I. Gurr
Vale View Cottage, St. Mary's, Isles of Scilly, TR21 0NU, UK

I. C. Hart
American Cyanamid Co., Agricultural Research Division, PO Box 400, Princeton, NJ 08543-0400, USA

W. C. Heird
Children's Nutrition Research Center, Medical Towers Building, 6608 Fannin, Suite 601, Houston, Tx 77030, USA

D. F. Hollingsworth
The Close, Petts Wood, Orpington, Kent BR5 1JA, UK

A. A. Jackson
Department of Human Nutrition, University of Southampton, Bassett Crescent East, Southampton SO9 3TU, UK

W. P. T. James
Rowett Research Institute, Greenburn Road, Bucksburn, Aberdeen AB2 9SB, UK

D. Lister
CAB International, Wallingford, Oxon OX10 8DE, UK

A. Lucas
MRC Dunn Nutrition Unit, Downham's Lane, Milton Road, Cambridge CB4 1XJ, UK

I. A. Macdonald
Hillside, Fountain Drive, London SE19 1UP, UK

C. F. Mills
Rowett Research Institute, Greenburn Road, Bucksburn, Aberdeen AB2 9SB, UK

R. Passmore
54 Newbattle Terrace, Edinburgh EH10 4RX, UK

A. M. Prentice
MRC Dunn Nutrition Unit, Downham's Lane, Milton Road, Cambridge CB4 1XJ, UK

A. Ralph
Rowett Research Institute, Greenburn Road, Bucksburn, Aberdeen AB2 9SB, UK

P. J. Reeds
Children's Nutrition Research Center, Medical Towers Building, 6608 Fannin, Suite 601, Houston, Tx 77030, USA

J. J. Robinson
Rowett Research Institute, Greenburn Road, Bucksburn, Aberdeen AB2 9SB, UK

M. F. Robinson
42 Prestwick Street, Maori Hill, Dunedin NW1, New Zealand

G. A. Rose
London School of Hygiene and Tropical Medicine, Keppel Street, London WC1E 7HT, UK

D. A. T. Southgate
AFRC Food Research Institute, Colney Lane, Norwich NR4 7UA, UK

M. J. Stock
Department of Physiology, St George's Hospital Medical School, Tooting, London SW17 0RE, UK

J. C. Waterlow
15 Hillgate Street, London W8 7SP, UK

A. J. F. Webster
Department of Animal Husbandry, The University of Bristol, Langford House, Langford, Bristol BS18 7DU, UK

E. F. Wheeler
Centre for Human Nutrition, London School of Hygiene and Tropical Medicine, 2 Taviton Street, London WC1H 0BT, UK

R. G. Whitehead
MRC Dunn Nutrition Unit, Downham's Lane, Milton Road, Cambridge CB4 1XJ, UK

E. M. Widdowson
9 Boot Lane, Barrington, Cambridge CB2 5RA, UK

Preface

In 1941 the following letter was circulated to people in different disciplines involved in work on nutrition.

'Just before the outbreak of war a suggestion was made by several people interested in research on nutrition that a Nutrition Society should be formed. Owing to the outbreak of war the idea was abandoned. The question has, however, again been raised and there are a considerable number of research workers and others in favour of holding meetings to discuss nutritional problems. Such meetings would serve a useful purpose, especially in enabling workers studying different aspects of the same problem in agricultural and medical institutions to meet and help each other with information and constructive criticism'.

The letter was signed by Sir Joseph Barcroft, Dr Harriette Chick, Professor J. C. Drummond, Dr John Hammond, Dr L. J. Harris, Sir Frederick Gowland Hopkins, Professor H. D. Kay, Sir Charles Martin, Sir Edward Mellanby, Sir John Orr and Professor R. A. Peters. It met with an enthusiastic response, and a preliminary business meeting was held in London in July 1941. It was agreed that a Nutrition Society should be formed on the lines of the Physiological and Biochemical Societies, and the first scientific meeting was held in Cambridge in October 1941. It took the form of a symposium on 'Evaluation of nutritional status'. The Society has flourished, the original membership of 179 has risen to 1629 and in 1991 it reached its Golden Jubilee. To celebrate the occasion a symposium was held, again in Cambridge, on 'The contribution of nutrition to human and animal health'. Older and younger members were invited to present papers so that founder members could speak of their experiences in wartime and after and younger scientists could review the great progress that has been made over the past 50 years as illustrated by the subject of their research. This book contains the 35 papers presented at the meeting.

It has always been the policy of the society to concern itself with both human and animal nutrition, and this is evident in the contributions to this symposium. The subject matter is divided into seven sections; the first three deal with the metabolism of energy and nutrients. The fourth and fifth sections cover special situations, pregnancy, lactation, growth and the response of the body to energy and protein deficiencies. The sixth section deals with food policy in UK over the past 50 years and tentative moves towards an integrated food and nutrition policy, and the final one with the topical subjects of food composition, nutrition education and the role of the food industry.

In a three-day symposium it was impossible to cover all aspects of nutrition and health and, in particular, the complex and controversial relationships between nutrition and disease were only briefly touched upon. When the centenary meeting of the Nutrition Society is held in 2041, much of today's uncertainty about these relationships will, we hope, have been clarified. The resolution of these and other nutritional problems will require the concerted effort of scientists from many disciplines, with the Nutrition Society continuing to provide the forum for exchange of information and constructive criticism foreseen by its founders.

Elsie M. Widdowson
John C. Mathers
January 1992

Abbreviations

BAT	brown adipose tissue
BMR	basal metabolic rate
CHD	coronary heart disease
DAPA	diaminopimelic acid
DAG	diacylglycerol
DEXA	dual X-ray absorptiometry
DLW	doubly labelled water
DOM	digestible organic matter
DP	degree of polymerisation
DQ	developmental quotient
EFA	essential fatty acids
H	metabolic heat production (also hydrogen)
HDL	high density lipoproteins
HIF	heat increment of feeding
IGF	insulin-like growth factors
IP_3	inositol triphosphate
LDL	low density lipoproteins
ME	metabolisable energy
MRI	magnetic resonance imaging
NAN	non-ammonia nitrogen
NE	net energy
NSP	non-starch polysaccharide
PAL	physical activity level
PEM	protein-energy malnutrition
PL	placental lactogen
PRL	prolactin
PUFA	polyunsaturated fatty acids

RS	resistant starch
SCFA	short chain fatty acids
SDS	slowly digestible starch
SFA	saturated fatty acids
TOBEC	total body electrical conductivity
TRH	thyrotropin-releasing hormone
TS	total starch
VFA	volatile fatty acids
VLDL	very low density lipoproteins

Part one

Energy intake and expenditure

1

Control of energy balance in experimental animals

MICHAEL J. STOCK

Given the expansion in experimental research, and the almost exponential rise in the scientific literature over the past 50 years, it is clearly impossible to give a thorough and exhaustive review of all the developments in the understanding of the control of energy balance in experimental animals. Thus, instead of attempting to give a semi-historical catalogue of advances, the emphasis will be given to contrasting the shifting interest shown in controls operating on intake and expenditure, and showing how new ideas arose out of the imaginative and ingenious use of different techniques, species and experimental paradigms. However, the first problem to resolve is to decide what is meant by 'experimental animals' in the title of this chapter, and why they should be treated differently from the other animals (including humans) that are covered in the chapters that follow.

There is little doubt that the most studied animals are laboratory rats and mice (the Home Office statistical returns on animal experiments confirm this), and much knowledge of the basic mechanisms of energy balance regulation stems from these two species. However, as Otto Edholm once frustratedly expostulated, 'Man is not a rat!', and the relevance (or irrelevance) of rodent energy balance to that in humans has been a more or less constant refrain throughout the history of this Society. Similar 'specist' arguments have been heard coming from farm-animal nutritionists, and the rodent nutritionists have often found themselves caught between these two camps. Justifiably, the human and farm-animal nutritionists can point to the social and economic implications and applications of the research on their respective species. The 'rat nutritionist's' response to this is to draw attention to the use and relevance of advances in basic knowledge resulting from laboratory studies and to the fact that biologists should be concerned with species other than our own or the food we eat. Moreover, it could be argued that man is much more like

3

a rat than Edholm thought, and that energy balance studies on rodents can be carried out on much larger numbers, with greater precision and in more diverse experimental situations than on most farm animals.

It would be quite wrong to get the impression from the above that the only experimental animals that have been used for energy balance studies are rats and mice. Over the years, researchers have come to realise the value of choosing the most appropriate species for particular problems, and, in addition to the other common laboratory species (hamsters, guinea-pigs, rabbits, cats, dogs), researchers have turned to a variety of often unusual or exotic species to study certain aspects of energy balance regulation. Examples, such as the spiny mouse, edible doormouse, woodchuck, wallaby, kestrel and fruit-eating bat, exhibit the diverse energetic strategies available to meet a variety of nutritional and environmental challenges. If nothing else, they warn of the dangers of relying on a fixed, mechanistic view of energy balance regulation based on detailed, but largely empirical, observations on a few domesticated species. The possibility that humans (or some humans) may have a metabolism more akin to that of the desert spiny mouse, or the wild farm rat, than that of the domesticated farm pig, is one that is beginning to emerge from studies on a variety of experimental animals.

Research on energy balance shows a somewhat fragmented history due to shifting fashions in the emphasis given to energy intake or expenditure. In the early 1940s, there was relatively little work being carried out on energy expenditure in laboratory animals. This area was dominated by the farm-animal nutritionists (e.g. Kleiber, Brody and others), who were developing new methods and concepts that eventually were to be taken up by the small-animal researchers. On the intake side, however, the pace was being set mainly by work on rats. Adolph's (1947) observations on the constancy of energy intake in young rats fed diets of differing energy density set in motion a search for the signals, detectors and integrating mechanisms responsible for this apparently precise control. That search is dotted with important contributions from notable researchers such as Brobeck, Ransome, Kennedy, Mayer and LeMagnen, and continues today in the groups of Leibowitz, Smith, Morley, Sclafani and others. For much of the past 50 years these workers (mainly from outside the UK) and their ideas dominated our view of energy balance regulation, and it is only in the past 10–15 years that the importance of controls on energy expenditure have begun to receive attention, and this is mainly due to the efforts of British researchers.

Most researchers working with laboratory species would now concede that there is a complex interaction between controls operating on intake and expenditure, but it is instructive to look back to see why the intake theories of energy balance regulation were once so dominant and exclusive. One possible reason could be that investigators restricted themselves to measurements (often short-term) of food intake (often the weight only), without attempting to assess any of the other variables, such as metabolisable energy, body weight and composition, or energy expenditure. Many of these workers were behavioural, or physiological psychologists, and often displayed a naive, or non-existent knowledge of mammalian energetics. Constancy of intake was usually taken as evidence of energy balance regulation, but it is now known there are situations where there can be marked alterations in energy balance without changes in energy intake. One example is the golden hamster, that manages to meet the entire cost of pregnancy without any increase in energy intake (Quek & Trayhurn, 1990). Another example is the rat, which when tubefed varying fractions of its daily energy intake, adjusts its voluntary food intake to match that of the free-feeding controls – an apparently clear demon- stration of the rat's robust and precise control of energy intake. Unfortunately for the proponents of the intake theory, these tubefed rats are no longer in energy balance, and become obese (Rothwell & Stock, 1978). If the experimental approach of those workers studying energy expenditure is compared to that of those interested in intake, it is seen that the former invariably assess intake, as well as other energy balance parameters. Indeed, the comparative slaughter technique for estimating expenditure requires this, and the fact that it also requires measurements being made over several days or weeks means that the danger of placing too much significance on short-term, transient fluctuations or adjustments in intake is avoided.

If one is looking for significant changes that have occurred in the past 50 years, one of the encouraging trends has been the willingness to view and integrate information from both sides of the energy balance equation. Moreover, having contrasted the different approaches used by those interested in the control of intake or expenditure, it should be emphasised that, between them, they have produced a remarkable array of techniques, manipulations and situations for the experimental study of energy balance; most, but probably not all of these have been listed in Table 1.1. It should be stressed that many of these interventions are feasible only in small experimental animals, and some have been instrumental in developing current concepts of energy balance regulation.

The accumulation of knowledge obtained using these various models

Table 1.1. *Manipulation of energy balance*

Diet	Food restriction	*Surgery*	CNS lesions
	Feeding frequency		Vagotomy/sympathectomy
	Pair-feeding/yoke-feeding		'Endocrinectomy'[a]
	Pair-gain feeding		Lipectomy
	Nutrient composition/energy density		Portal/caval shunt
	Supplements (e.g. sucrose solutions)		Parabiosis
	'Cafeteria' feeding		Crossed intestine
	Enteral/parenteral feeding		
		Environment	Temperature
Activity	Running wheel/treadmill		Photoperiod
			Radiation
	Swimming		
	Housing density	*Pathology*	Infection
	Operant activity		Injury
			Cancer
Genetic	Inter- and intrastrain		
	Wild vs. domesticated	*Drug*	Central and peripheral agonists, and antagonists affecting hormones
	High vs. low gain		Neurotransmitters and enzymes
	Lean vs. obese		
	Diabetic and dystrophic		

[a] Endocrinectomy = adrenalectomy, thyroidectomy, etc.

means that we now have a very detailed understanding of the central and peripheral pathways and mechanisms controlling energy intake. Unfortunately, it is a very complex system, and far different from the original 'dual-centre' theory of hypothalamic control based on a simple reciprocal relationship between the ventromedial and lateral hypothalamus. The central pathways now involve over 20 discrete nuclei or areas, and over 16 different neurotransmitters, many of which involve interactions with several receptor subtypes. In addition to the central glucose-receptor and glucose-sensitive neurones, afferent information relating to feeding, digestion and nutrient influx arrives from a variety of peripheral sites, and also one has to account for the impact of other environmental (e.g. temperature, photoperiod) factors, as well as the social and psychological influences on intake. The amount of information is now so great, it almost transcends one's ability to assimilate it and place it in a coherent framework. Blundell (1991) has made a good attempt at this, but the interested reader who follows up this reference should be warned that it is still not easy to understand, in spite of its superficial attractiveness.

Some of the more fascinating advances in intake control relate to the role of glucocorticoids and the paraventricular nucleus in determining diurnal feeding patterns and nutrient selection (Leibowitz, 1991), and the link between plasma tryptophan, brain serotonin, carbohydrate preferences and mood (Wurtman & Fernstrom, 1976). However, this still leaves the problem of relating intake control to energy balance, and there are numerous theories that attempt to link the two. The most obvious are those based on indices of nutrient levels or fluxes – hence the glucostatic (Mayer, 1953), lipostatic (Kennedy, 1956), glucolipostatic (LeMagnen *et al.* 1973) and aminostatic (Mellinkoff *et al.*, 1956) theories. To these, one must add those based on some common currency of energy utilisation or availability. Thus, the list expands to include the thermostatic (Brobeck, 1948; recently resurrected in an unconvincing, and contrived fashion by Rampone & Reynolds, 1991), the energostatic (Booth, 1972), and a variant of this, with impeccable Greek etymology, the ischymetric theory (Nicolaidis, 1987).

Given a plethora of theories, all with a degree of experimental support and each capable of explaining certain features of energy balance, it is tempting to construct a control scheme that includes elements from all of them. This sounds a little like an intellectual 'cop-out' designed to avoid offending the proponents of any one theory, but it is not unreasonable to assume that any system for controlling something as important as energy balance will have multiple inputs, even though some may now be vestigial remnants of mammalian evolution. Biological experience also tells us that it is unlikely that the regulation of anything as important as energy balance would rely entirely on input controls, and the most efficient and precise way to achieve balance would be to control both intake and output. However, there is nothing like the equivalent of the various intake control theories listed above to explain the control of expenditure. Indeed, the prevailing dogma has been that, in most defined situations, energy expenditure is fixed, predictable and not subject to central, neural control.

The ability to partition and predict the fate of metabolisable energy has been the major aim of the farm-animal nutritionists, and their success in this is attested by the systems for feed and energy requirements they have formulated. As a result, most of the methods, terminology and concepts are due to them, and those working with experimental animals have had little to add. However, the nutritionists interested in large animals are restricted to a few, highly selected and notably efficient species, whereas the range of laboratory species and experimental situations (see Table 1.1) available provides the small-animal nutritionist with a much broader insight into biological diversity and adaptability. As a result, some of the more provocative ideas to emerge in the past 50 years have come from such studies as those on hibernators and cold-adapted, 'cafeteria-fed' and genetically obese rodents. One particular development concerns adaptive (or facultative) forms of heat production.

This is not the place to go into the details and evidence for adaptive forms of thermogenesis, such as non-shivering and diet-induced thermogenesis, or the role of the sympathetic nervous system and brown adipose tissue in energy balance regulation; these topics are reviewed in Trayhurn & Nicholls (1986), Stock & Rothwell (1987) and in a Nutrition Society symposium (Nutrition Society, 1989). However, as an interested participant in this area, the opportunity to make some general comments cannot be passed up.

Firstly, the existence of a variable, adaptive component, such as diet-induced thermogenesis, introduced into nutritional energetics the concept that apparently 'wasteful' mechanisms of energy utilisation could play an important role in energy balance regulation, although Kleiber (1961) had already coined the phrase 'homeostatic waste' to describe thermogenic adaptions to nutrient imbalances. Moreover, the same, or similar thermogenic mechanisms appear to operate in various catabolic states, such as fever, trauma, sepsis and cachexia (Rothwell, 1990). The concept of a 'wasteful', or thermogenic genotype complements that of the 'thrifty genotype', used to describe genetically obese rodents (Coleman, 1978) and humans (O'Dea & Hopper, 1991) which, at least in the rodent models, is mainly expressed as a thermogenic defect. It is worth noting that the physiological and biochemical basis of the thermogenic defect in both genetic and experimental forms of obesity is relatively well described, whereas a specific pathway or lesion has yet to be shown to account for the hyperphagia exhibited by these obese rodents. The importance of diet-induced thermogenesis was not fully recognised until the turn of the last decade, but resulted in a rapid expansion in research activity in the 1980s that continues today. However, what is difficult to understand is that, although British researchers led the world in this area, there was little recognition of their efforts in UK nutrition circles. As Trayhurn (1991) points out, it was not until 1988 that the Nutrition Society recognised the topic by holding a symposium, long after those organised by other UK and international societies.

The precise role and mechanisms of diet-induced thermogenesis and other adaptive forms of energy expenditure in the regulation of energy balance have yet to be fully elucidated, but the same can also be said for energy intake. In fact, it is now becoming obvious that the two sides of this balance operate through common, central (i.e. hypothalamic) mechanisms, and many of those theories of intake control mentioned earlier (glucostatic, lipostatic, etc) are probably equally applicable to the control of ex-penditure. Thus, the main challenge facing future workers is, having identified the afferent signals, central pathways and neurotransmitters involved, to produce a coherent, integrated scheme of energy balance regulation that accounts for the quantitative and temporal actions and interactions between the controls operating on intake and expenditure. This is a daunting task, but one that could be made much easier if the gene (e.g. the 'obese', or 'fatty' gene) responsible for the profound disturbances in energy balance seen in genetically obese rodents could be identified.

Finally, the contribution to the health and welfare of humans and other animals resulting from energy balance studies in experimental animals has to be considered. One has to extrapolate between species and the 'Man is not a rat' problem, by which one presumes man is neither a mouse, nor a dog, nor any other animal. Whilst recognising the obvious differences between animals, the distinction between humans and other animals is a dangerous form of 'specism' that (*a*) ignores common biological traits, and (*b*) opens the door to the anti-vivisectionists and similar groups who would argue that animal research has no relevance to humans. In fact, Edholm's 'Man is not a rat' exclamation resulted from the mistaken belief that food intake in rats was precisely controlled to meet physiological requirements and, unlike humans, was unaffected by social and psychological influences. However, it is now known that rodents respond much like ourselves to varied and palatable food (e.g. cafeteria diets, sucrose solutions) and stress (e.g. tail-pinch). They exhibit neophobia and social facilitation, and can even 'teach' each other to overcome aversion to unpalatable diets (Galef, 1989). In terms of expenditure, it is also known that the thermoneutral temperature for rats (29 °C) can be extended down to 18 °C if they are given the freedom to indulge in behavioural thermoregulation (Poole & Stephenson, 1977). These, and examples from other laboratory species, show that there are many more physiological, nutritional and behavioural similarities between experimental animals and humans than the 'specists' are aware of. While these similarities do not remove the inherent dangers of inter-specific extrapolation, they certainly justify the continued use of experimental laboratory species for research that is both basic and relevant to human health and welfare.

Recent examples include the development of serotonergic appetite-suppressant drugs for weight reduction which, as predicted from animal studies, also influence carbohydrate preference. Another is the development of the novel thermogenic anti-obesity drugs, which originates from, and depends on, studies on brown adipose tissue in rodents (Arch, 1989) and dogs (Holloway et al., 1985). This development also illustrates how research in an obscure area of rodent physiology (brown fat thermogenesis), which many considered pointless and irrelevant, had far-reaching consequences. It led to the identification of a third, or β_3-adrenoceptor (Arch et al., 1984), which has since been shown to exist in the human genome (Emorine et al., 1989), and has opened up many new avenues for studying the autonomic control of metabolism. Likewise, the 'repartitioning' effects of certain β_2-selective adrenergic agonists (e.g. clenbuterol, fenoterol) were first noticed (Emery et al., 1984) during investigations into the sympathetic control of thermogenesis. Notwithstanding the EEC legislative restrictions on the use of these compounds in commercial livestock production, they offer the potential for manipulating body composition in both animals and humans, and indicate that there still is much to learn about the adrenergic control of body composition. Finally, and for the future, there is intense research activity centred around the role of cytokines and other mediators in the hypermetabolic responses seen in animal models of trauma, sepsis and cachexia. Unlike some others, the relevance of these animal studies to the human condition is readily recognised by clinical colleagues. Hopefully this recognition can continue to be justified and they can be helped to develop a better understanding and new methods of controlling these debilitating conditions.

References

Adolph, E. F. (1947). Urges to eat and drink in rats. *American Journal of Physiology*, **151**, 110–25.

Arch, J. R. S. (1989). The brown adipocyte β-adrenoceptor. *Proceedings of the Nutrition Society*, **48**, 215–23.

Arch, J. R. S., Ainsworth, A. T., Cawthorne, M. A., Piercy, V., Sennit, M. V., Thody, V., Wilson, C. & Wilson, S. (1984). Atypical β-adrenoceptor on brown adipocytes as target for anti-obesity drugs. *Nature*, **309**, 163–5.

Blundell, J. (1991). Pharmacological approaches to appetite suppression. *Trends in Pharmacological Science*, **12**, 147–57.

Booth, D. A. (1972). Postabsorptively induced suppression of appetite and the energostatic control of feeding. *Physiology and Behaviour*, **9**, 199–202.

Brobeck, J. R. (1948). Food intake as a mechanism of temperature regulation. *Yale Journal of Biological Medicine*, **20**, 545–52.

Coleman, D. L. (1978). Diabetes and obesity: thrifty mutants? *Nutrition Reviews*, **36**, 129–32.

Edholm, O. G. (1973). Energy expenditure and food intake. In *Energy Balance in Man*, Apfelbaum, M. & Miller, D. S., eds, pp. 51–60, Paris: Masson.

Emery, P. W., Rothwell, N. J., Stock, M. J. & Winter, P. D. (1984). Chronic effects of β_2-adrenergic agonists on body composition and protein synthesis in the rat. *Bioscience Report*, **4**, 83–91.

Emorine, L. J., Marullo, S., Briend-Sutren, M. M., Patey, G., Tate, K., Delavier-Klutchko, C. & Strosberg, A. D. (1989). Molecular characterisation of the human β-adrenoceptor. *Science*, **245**, 1118–21.

Galef, B. G. (1989). Enduring social enhancement of rats' preferences for the palatable and piquant. *Appetite*, **13**, 81–92.

Holloway, B. R., Stribling, D., Freeman, S. & Jamieson, L. (1985). The thermogenic role of adipose tissue in the dog. *International Journal of Obesity*, **9**, 423–32.

Kennedy, G. C. (1956). The role of depot fat in the hypothalamic control of food intake in the rat. *Proceedings of the Royal Society of London, B*, **140**, 578–92.

Kleiber, M. (1961). *The Fire of Life*. London: Wiley, 454 pp.

Leibowitz, S. F. (1991). Neurochemical control of macronutrient intake. In *Progress in Obesity Research*, Oomura, Y., Tarui, S., Inoue, S. & Shimazu, T. eds, pp. 13–18, London: Libbey.

LeMagnen, J., Devos, M., Gandillière, J-P., Louis-Silvestre, J. & Tallon, S. (1973). Role of the lipostatic mechanisms in regulation by feeding of energy balance in rats. *Journal of Comparative Physiological Psychology*, **84**, 1–23.

Mayer, J. (1953). Regulation of energy intake and body weight: the glucostatic theory and lipostatic hypothesis. *Annals of the New York Academy of Sciences*, **63**, 15–42.

Mellinkoff, S. M., Frankland, M., Boyle, D. & Greipel, M. (1956). Relationship between serum amino-acid concentration and fluctuation in appetite. *Journal of Applied Physiology*, **8**, 535–8.

Nicolaidis, S. (1987). What determines food intake? The Ischymetric Theory. *NIPS*, **2**, 104–7.

Nutrition Society. (1989). Brown adipose tissue – role in nutritional energetics. *Proceedings of the Nutrition Society*, **48**, 165–256.

O'Dea, K. & Hopper, J. (1991). Obesity and non-insulin-dependent diabetes in

Australian Aborigines. In *Progress in Obesity Research*, Oomura, Y., Tarui, S., Inoue, S. & Shimazu, T., eds, pp. 645–648, London: Libbey.

Poole, S. & Stephenson, J. D. (1977). Body temperature regulation and thermoneutrality in rats. *Quarterly Journal of Experimental Physiology*, **62**, 143–9.

Quek, V. S-H. & Trayhurn, P. (1990). Calorimetric study of the energetics of pregnancy in golden hamsters. *American Journal of Physiology*, **259**, R807–12.

Rampone, A. J. & Reynolds, P. J. (1991). Food intake regulation by diet-induced thermogenesis. *Medical Hypotheses*, **34**, 7–12.

Rothwell, N. J. (1990). Neuroendocrine mechanisms in the thermogenic responses to diet, infection and trauma. In *Circulating Regulatory Factors and Neuroendocrine Function*, Porter, J. C. & Jezova, D., eds, New York: Plenum Press.

Rothwell, N. J. & Stock, M. J. (1978). A paradox in the control of energy intake in the rat. *Nature*, **273**, 146–7.

Stock, M. J. & Rothwell, N. J. (1987). Criteria and experimental evidence for luxoskonsumption. In *Recent Advances in Obesity Research* vol 5, Berry, E. M., Blondheim, S. H., Eliahou, H. E. & Shafrir, E., eds, pp. 124–130, London: Libbey.

Trayhurn, P. (1992). My favourite paper. *BNF Bulletin*, **64**, 58–60.

Trayhurn, P. & Nicholls, D. G. (1986). *Brown Adipose Tissue*. London: Arnold.

Wurtman, R. J. & Fernstrom, J. D. (1976). Control of brain neurotransmitter synthesis by precursor availability and nutritional state. *Biochemical Pharmacology*, **25**, 1691–6.

2

Control of energy intake in farm animals

J. M. FORBES

The situation in 1941

At the time of the founding of the Nutrition Society, very little was known about how food intake is controlled. Hetherington & Ranson (1940) had just published their observations on the effects of hypothalamic lesions on body fatness, and Adolph's demonstration that rats compensate for dietary dilution was soon to follow (Adolph, 1947). As far as farm animals are concerned, there was a realisation that ruminants ate more of a high-quality forage than of a poorer material (see Balch & Campling, 1962).

The last 50 years

Since the founding of the Society there have been great advances, including many by members, some first published in Abstract form in the *Proceedings of the Nutrition Society* and then more fully in the *British Journal of Nutrition*. Advances have stemmed particularly from work with laboratory animals, in which category the pig must now be included.

Simple-stomached animals
Dietary influence

Of necessity, there is a great deal of interest in the efficiency with which farm animals utilise their food in order to optimise economic returns. It is therefore not surprising that effects of diet quality on voluntary intake have been studied in detail. As is the case with laboratory rodents, both pigs (Owen & Ridgman, 1967) and poultry (Hill & Dansky, 1954) vary their intake inversely with the yield of digestible nutrients per kilogram of food. Further study showed that this compensation was not exact and that

13

there was a positive relationship between digestible energy concentration and intake of digestible energy. In commercial practice, fat is included in poultry layer diets, where maximum intake is required.

In the search for mechanisms involved in the control of food intake, the digestive tract has been of particular interest. Loading the stomach of young pigs with glucose solution reduced the rate of emptying to such an extent that gastric distension was thought to have been involved in meal termination (see Rayner & Gregory, 1989). Infusion of 38 g of glucose in solution into the duodenum of hungry growing pigs shortly after the start of their daily meal significantly depressed intake while prior bilateral thoracic vagotomy prevented the effect (Stephens, 1985), confirming that the feedback information in this case was via a neural link with the CNS. In view of the evidence from laboratory animals that the liver plays an important role in the control of intake (see Forbes, 1988), Stephens & Baldwin (1974) infused glucose or amino acids into the hepatic portal vein of pigs but failed to affect subsequent food intake.

In chickens also, infusions of nutrient solutions into the crop depressed food intake (Shurlock & Forbes, 1981a) and hepatic portal vein infusion of glucose or amino acid solutions reduced intake in a dose-dependent manner (Shurlock & Forbes, 1981b; Rusby & Forbes, 1987), these effects also being attenuated by vagotomy (Rusby et al., 1987).

Central nervous control

Intake control is centred in the brain, and most studies have used injections of neural transmitters or pharmacological agents which modify the release or action of these transmitters. In sheep, cattle and pigs, noradrenaline (an α-adrenergic agonist) injected into the hypothalamus stimulated feeding, agreeing with earlier observations with rats. Cholecystokinin (CCK) has been proposed as having a major role in the control of feeding, both peripherally and centrally. In pigs injected with CCK into the lateral ventricles at doses thought to be within the physiological range, based on concentrations of CCK found in human cerebrospinal fluid, a dose-dependent reduction in food intake was observed, cessation of feeding appearing to be similar to normal satiety, with no effect on drinking (Parrott & Baldwin, 1981). A CCK blocker given intravenously caused a dose-related increase in food intake during the following two hours (Ebenezer, De La Rive & Baldwin, 1990), suggesting that endogenous CCK is involved in the normal control of feeding.

Neuropeptide Y (NPY) is perhaps the most potent brain substance in stimulating intake. In the only reported work with pigs (Parrott, Heavens & Baldwin, 1986) 25 to 100 μg of NPY injected into the lateral ventricles stimulated feeding in a dose-related manner, the highest dose causing a 12-fold increase in the number of reinforcements obtained in the 30 min following injection.

There is evidence that the brain is sensitive to energy availability. Food intake was stimulated by cerebroventricular injection of 2-deoxy-D-glucose, which blocks the uptake of glucose into cells (Parrott & Baldwin, 1978).

Ruminants

Until 25 years ago it was considered that the amount of food eaten by ruminants was limited by the physical capacity of the digestive tract, especially the rumen, and the rate of disappearance of digesta (Blaxter, 1962). Balch & Campling (1962) performed experiments with cows, including inflation of balloons in the rumen, and showed the importance of the physical limit imposed on intake by the capacity of the rumen. The animals were trained to have access to hay for only 4 hours per day, however, so they had to eat a large amount in that period, which led to an over-emphasis of physical control. It is still thought that physical limitation of intake is especially important when nutrient requirements are high, as in late pregnancy and during lactation. Subsequent work has shown that there are some circumstances where intake is negatively related to digestible organic matter (DOM) content of the feed, implying a regulation of the intake of energy rather than bulk (Baumgardt, 1970). In view of the large amounts of short chain fatty acids (SCFAs) produced in the rumen there has been a large number of studies on their action as negative feedback signals. There are receptors in the rumen epithelium sensitive to acids, as well as tactile stimuli, and it was assumed that these are involved when infused salts of SCFAs are observed to depress intake (Baile & Forbes, 1974). However, de Jong (1986) said that such infusions raise blood sodium levels to well above normal and Grovum (1987) has pointed out that such effects could just as well be due to the osmotic effects of infusing salts, although osmoreceptors have not been identified in the rumen with certainty. Perhaps Grovum's emphasis on osmolality as a major controller of intake is linked to the fact that in some experiments water was withheld during the experimental periods. Drinking is a natural response to increased osmolality, and preventing this does not allow the animal to correct the disturbance induced by salt infusions. Access to water alleviates, to some extent, the intake-depressing effects of raised osmolality of rumen contents (Barrio, Bapat & Forbes, 1991). Clearly, further research is needed to elucidate the relative roles of acids and osmolality in the control of feed intake in the ruminant.

In parallel with studies on the role of the liver in the control of intake in simple-stomached animals, it was shown that propionate infused into the hepatic portal vein of sheep had a much greater effect than when given into the general circulation and that this effect was prevented by local denervation of the liver (Anil & Forbes, 1980). As propionate is taken up almost completely by the liver to be used in gluconeogenesis, the effect is similar to that of glucose in the rat and chicken. Although they are not fully understood, there are clearly mechanisms whereby intake of highly digestible feeds is limited by metabolic means before the physical limit to intake is reached, otherwise, there would be gross overeating of digestible nutrients when ruminants were fed on such diets.

However, any one treatment, such as experimental rumen distension or infusion of one of the SCFAs, has to be given at a level much greater than that occurring in the normal animal in order to depress intake significantly; intake could not be said to be controlled by any single factor. To test the hypothesis that feedback signals are additive in their effect on intake, Mbanya and colleagues (Anil, Forbes & Mbanya, 1987; Mbanya, Anil & Forbes, 1989)) infused acetate, infused propionate, and inflated balloons in the rumen of lactating cows in all combinations of treatments and found approximately additive effects on the intake of hay or silage. It seems likely, therefore, that feeding is controlled by a combination of small changes taking place in the digestive tract and in the body during and between meals.

The current situation

The Food Industry in the developed world is as much concerned with adding value to its products and satisfying customers' whims (often generated by advertising) as it is with satisfying nutrient requirements. To a lesser extent, the same is becoming true of the Animal Feed Industry, partly to disguise the use of unpalatable ingredients and partly to take advantage of animals' ability to control their intake of more than one nutrient at once, if given the chance. More attention is being paid to monitoring feeding behaviour as well as recording daily intakes, and feed intakes of individual animals, monitored automatically, are being used by animal breeders to select more efficient stock.

Flavour enhancers

In adult animals offered a single food, there is no long-term effect of manipulating the flavour of that food. However, there are some situations in which flavour improvement can stimulate intake in the short term.

Young pigs are quite sensitive to taste, and their preference for glucose or sucrose solutions increases with the logarithm of concentration in aqueous solution up to 0.1 M (Kennedy & Baldwin, 1972). The preference for saccharin solutions is not as marked, but Talin, a natural sweetener and flavour enhancer, increases the intake of food when it is included in the drinking water.

Talin, when included with other citrus flavouring agents in compound feeds for dairy cows, increased the rate of eating, especially when the compound feed contained bitter-tasting oilseed rape meal (Frederick, Forbes & Johnson, 1988). This is as significant to the farmer as to the cow because this product masks the change in taste occurring when one batch of compound is formulated with different proportions of raw materials from the previous one to which the cows (and the farmer) had become accustomed.

Choice feeding

Food intake is not always controlled in order to balance energy input with energy output, and intake is depressed by diets which are deficient in protein, essential amino acids, minerals or vitamins. Growing pigs showed aversion to a feed with an imbalanced amino acid composition compared to one with protein containing a balanced mixture of amino acids or a protein-free feed (Devilat, Pond & Miller, 1970). It took approximately 24 h for pigs to recognise an imbalanced diet which is consistent with a learned aversion to a feed which causes *Malaise*. It has been shown that pigs (Kyriazakis, Emmans & Whittemore, 1990) and poultry (Shariat-madari & Forbes, 1990) can regulate their protein intake independently of energy intake under these conditions, as long as they are given the opportunity to learn the differences between the yields of nutrients from the different foods. There is some evidence to suggest that ruminants can also make sensible selections from different foods, and that appetites for other nutrients can also be developed under the right conditions. Although there has been commercial interest in choice feeding before, the improved understanding of diet selection warrants a new look. Development of equipment to deliver two or more feeds from which trained animals can make selections will allow free-choice feeding to be used in farming practice to improve the efficiency of utilisation of the diet while allowing animals a more varied environment.

Automatic monitoring of feed intake

Developments in electronics have enabled robust equipment to be developed to monitor feed intakes by identifying animals as they eat and recording the size of each meal. For example, the system developed for cattle at Leeds (Forbes *et al.*, 1987) has now been brought up to date and is being used for nutrition research in Northern Ireland and for selection of breeding stock in Northumberland. Similar equipment is also available for pigs (Brown & Henderson, 1989). In so far as the control of food intake is concerned, such equipment has been used for individual animals and has shown that denervation of the liver, while not affecting daily intake, does result in fewer but larger meals, both in sheep (Anil & Forbes, 1980) and in chickens (Rusby *et al.*, 1987). This is evidence of an important role for the liver in the control of intake, denied by some who have quoted the lack of effect of liver denervation on daily intake.

Attempts to integrate current knowledge by means of computer simulation have shown that understanding of the control of intake is still not complete (e.g. Forbes, 1980; Ilius & Gordon, 1991).

The next five years

It is clearly impossible to predict what will happen to improve understanding of how food intake is controlled because research is, by its very nature, unpredictable. However, there are a few areas in which it is possible to speculate about developments; breakthroughs are not so easy to forecast.

Feeding behaviour

The use of automated equipment will spread and will allow us to study diet selection and feeding-related phenomena such as social dominance order (Rutter *et al.*, 1987).

Development of new hypotheses

Models of rumen function and metabolism will be incorporated in intake models as hypotheses of intake control arise to be tested. Most models of digestion and metabolism work on fixed iteration intervals and cannot be used in models which attempt to predict meal size and timing.

It is refreshing to have a totally new approach to a difficult problem, and such has been provided for intake control in ruminants by Ketelaars &

Tolkamp (1991). They propose that the intake of forages is not limited by their physical bulk but by their efficiency of utilisation. According to the authors' theory, the benefits from the nutrients becoming available through the digestion of a feed are balanced against the oxygen consumed in the assimilative processes. They point out that the predictions by the Agricultural Research Council (1980) concerning the relationship between dietary net energy supply and oxygen consumption on the one hand, and the level of voluntary feed intake on the other, show that the weight of feed eaten voluntarily coincides with the level of feeding which gives maximum efficiency. However, the shape of the curve relating efficiency of utilisation to yield of net energy must be uncertain at this point because, by definition, animals do not eat more than that amount so that metabolic studies cannot be carried out at such high levels of intake. In speculating on a possible mechanism for relating voluntary intake to efficiency. Ketelaars and Tolkamp suggest that intracellular pH could be monitored to fulfil this function. However, because pH is such a universal property it is unlikely to have an absolute role in the control of any single function, unlike specific messengers such as cyclic AMP. It is as yet uncertain, therefore, to what extent this interesting hypothesis will provide an answer to the problem of intake control.

Molecular biology

The use of antisera and specific agonists and antagonists has already led to some insights into the central nervous mechanisms controlling intake. The possibility of making such tools to order will allow a finer dissection of these mechanisms. The ultimate aim might be seen as the ability to manipulate the 'set-point' for intake control. However, as food intake is, to a large extent, controlled by the animal's requirements for nutrients, it would seem more fruitful to seek to control processes such as growth and milk composition. If large increases in production were to be achieved, animals would be pushed closer to their physical capacity to store and digest food and a better knowledge of the physical aspects of control will then become important. Significant stimulation of milk yield by dairy cows is now possible, using bovine somatotrophin (BST), and this is compensated for by increased feed intake, as long as the quality of the feed is sufficiently good so that gut capacity is not exceeded. This capacity is likely to be effectively increased in BST-treated animals, in which the potential to remove nutrients from the blood and gut is increased so that distension can become greater before the total of the various negative feedback signals is large enough to cause satiety.

Conclusion

Despite the large amount of research into this important field over the last 50 years, there are still fundamental gaps in understanding of what controls food intake. Progress will be made by pursuing studies in a range of disciplines and integrating the available information and hypotheses by means of quantitative models.

References

Adolph, E. F. (1947). Urges to eat and drink in rats. *American Journal of Physiology*, **151**, 110–25.

Agricultural Research Council. (1980). *The Nutrient Requirements of Ruminant Livestock*. Slough: Commonwealth Agricultural Bureaux, 351 pp.

Anil, M. H. & Forbes, J. M. (1980). Feeding in sheep during intraportal infusions of short-chain fatty acids and the effect of liver denervation. *Journal of Physiology*, **298**, 407–14.

Anil, M. H., Forbes, J. M. & Mbanya, J. N. (1987). Additive effects of acetate, propionate and distension of the rumen on hay intake by lactating cows. *Journal of Physiology*, **386**, 61P.

Baile, C. A. & Forbes, J. M. (1974). Control of feed intake and regulation of energy balance in ruminants. *Physiological Reviews*, **54**, 160–214.

Balch, C. C. & Campling, R. C. (1962). Regulation of voluntary food intake in ruminants. *Nutrition Abstracts and Reviews*, **32**, 669–86.

Barrio, J. P., Bapat, S. T. & Forbes, J. M. (1991). The effect of drinking water on food-intake responses to manipulations of rumen osmolality in sheep. *Proceedings of the Nutrition Society*, **50**, 98A.

Baumgardt, B. R. (1970). Regulation of feed intake and energy balance. In *Physiology of Digestion and Metabolism in the Ruminant*, Phillipson, A. T., ed., pp. 235–253, Newcastle upon Tyne: Oriel Press.

Blaxter, K. L. (1962). *The Energy Metabolism of Ruminants*. London: Hutchinson, 329 pp.

Brown, A. N. R. & Henderson, M. (1989). Development of an *ad libitum* food intake recording system for pigs. In *The Voluntary Food Intake of Pigs*, Forbes, J. M., Varley, M. A. & Lawrence, T. L. J., eds, Occasional Paper No. 13, p. 111, British Society of Animal Production.

de Jong, A. (1986). The role of metabolites and hormones as feedbacks in the control of food intake in ruminants. In *Control of Digestion and Metabolism in Ruminants*, Milligan, L. P., Grovum, W. L. & Dobson, A., eds, pp. 459–478, Englewood Cliffs, NJ: Prentice-Hall.

Devilat, J., Pond, W. G. & Miller, P. D. (1970). Dietary amino acid balance in growing-finishing pigs – effect on diet preference and performance. *Journal of Animal Science*, **30**, 536–43.

Ebenezer, I. S., De La Rive, C. & Baldwin, B. A. (1990). Effects of the CCK receptor antagonist MK-329 on food intake in pigs. *Physiology and Behavior*, **47**, 145–8.

Forbes, J. M. (1980). A model of the short-term control of feeding in the ruminant: effects of changing animal or feed characteristics. *Appetite*, **1**, 21–41.

Forbes, J. M. (1988). Metabolic aspects of the regulation of voluntary food intake and appetite. *Nutrition Research Reviews*, **1**, 145–68.

Forbes, J. M., Jackson, D. A., Johnson, C. L., Stockill, P. & Hoyle, B. S. (1987). A method for the automatic monitoring of food intake and feeding behaviour of individual cows kept in a group. *Research and Development in Agriculture*, **3**, 175–80.

Frederick, G., Forbes, J. M. & Johnson, C. L. (1988). Masking the taste of rapeseed meal in dairy compound food. *Animal Production*, **46**, 518.

Grovum, W. L. (1987). A new look at what is controlling food intake. In *Symposium Proceedings, Feed Intake by Beef Cattle*, Owens, F. N., ed., pp. 1–40, Oklahoma State University: Stillwater, Oklahoma.

Hetherington, W. & Ranson, S. W. (1940). Hypothalamic lesions and adiposity in the rat. *Anatomical Record*, **78**, 149–72.

Hill, F. W. & Dansky, L. M. (1954). Studies of the energy requirements of chickens. 1. The effect of dietary energy level on growth and feed consumption. *Poultry Science*, **33**, 112–19.

Ilius, A. W. & Gordon, I. J. (1991). Prediction of intake and digestion in ruminants by a model of rumen kinetics integrating animal size and plant characteristics. *Journal of Agricultural Science*, in press.

Kennedy, J. M. & Baldwin, B. A. (1972). Taste preferences in pigs for nutritive and non-nutritive sweet solutions. *Animal Behaviour*, **20**, 706–18.

Ketelaars, J. & Tolkamp, B. (1991). Toward a new theory of feed intake regulation in ruminants. Doctoral thesis, Agricultural University Wageningen, The Netherlands, 254 pp.

Kyriazakis, I., Emmans, G. C. & Whittemore, C. T. (1990). Diet selection in pigs: choices made by growing pigs given foods of different protein concentrations. *Animal Production*, **51**, 189–99.

Mbanya, J. N., Anil, M. H. & Forbes, J. M. (1989). Combined effects of intraruminal application of acetate, propionate and distension on silage intake by dairy cows. *Animal Production*, **48**, 639.

Owen, J. B. & Ridgman, W. J. (1967). The effect of dietary energy content on the voluntary feed intake of pigs. *Animal Production*, **9**, 107–13.

Parrott, R. F. & Baldwin, B. A. (1978). Effects of intracerebroventricular injections of 2-deoxy-D-glucose, D-glucose and xylose on operant feeding in pigs. *Physiology and Behavior*, **21**, 329–31.

Parrott, R. F. & Baldwin, B. A. (1981). Operant feeding and drinking in pigs following intracerebroventricular injection of synthetic cholecystokinin octapeptide. *Physiology and Behavior*, **26**, 419–22.

Parrott, R. F., Heavens, R. P. & Baldwin, B. A. (1986). Stimulation of feeding in the satiated pig by intracerebroventricular injection of neuropeptide Y. *Physiology and Behavior*, **36**, 523–5.

Rayner, D. V. & Gregory, P. C. (1989). The role of the gastrointestinal tract in the control of voluntary food intake. In *The Voluntary Food Intake of Pigs*, Forbes, J. M., Varley, M. A. & Lawrence, T. L. J. Occasional Publication No. 13, pp. 27–39, British Society of Animal Production.

Rusby, A. A., Anil, M. H., Chatterjee, P. & Forbes, J. M. (1987). The effects of intraportal infusion of glucose and lysine on the food intake of intact and hepatic vagotomised chickens. *Appetite*, **9**, 65–72.

Rusby, A. A. & Forbes, J. M. (1987). Effects of infusions of lysine, leucine and ammonium chloride into the hepatic portal vein of chickens on voluntary food intake. *British Journal of Nutrition*, **58**, 325–31.

Rutter, S. M., Jackson, D. A., Johnson, C. L. & Forbes, J. M. (1987).

Automatically recorded competitive feeding behaviour as a measure of social dominance in dairy cows. *Applied Animal Ethology*, **71**, 41–50.

Shariatmadari, F. & Forbes, J. M. (1990). Growth and food intake responses of broiler and layer chickens to diets of different protein contents, and a choice of protein content. *Proceedings of the Nutrition Society*, **49**, 217A.

Shurlock, T. G. H. & Forbes, J. M. (1981*a*). Factors affecting food intake in the domestic chicken. The effect of infusions of nutritive and non-nutritive substances into the crop and duodenum. *British Poultry Science*, **22**, 323–31.

Shurlock, T. G. H. & Forbes, J. M. (1981*b*). Evidence for hepatic glucostatic regulation of food intake in the domestic chicken and its interaction with gastrointestinal control. *British Poultry Science*, **22**, 333–46.

Stephens, D. B. (1985). Influence of intraduodenal glucose on meal size and its modification by 2-deoxy-D-glucose or vagotomy in hungry pigs. *Quarterly Journal of Experimental Physiology*, **70**, 129–35.

Stephens, D. B. & Baldwin, B. A. (1974). The lack of effect of intrajugular or intraportal injections of glucose or amino-acids on food intake of pigs. *Physiology and Behavior*, **12**, 923–9.

3

Energy expenditure: studies with animals

A. J. F. WEBSTER

Over the last 50 years most studies of energy metabolism with farm animals have concentrated on producing comprehensive and reliable sets of numbers and coefficients which can be incorporated into national standards for the energy requirements of farm animals (e.g. Agricultural Research Council, 1980). This short chapter cannot begin to consider the fine details of these numbers (but see Blaxter, 1989) and will, instead, concentrate on the development of biological and practical concepts underlying the continuing study of energy metabolism.

Traditional calorimetric studies with farm animals have measured two components of the energy balance equation and predicted the third, i.e.

$$I_{ME} = H + R_E$$

where I_{ME} is metabolisable energy (ME), H is metabolic heat production and R_E is energy retention. Research has taken two forms: 1) characterisation of feedstuffs in terms of their capacity to supply ME and 2) measurement and analysis of factors affecting energy expenditure (H). Characterisation of feeds is largely outside the scope of this chapter. Briefly, the UK has adopted Blaxter's (1962) proposal that ME constitutes a precise, measurable, operational definition of the supply of energy-yielding substrates to the tissues of a given species. Differences in the efficiency of utilisation of ME for different purposes (maintenance, lactation, protein and fat deposition, etc) are defined by coefficients (k_m, k_l, k_p and k_f respectively). Different national feeding systems based variously on ME or Net energy (NE) tend to differ in their estimates of energy requirement (Van der Honing & Steg, 1990) but these differences are not so much conceptual as a consequence of the experiments on which they were based (QV).

So far, therefore, farm-animal calorimetry has been extremely useful but largely empirical. Future developments in the science of energy metabolism require a progression from empirical to mechanistic models of the supply and utilisation of energy-yielding substrates (e.g. Gill, Beever & France, 1989), but only if they can ensure, at least, no loss of precision.

The three most important limitations of ME (or NE) as a description of the input to energy metabolism are:

1. It does not distinguish between different absorbed nutrients used for energy metabolism, e.g. amino acids, lipids, glucose, C-2 and C-3 volatile fatty acids (VFA), etc, so can only account for differences in the efficiency of utilisation of ME in an empirical way.
2. It cannot predict effects of substrate supply on the composition of milk or body gains.
3. It does not, in herbivores, distinguish between fermented and non-fermented sources of ME. This does not affect energy metabolism when considered in isolation, but precludes proper consideration of energy/protein relationships.

However, if complex mechanistic models of the supply and metabolism of energy-yielding nutrients are to be useful, they will always have to be calibrated against standards based on simple energy conversions (i.e. $I_{ME} = H + R_E$). The joule is likely to remain as the absolute unit of account, and values for the supply and turnover of individual substrates stated first in relative terms, then scaled to conform with I_{ME} and H as measured by conventional calorimetry.

Measurement of energy expenditure

Much of calorimetric research over the last 50 years has been devoted to the development and refinement of methods for measuring or estimating energy expenditure. All methods are based on the central, classic premise of Lavoisier & La Place (1783) that the heat production of an animal is quantitatively related to its respiratory exchange. The exact nature of this relationship has been reviewed by Blaxter (1989) and McLean & Tobin (1987).

The success of respiration calorimetry has largely removed the need for direct calorimeters. However, both share the constraint that the animal is confined, often in isolation. The choice of method for estimating energy expenditure under 'natural' conditions depends on whether one requires a dynamic or an integral method. For dynamic purposes, the most effective approach is to measure blood flow and the difference in oxygen content between arterial and venous blood. This is not easy, but new techniques for measurement of blood flow by transit-time ultrasound and *in situ* measurement of venous O_2 saturation by fibre optics oximetry have enormous potential (Giles & Gooden, 1991).

Over longer time periods, it is possible to estimate CO_2 production (and thus H after correction for respiratory quotient) from measurement of CO_2 flux (McLean & Tobin, 1987) either by continuous infusion of $^{14}CO_2$ or by single injection of doubly labelled water ($^2H_2{}^{18}O$) on the basis that ^2H is lost only as water but ^{18}O is lost both as water and carbon dioxide (Coward, 1988). The doubly labelled water method is expensive and inherently lacks precision but has the considerable merits of being both non-invasive and non-intrusive.

As one integrates over progressively longer periods (e.g. 1 year) then food intake and changes in body mass, suitably converted into energy units, become the most reliable indicators of energy exchange. Whether or not this is good news depends on one's point of view. All students of energy metabolism should be aware of the parable of the Narcissus and the Slob. The Narcissus, who, by dint of extreme self-absorption, restricts weight gain to 5 kg between the ages of 20 and 40 years, balances ME to H with a precision better than 1:1000. The Slob, who deposits 40 kg of pure fat over this time, still consumes only 1.3% more ME than he expends as heat. An error term of 1.3% may just be measurable in a calorimeter but not in conditions that could be extrapolated for 20 years. It is certainly beyond the limits of resolution of the doubly labelled water technique.

Analysis of energy expenditure

There have been four quite distinct approaches to the analysis of energy expenditure in animals. These are:

1. Whole-body variables; size, heat increment of feeding (HIF), activity, cold thermogenesis.
2. Substrate supply (carbohydrates, fats, VFAs, etc).
3. Energetics of specific reactions; protein and glucose turnover, Na^+K^+-ATPase dependent respiration (etc).
4. Organ and tissue-specific measurements of H.

All four approaches are necessary and complementary.

Whole-body analysis

This approach constitutes the majority of calorimetry over the last 50 years (Blaxter, 1989). Most workers now accept that the effect of size on H, both between and within species, can, as a first approximation, be scaled according to W (kg)$^{0.75}$. Under standard conditions in a calorimeter where activity and thermoregulation are minimal, H has been conventionally defined by basal metabolic rate (BMR) and HIF, terms which merely describe the intercept and slope of the line relating H (or R_E) to I_{ME}. These definitions are useful for practical feeding standards but have little biological meaning.

There are two serious concerns about the use of calorimetric studies to predict the energy requirements of farm animals. The first relates to ME requirement for maintenance. For example, most allowances for cattle based on calorimetry range between 450 to 500 kJ $ME/\mathrm{kg}^{0.75}$ d (ARC, 1980). Most estimates of the energy expenditure of cattle based on food intake required to maintain body mass over extended periods range from 550 to 650 kJ $ME/\mathrm{kg}^{0.75}$ d (Webster, 1989), a discrepancy rather greater than one would predict from the factorial approach which sums the costs of BMR, HIF, activity and cold thermogenesis. Differences between the energy expenditure of free-ranging animals and those confined in calorimeters have not yet been fully explained and will require not only more studies of H on free range but also a more complete, simultaneous description of a wide range of variables in the external and internal environment, i.e. not only temperature, wind speed, distance walked, etc, but also less tangible concepts such as anxiety and state of alertness.

The other major worry derives from the fact that measurements of k_f, the efficiency of utilisation of ME for growth and fattening, based on calorimetry tend to be greater than those based on comparative slaughter (Beever et al., 1988). This may be because calorimetric trials are usually based on short-term changes in plane of nutrition whereas in slaughter trials each individual in usually kept on one plane of nutrition for the whole of the experiment. The implication of these two observations is that many calorimetric trials may underestimate the ME requirements for both maintenance and growth in many farm animals.

Effects of substrate supply on energy expenditure

The notion that H is dependent on the composition of absorbed nutrients dates back to Rubner (1902). It is now possible to describe the energy losses associated with, e.g. the synthesis of fats, peptides, etc, from different substrates stoichiometrically (Milligan, 1971; Blaxter, 1989). These estimates agree reasonably well with *in vivo* measurements of k_f in animals fed balanced diets and depositing energy primarily as fat implying, in these circumstances, that synthesis equals deposition, i.e. negligible turnover.

Partition of the efficiency of retained energy between protein and fat deposition (k_p and k_f, Pullar & Webster, 1977) once again revealed a consistent pattern, although k_p (0.45 for pigs and rats fed a predominantly carbohydrate diet) is substantially less than the theoretical energetic efficiency of protein synthesis. This reflects protein turnover, although gives no indication of its magnitude since real biological processes like protein synthesis can only be partitioned arbitrarily between k_p and maintenance.

The longest running debate in farm-animal calorimetry has concerned the efficiency of utilisation of VFA absorbed from the rumen. The origin of this debate was the unquestioned observation that, in ruminants, k_f for forage diets is lower than that for cereals. Armstrong & Blaxter attributed this to the ratio of acetate to propionate in the end products of fermentation (see Blaxter, 1962). Ørskov was unable to reproduce their results, and in an equally classic and increasingly elegant set of infusion experiments lasting to this day, Ørskov & MacLeod (1990) have demonstrated no significant differences in k_f at acetate:propionate ratios ranging from 850:50 to 450:450. The most constructive attempt to reconcile these differences was made by MacRae & Lobley (1982). Summarising their argument over-simplistically, increasing the acetate:propionate (i.e. C2:C3) ratio will not reduce efficiency so long as there is adequate NADPH and glycerol-3-phosphate to allow the animal to convert acetate into fatty acids and triglycerides. Normally this would be provided by propionate, but if not, other substrates such as glucogenic amino acids would become necessary. This may stimulate substrate cycles and would certainly increase energy expenditure in urea synthesis.

Lobley (1991) has reviewed the interactions between metabolism of amino acids and energy-yielding substrates in ruminants. It is hard to escape the conclusion that the relatively low efficiency of the ruminant with respect to pigs and poultry is not only attributable to obvious things like energy losses during fermentation but also to the fact that the processes of ruminant digestion often generate a seriously unbalanced diet. The advent of improved techniques for the quantitative, reasonably precise, *in vivo* measurement of specific substrate metabolism in specific organs and tissues offers exciting possibilities for a new generation of good and useful science in ruminant metabolism.

Energetics of specific reactions

In recent years, as new techniques have become available, several attempts have been made to relate thermogenesis to specific metabolic processes.

A. J. F. Webster

Table 3.1. *Estimates of the contribution of different metabolic processes to visceral and whole-body thermogenesis in sheep*

	Proportion of total O_2 consumption (J/kJ)	
	Gut + liver	Whole body
Metabolism in gut and liver		
Protein synthesis	177	71
Protein degradation	68	27
Na^+K^+-ATPase	255	102
Substrate cycling	90	36
Urea synthesis	125	50
Total	715	286

From Huntington & McBride, 1988.

Estimates by Huntington & McBride (1988), summarised in Table 3.1, account for 715 J/kJ *H* within the gut and liver of sheep, the principal contributors being protein turnover (synthesis plus degradation) 245 J/kJ and Na^+K^+-ATPase dependent respiration 255 J/kJ. Their results also imply that *H* in gut and liver contributes 400 J/kJ (286/0.715) to total *H*. This overall result agrees well with direct measurements of *H* in the gut and liver (q.v.) but the individual values, based largely but not entirely on *in vitro* studies, need to be treated with some caution. Discrepancies between *in vitro* and *in vivo* measurements of *H* are well recognised. More seriously, Coulson & Herbert (1981) have stressed the absurdity that, when *in vitro* measurements of *H* are compared on a between-species basis, *H* is proportional to tissue mass$^{1.0}$, not mass$^{0.75}$. Between-species comparisons of *in vitro* H can give estimates that are ludicrously at variance with the concept of metabolic body size ($W^{0.75}$). This reflects the fact that metabolic rates *in vivo* are constrained less by the capacity of enzymes to drive reactions in an ideal medium than by the rate at which the circulation can supply substrates and support tissue respiration.

Organ thermogenesis

The classical approach to the measurement of organ thermogenesis *in vivo* is to measure blood flow and the arterio-venous difference in O_2 concentration, $\Delta[O_2]$. Recent *in vivo* measurements summarised by Huntington & McBride (1988) suggest that, in sheep, the portal-drained viscera and liver contribute, on average, respectively 20 and 25% to whole body thermogenesis. Since it is known that the mass of these metabolically hyperactive tissues changes greatly with changes in plane of nutrition, it follows that they must make a far greater contribution to HIF. Koong, Farrell & Nienaber (1985) confirmed this hypothesis in an elegant experiment which compared weights of gut and liver and BMR in pigs reared to 40 kg on low:high (LH) and high:low (HL) planes of nutrition. On average, the ratios (LH:HL) were 1.36 for gut and liver weight and 1.41 for BMR, despite the fact that the viscera only contributed about 4.4 and 5.9% to total body mass in the two groups.

These large differences are consistent with the assumption that gut and liver contribute about 40% to total *H*. Very recently, Taylor & Murray (1991) have been able to relate differences in maintenance *H* of cattle associated both with genotype and plane of nutrition to differences in the relative weights of different organs. It is possible (although unnecessary) to speculate that *all* the observed differences in *H* can be related to organ mass, i.e. thermogenesis per unit mass within each organ remains the same.

Resynthesis of whole-animal thermogenesis

Having analysed thermogenesis in four different, complementary ways, an attempt must be made to reassemble the pieces, not in the expectation of creating a grand, mechanistic model of energy exchanges in farm animals, but to examine where the last 50 years of research have got to and what happens next.

It is probably fair to conclude that, for simple-stomached species, pigs and poultry, measurements of *ME* and *NE* in feedstuffs are nearing the practical limits of refinement. For ruminants, however, there remain substantial areas of uncertainty relating to differences in *NE*, e.g. between forages and concentrates and between forages harvested at different seasons. If these are to be predicted in a practically reliable way a satisfactory mechanistic explanation is needed that incorporates differences in the work of digestion (eating, fermentation, etc – see Webster, 1989), differences in visceral mass attributable both to quantity and quality of diet, differences in substrate supply and differences in substrate cycling. These are not mutually exclusive.

The extent to which thermogenesis is determined by the partition of retained nutrients into protein, fat (and lactose) in body tissues and milk has been reasonably well defined, although only in an empirical way. It is possible to construct models which predict the destination of energy-

Table 3.2. *Intake* (ME) *and expenditure* (H) *of energy* $(kJ/kg\ W^{0.75}$ per day) *by man and animals during growth, lactation and different forms of labour*

	Energy exchange (kJ/kg $W^{0.75}$ per d)	
Work and species[a]	ME	H
Labour, man,		
clerk	520	520
miner	625	625
cyclist (*Tour de France*)	985	1510
herbivores, on range	700	700
passerine birds, feeding young	1580	1580
Growth, pig (20 kg)	1200	800
broiler fowl (2 kg)	1000	600
Lactation, dairy cow (35 l/day)	1860	1020
sow (12 piglets)	1680	900
woman (one child)	720	590

[a] Original references given in Webster (1988) except for the cyclist (Westerterp *et al.*, 1986).

yielding and other substrates (Gill *et al.*, 1989; Oldham & Emmans, 1989), but these have yet to be tested by large-scale experimentation.

The major area of uncertainty relates to those aspects of thermogenesis which cannot be attributed to size (as defined by $W^{0.75}$) or to the quantity and quality of the feed (i.e. HIF). There are clear, substantial differences in maintenance H between confined and free-living animals that are inadequately described by summing the predicted effects of environmental variables such as distance walked, air temperature, etc. It may be possible to explain the large differences in 'maintenance' attributable to sex or genotype by: 1) differences in 'activity' (broadly defined to include such things as alertness) and 2) differences in the relative mass of the major organs and tissues having different metabolic rates.

Finally, since farm animals are sentient creatures and not just heat engines, it is appropriate to ask just how much work we should expect of them. Table 3.2, updated from Webster (1988), compares 24-h energy expenditure (kJ/kg $W^{0.75}$ d) in man, free-living animals and domestic animals engaged in the work of growth and lactation. Growth in intensively reared domestic animals is comparable to energy costs of maintenance for an animal on fairly extensive free-range or heavy manual labour for man (forestry). Lactation, even given the quantitatively modest yield of the human female, carries a work load intermediate between that of the miner and the forester. For the high-yielding dairy cow, the sustained energy demands of lactation exceed almost everything but the frenetic (and transient) activities of passerine birds feeding their young or cyclists engaged in that unique act of masochism, the *Tour de France* (Westerterp *et al.*, 1986). It is not surprising therefore that many of the serious production diseases of cattle can be linked to the high metabolic demands of lactation. Energy metabolism is only a part (a big part) of the contribution of nutrition to human and animal health. It can, however, be used, in part, to quantify not only the efficiency of conversion of animal feed into animal produce, but also the acceptable bounds of humanity in the pursuit of this end.

References

Agricultural Research Council (1980). *The Nutrient Requirements of Farm Livestock, No. 2. Ruminants.* 2nd edn. Farnham Royal: Commonwealth Agriculture Bureau.

Beever, D. E., Cammell, S. B., Thomas, C., Spooner, M. C., Haines, M. J. & Gale, D. L. (1988). The effect of date of cut and barley substitution on gain and on the efficiency of utilisation of grass silage by grazing cattle. 2. Nutrient supply and energy partition. *British Journal of Nutrition*, **60**, 307–19.

Blaxter, K. L. (1962). *The Energy Metabolism of Ruminants.* Hutchinson, London.

Blaxter, K. L. (1989). *Energy Metabolism in Animals and Man.* Cambridge: Cambridge University Press.

Coulson, R. A. & Herbert, J. D. (1981). Relationship between metabolic rate and various physiological and biochemical parameters. A comparison of alligator, man and shrew. *Comparative Biochemistry and Physiology*, **69**, 1–13.

Coward, W. A. (1988). The doubly-labelled water ($^2H_2{}^{18}O$) method: principles and practice. *Proceedings of the Nutrition Society*, **47**, 209–18.

Giles, L. R. & Gooden, J. M. (1991). New approaches to the measurement of energy expenditure in pigs. *Recent Advances in Animal Nutrition in Australia*, pp. 215–220, Armidale: University of New England.

Gill, M., Beever, D. E. & France, J. (1989). Biochemical bases needed for the mathematical representation of whole animal metabolism. *Nutrition Research Reviews*, **2**, 181–200.

Huntington, G. B. & McBride, B. W. (1988). Ruminant splanchnic tissues: energy costs of absorption and net metabolism. In *Biomechanisms regulating growth and development*, Steffens, G. L. & Rumsey, T. S., eds, pp. 313–328, Boston: Kluwer.

Koong, L. J., Farrell, C. L. & Nienaber, J. A. (1985). Assessment of the interrelationships among levels of intake and production, organ size and fasting heat production in growing animals. *Journal of Nutrition*, **115**, 1383–90.

Lavoisier, A. L. & La Place, P. S. (1783). Memoire sur la chaleur. *Memoires de l'Academie des Sciences*, pp. 494–531.

Lobley, G. E. (1991). The importance of interactions on protein and amino acid metabolism. *Proceedings of 6th International Symposium, Protein and Metabolism.* EAAP Publ. No. 59, pp. 66–79.

McLean, J. A. & Tobin, G. (1987). *Animal and Human Calorimetry*. Cambridge: Cambridge University Press.

MacRae, J. C. & Lobley, G. E. (1982). Some factors which influence thermal energy losses during the metabolism of ruminants. *Livestock Production Science*, **9**, 447–56.

Milligan, L. P. (1971). Energetic efficiency and metabolic transformations. *Federation Proceedings*, **30**, 1454–8.

Oldham, J. D. & Emmans, G. C. (1989). Prediction of responses to required nutrients in dairy cows. *Journal of Dairy Science*, **72**, 3212–29.

Ørskov, E. R. & MacLeod, N. A. (1990). Dietary-induced thermogenesis and feed evaluation in ruminants. *Proceedings of the Nutrition Society* **49**, 227–37.

Pullar, J. D. & Webster, A. J. F. (1977). The energy costs of protein and fat deposition in the rat. *British Journal of Nutrition*, **37**, 355–63.

Rubner, M. (1902). *Die Gesetze des Energie verbrauchs bei de Ernahrung.* Leipzig, p. 109.

Taylor, St. C. S. & Murray, J. T. (1991). Effect of feeding level, breed and milking potential on body tissues and organs of mature, non-lactating cows. *Animal Production*, **53**, 27–38.

Van der Honing, Y. & Steg, A. (1990). Comparisons of energy evaluation systems of feeds for ruminants. In *Feedstuff Evaluation*, Wiseman, J. & Cole, D. J. A. eds, pp. 1–20, London: Butterworths.

Webster, A. J. F. (1988). Comparative aspects of the energy exchange. In *Comparative Nutrition*, Blaxter, K. L. & MacDonald, I., eds, pp. 37–53, London: Libbey.

Webster, A. J. F. (1989). Bioenergetics, bioengineering and growth. *Animal Production*, **48**, 249–69.

Westerterp, K. R., Saris, W. H. M., Van Es, A. & Ten Hoor, R. (1986). Use of the doubly-labelled water technique in humans during heavy sustained exercise. *Journal of Applied Physiology*, **61**, 2162–7.

4

Energy expenditure of man: earlier studies

R. PASSMORE

I am going to discuss experimental techniques, field surveys, committees and the general climate of opinion with all of which I was concerned 35 to 50 years ago. This period can now be considered as a sort of twilight zone. It is certainly not current affairs but I do not like to think of it as history. Throughout this period the main concern of nutritionists was with the insufficiency of the food supply in almost all countries. World War II had curtailed food production throughout Europe and in many other parts of the world and, more importantly, had destroyed much of the transport needed for its distribution. After the war had ended, there were not the ships to carry grain from the granaries in North America and Australia to Europe. In the United Kingdom, people had accepted rationing of butcher's meat, bacon, milk, cheese, sugar and fats as necessary for the country's survival in wartime and looked forward to the removal of these restrictions when hostilities ceased. Instead, they were subjected, for the first time, to bread rationing in 1946, and in 1947 to potato rationing owing to a partial collapse of the crop. Housewives had greater difficulty in finding sufficient foods to feed their families during the winter of 1947–48 than at any time during the war. It was not until 1953 that all rationing was removed. In the early days of our Society, food requirements in relation to energy demands was a prime concern for both housewives and nutritional scientists.

The validity of calculating rates of energy expenditure from measurements of oxygen consumption (indirect calorimetry) had been established in 1899 using the Atwater–Rosa human calorimeter (Atwater & Benedict, 1899). Thereafter, rates over short periods under laboratory conditions were readily determined using the Douglas bag and Haldane gas analysis apparatus, but studies under field conditions were limited by the Douglas bag being cumbersome and only usable for short periods. All estimates of

33

human energy requirements were based on measurements of energy intake in food. In 1940, a light portable apparatus for measuring the respiratory exchanges was described by two Hungarians (Kofranyi & Michaelis 1941). This consisted of a dry gas meter which automatically measured the volume of the expired air and, at the same time, collected an aliquot sample. This sample, in volume from 0.2 to 0.7% of the air passing through the meter, was stored in a rubber bag and was available for analysis.

The apparatus weighed less than 4 kg and could be carried on the back like a haversack. It was used in wartime Germany, where it was renamed the Max Plank respirometer, to measure energy expenditure during whole shifts of work in factories and mines (Lehmann, Müller & Spitzer, 1950). The findings of their surveys were considered in allocating rations to industrial workers. But the Germans studied rates of energy expenditure only during occupational work and not in the home and during recreational activities. After the war, British workers measured, for the first time, rates for men and women over whole 7-day periods, whilst they carried out their normal daily life. The groups studied were coal miners and colliery clerks in Fife, military cadets at Sandhurst and middle-aged housewives and their working daughters in Glasgow. Before discussing the findings of these surveys, and the use of the results, let us consider how these results were obtained.

Hugh Magee initiated his work when, soon after hostilities had ceased, he went to Germany as a nutritionist on the staff of the Ministry of Health and brought back to London a Kofranyi-Michaelis respirometer or KM as we called it. Hugh was an old friend of mine. We had first met in 1936 on a cruise down the Volga to Stalingrad with our wives, and also with Hugh Sinclair, after attending the 15th International Congress of Physiology in Leningrad. Hugh was a good-hearted Ulsterman, a Catholic who remained, throughout his life, attached to the family farm in County Down. He was, when we first met, physiologist at the Rowett Institute under John Boyd Orr. At a meeting of the Physiological Society after the war he told me that he had a KM in his office and asked if I would like to have it in Edinburgh to see if it worked. These two chance meetings with Hugh determined a great part of my professional life. In Edinburgh, we soon found that under laboratory conditions we got the same results using the KM as with Douglas bags.

This technical development, coming at a time when there was much general interest in whether or not people in this country were getting enough to eat, led the Medical Research Council to appoint in 1951 a Diet and Energy Committee. The Committee decided that, for a reassessment of energy demands on workers, studies should include both dietary investigations and a detailed examination of energy expenditure throughout the entire 24 hours. The Committee was made up of R. C. Garry (Chairman), G. P. Crowden, D. J. C. Cunningham, D. P. Cuthbertson, C. G. Douglas, O. G. Edholm, A. Hemingway, Esther M. Killick, H. E. Magee, J. B. de V. Weir and R. Passmore (Secretary). It was a group of human physiologists interested in exercise and nutrition. The absence of the names of R. A. McCance and Elsie M. Widdowson was due to their being then heavily engaged in Wuppertal on their classical study of the state of nutrition of the hungry people in post-war Germany.

The first task of the Committee was to organise a pilot study in which food intake and energy expenditure would be measured over several days in subjects living an artificially controlled life. This was carried out in Edinburgh on five male medical students who slept and were fed in the University's Department of Public Health for 13 days. During the first 3 and last 5 days they led a sedentary life and did not leave the building except on a few occasions to go on small errands. In the intermediate 5 days they walked up to 20 miles daily on a track at the University sports ground. Overall energy expenditure was calculated from a minute by minute record of activities, kept by each subject in a small notebook, and from over 30 measurements on each subject of the cost of activities. Over the 13 days there was for each subject a satisfactory agreement between the estimated energy expenditure and the energy value of the food eaten (Passmore, Thomson & Warnock, 1952). This result encouraged the Committee to go on to support field surveys.

The Chairman of the Committee, Robert Garry, who was Professor of Physiology in Glasgow, sent over to Edinburgh on one or two days a young medical graduate who had recently joined his department to observe this pilot study. This was my introduction to John Durnin 40 years ago, and may be said to be the start of his distinguished career.

Robert Garry was a pupil of E. P. Cathcart in the Department of Physiology at Glasgow. Cathcart had himself a deft hand with Douglas bags and the Haldane apparatus, and two of his pupils studied energy expenditure in man. The first, J. B. Orr, measured the energy used by infantry recruits in training (Cathcart & Orr, 1919) and the second, Miss E. M. Bedale, carried out a classical study on women carrying loads in different ways which I commend to you (Bedale, 1924). Cathcart, like Atwater, Rubner and Lusk and many others, was a pupil of Voit in Munich. Voit was a pupil of Liebig in Giessen, and Liebig had developed his interest in nutrition in Paris from Lavoisier's pupils. So now I can give you a genealogy in the language of the *Pentateuch*. Antoine Lavoisier begat Justus von Liebig, who begat Carl von Voit, who begat Edward Cathcart, who begat Robert Garry, who begat John Durnin.

Cathcart came to be a pupil of Voit in the following manner. After qualifying in medicine, he decided on a career in obstetrics and was advised by Robert Muir, the distinguished Glasgow pathologist, that Munich was the best place to go to for postgraduate studies. Armed with appropriate credentials and an introduction, he arrived in Munich and on his first morning he set out from his hotel to find the Institute of Obstetrics. He entered an impressive building to ask the way. In the hall he met a man who told him that he was in the Institute of Hygiene and that he was talking to its director, Carl von Voit. The conversation continued and Cathcart never got to the Institute of Obstetrics. This story was told me many years ago by Robert Garry late in the evening after a meeting of the Nutrition Society. I do not vouch for its accuracy, but it illustrates how chance determines the career of so many scientists.

The pilot survey encouraged the planning of the field surveys on coal miners and colliery clerks, in East Fife, on military cadets at Sandhurst and on Glasgow housewives and their daughters (Garry *et al.* 1955; Widdowson *et al.*, 1954; Edholm *et al.*, 1955; Durnin, Blake & Brockway, 1957). Each of these required organisation on a large scale; for instance 36 people were engaged in East Fife for 6 weeks in collecting and analysing the data from 19 miners and 10 clerks.

These surveys established that daily rates of energy expenditure of individuals could be determined either from measurements of daily food intake or by indirect calorimetry combined with recording of activities. They aroused much interest at the time and many similar surveys have since been carried out on different groups of individuals in the United Kingdom and in other countries (Davidson & Passmore, 1986). But how valuable have the results been and have they been worth the large amounts of the investigators' time and of public money used to obtain them? I look back on these studies carried out over 35 years ago, sometimes with my critical scientific faculties, and sometimes with nostalgia.

When in a critical mood I can only conclude that the results are of very limited value. The only physiological fact established was that food intakes do not match energy expenditure on a daily basis. An analysis by Durnin (1961) of the records of 69 subjects in those early experiments showed in only 4 a significant correlation between daily intake and output of energy, although over the whole 7 days in the majority there was a close agreement between the two. This is important as it shows that changes in gastro-intestinal activity and in concentrations of hormones and metabolites in the blood, arising directly after a meal, cannot provide a full explanation of feeding behaviour and so of the regulation of body weight. It is appropriate at this Jubilee Celebration to recall the name of G. C. Kennedy, a contemporary of mine whose early death was a great loss to our Society. His paper (Kennedy, 1953), based on experiments on rats, suggesting a long-term regulating mechanism that depends on information on the size of fat stores, has been often overlooked and his suggestion needs further studies.

Some points of at least local interest were established. Thus the colliery clerks' expenditure of energy when off duty at home and in active recreations did not differ from that of the coal face miners, although at work, the latter expended 860 kcal a day more. Thus the sedentary workers showed no tendency to compensate for their relatively small expenditure of energy during working hours by vigorous leisure-time activity.

The military cadets spent more of their time and energy in dressing and cleaning their uniforms than in sport or in military training. The Glasgow housewives utilised only a small amount of their total daily energy in carrying out domestic work. These findings are but a small reward for the effort and expense in obtaining them.

In one respect these early surveys were, in my opinion, misleading and had unfortunate consequences. They encouraged attempts to draw up tables of recommended dietary allowances or intakes (RDA or RDI). The first of these was published in the USA in 1943. After the war, enthusiasts (and I was one of them) saw them as a means of giving sound advice based on scientific evidence to administrators responsible for national diets. Committees sprang up and flourished. Soon after the results of the East Fife Survey became available the FAO Committee on Caloric Requirements was convened in Rome (FAO, 1957) with Professor Garry, Dorothy Hollingsworth and myself as members. The Committee's report has a long appendix that describes and discusses the use of energy costs of activities as a guide to recommendations for energy requirements and concludes that 'further work in this field will enable requirements to be assessed on a firmer basis'. Membership of two FAO and three UK committees on RDAs has gradually convinced me that this was a vain hope. Uncertainties in how representative is the scientific data and differences in its interpretation by scientists undermine confidence in the recommendations. They continue to be misused by applying them to individuals for which they are never intended. Delays in publication of the reports of the latest USA and UK Committees suggests that RDAs are passing into the twilight zone. Hopefully, they will soon become history.

Despite my present doubts of the scientific value of this early work, I look back on it with nostalgia. This is because the men and women taking part as organisers or field workers and also as subjects all seemed to be enjoying it. In Fife, one of our field workers was Jean Marr. She took a personal interest in the subjects, and this is, in my opinion, the most important factor in collecting accurate data. The Fife study led Jean to go into nutritional research where she has had a distinguished career. This enjoyment of fieldwork arises, I suspect, out of the interest inherent in all mysteries. This has been clearly expressed in a great American novel, *Main Street*, written by Sinclair Lewis

The greatest mystery about a human being is not his reaction to sex or praise, but the manner in which he contrives to put in twenty four hours a day. It is this which puzzles the longshoreman about the clerk, the Londoner about the Bushman. It was this that puzzled Carol in regard to the married Vida.

We sometimes get partial solution to these puzzles which may be of practical use. For instance a civil servant in the Post Office from 1841 to 1867 acting as an official surveyor toured the rural areas of Ireland, and other regions, being concerned with how the local post office staff spent their time and energy, and how this affected the time taken for delivery of mails. Much of Trollope's own time was spent on horseback visiting sub-post offices and he used this time to draw up in his mind the characters and scenes of his stories. These he put down on paper between 5.30 and 8.30 a.m. before starting his official duties. He wrote 47 novels, most of them in this way. We have a clear picture (Mullen, 1990) of how, while pursuing effectively two careers, this one man spent his time and energies – but only in qualitative terms.

The surveys in the 1950s showed that it was possible to make quantitative measurements on some men and women – but only for a short period of time which may or may not have been representative of their usual way of living. Although these surveys now seem to me of little or no scientific value, as I have already said, they drew the attention to how much of the life of even apparently active persons was spent sitting. A shorter working week, mechanisation in industry, new domestic appliances and much more public and private transport, each were contributing to making the major part of people's time being spent sitting. In an essay on Caloric Requirements published in *The Lancet* in 1964 (Passmore, 1964), I suggested that *homo sapiens* was turning into *homo sedentarius* and that this was not wise. *Homo sedentarius* has often been advised by doctors to take more exercise. As long ago as 1760 Adam Smith wrote to Lord Shelburne: 'My friend Dr. Cullen took me aside on the street in Edinburgh and told me that he thought it his duty to inform me plainly that if I had any hope of surviving next winter I must ride at least five hundred miles before the beginning of September' (Barfoot, 1991). Over the years many papers have recorded data indicating that a sedentary way of life does not conduce to longevity and that it predisposes to obesity, diabetes and cardiovascular disease. The latest, and to me the most convincing is the report on the health of 10 314 civil servants working in Whitehall (Marmot *et al.*, 1991). As suggested in 1964 *homo sapiens* would be healthier if he became *homo sportivus*. To achieve this he has to be provided with the necessary education and facilities. For many this is the responsibility of government. Sadly, in our schools and universities, teachers of physical education were then and continue to be bottom of the staff pecking order. Too many sports fields continue to be ploughed up to create housing estates.

Plus ça change, plus c'est la même chose. A paper in the March issue of the *British Journal of Nutrition* of this year (Livingston *et al.*, 1991) reports a study on the energy expenditure of 16 men and 16 women in Belfast. Technically, the doubly labelled water method has made measurement of energy expenditure infinitely easier and perhaps more reliable. But the results will be no surprise to anyone who took part in the earlier surveys. The paper ends by welcoming attempts to promote sport in Northern Ireland and emphasising the value to health of leisure-time activities. There is no reference to the earlier surveys which seem to be now forgotten, but the tables of rates of energy expenditure of physical activities prepared at the time by Durnin and myself (Durnin & Passmore 1967; Passmore & Durnin, 1955) appear to be still useful. A safe bet is that at the Society's centenary meeting there will be a discussion on the problems of energy expenditure. Hopefully, some of those who will be taking part will have looked at some of the papers of those of us who in the 1950s found these problems to be of fascinating interest.

References

Atwater, W. O. & Benedict, F. G. (1899). Metabolism of matter and energy in the human body. *US Department of Agriculture Bulletin No. 69.*

Barfoot, M. (1991). Dr. William Cullen and Mr. Adam Smith: a case of hypochondriasis? *Proceedings of the Royal College of Physicians of Edinburgh*, 21, 204–14.

Bedale, E. M. (1924). Comparison of the energy expenditure of a woman carrying loads in eight different positions. *Medical Research Council Industrial Fatigue Research Board No. 29.*

Cathcart, E. P. & Orr, J. B. (1919). The energy expenditure of the infantry recruit in training. *His Majesty's Stationery Office.*

Davidson, L. S. P. & Passmore, R. (1986). *Human Nutrition and Dietetics.* 8th edn. p. 25. Edinburgh: Churchill Livingstone.

Durnin, J. V. G. A. (1961). Appetite and the relation between expenditure and intake of calories in man. *Journal of Physiology (London)*, **156**, 294–309.

Durnin, J. V. G. A., Blake, E. C. & Brockway, J. M. (1957). The energy expenditure and food intake of middle-aged Glasgow housewives and their adult daughters. *British Journal of Nutrition*, **11**, 85–94.

Durnin, J. V. G. A. & Passmore, R. (1967). *Energy, Work and Leisure*. London: Heinemann.

Edholm, O. G., Fletcher, J. G., Widdowson, E. M. & McCance, R. A. (1955). The energy expenditure and food intake of individual men. *British Journal of Nutrition*, **9**, 286–300.

Food and Agriculture Organization of the United Nations. (1957). Calorie Requirements. *FAO Nutritional Studies No. 15*, Rome.

Garry, R. C., Passmore, R., Warnock, G. M. & Durnin, J. V. G. A. (1955). Studies on expenditure of energy and consumption of food by miners and clerks, Fife, Scotland, 1952. *Medical Research Council, Special Report Series No. 289*. London: HMSO.

Kennedy, G. C. (1953). The role of depot fat in the hypothalamic control of food intake in the rat. *Proceedings of the Royal Society of London B* **140**, 578–92.

Kofranyi, E. & Michaelis, H. F. (1941). Ein tragbarer Apparat zur Bestimmung des Gasstoffwechsels. *Arbeitsphysiologie*, **11**, 148–50.

Lehmann, G., Müller, E. A. & Spitzer, H. (1950). Der Calorienbedarf bei gewerblicher Arbet. *Arbeitsphysiologie*, **14**, 166–235.

Livingston, M. B. E., Strain, J. J. & Prentice A. M. *et al.* (1991). Potential contribution of leisure activity to the energy expenditure patterns of sedentary populations. *British Journal of Nutrition*, **65**, 145–55.

Marmot, M. C., Smith, G. D., Stansfeld, S. *et al.* (1991). Health inequalities among British civil servants: the Whitehall II Study. *Lancet* **i**, 1387–93.

Mullen, R. (1990). *Antony Trollope, a Victorian in His World*. London: Duckworth.

Passmore, R. (1964). How many Calories? Food requirements reconsidered in relation to activity. *Lancet* **ii**, 853–4.

Passmore, R. & Durnin, J. V. G. A. (1955). Human energy expenditure. *Physiological Reviews*, **35**, 801–40.

Passmore, R., Thomson, J. G. and Warnock, G. M. (1952). A balance sheet of the estimation of energy intake and energy expenditure as measured by indirect calorimetry, using the Kofranyi–Michaelis calorimeter. *British Journal of Nutrition*, **6**, 253–64.

Widdowson, E. M., Edholm, O. G. and McCance, R. A. (1954). The food intake and energy expenditure of cadets in training. *British Journal of Nutrition*, **8**, 147–55.

5

Energy requirements of man: recent thinking

ANDREW M. PRENTICE and WILLIAM A. COWARD

Our assigned subtitle 'Recent Thinking' will be interpreted as covering the second 25 years of the Nutrition Society's history. This commences in 1966 when names such as Passmore, Edholm, Miller, Durnin, McCance, Widdowson, Southgate and others dominated the field of human energy expenditure. Compared to the pre-war years when indirect calorimetry was a common clinical tool for the diagnosis of thyroid disorders, and when there were an estimated 10000 calorimetry systems in existence in the United States, 1966 was the beginning of a period of relative quiescence. This was soon followed by a resurgence of interest in energy expenditure as the prevalence of obesity started to rise and as it assumed a more dominant position on the social, public health and scientific agenda.

In a paper of this length, full justice cannot possibly be done to the many important developments that have occurred. Our coverage will therefore be restricted to a rapid tour of the major foci of interest during the past 25 years (see Table 5.1), followed by a consideration of some of the major technological developments which have been so essential to progress, and finally by predictions of the areas where the most exciting developments are likely to occur in the near future. In doing so, those areas where Society members, both at home and abroad, have made a particular impact will be highlighted.

Energy requirements

The need to establish recommendations for dietary energy intakes has been a surprisingly influential factor in promoting research, and in the latest FAO/WHO/UNU RDAs, incorporated in the now famous 'Blue Book', British nutritionists played a leading role. Professor Waterlow was chairman, Professor Durnin and Dr Whitehead were members, and Professor James was an influential adviser. The document signalled a

Table 5.1. *Major areas of interest over the past 25 years*

Energy requirements	From conception to death
Reproduction	Pregnancy: birth outcome
	energy costs
	Lactation: milk output
	energy costs
Nutrition in	Metabolic adaptation
developing countries	Productivity
	Protein-energy malnutrition
Work and exercise	Sport & performance
	Slimming
	Cardiovascular fitness
	Other health correlates
Diet	Unavailable carbohydrates
	Novel foods & food substitutes
	Artificial sweeteners
	Alcohol
	Fat: carbohydrate ratio
	Dietary assessment techniques
Clinical states	Cancer cachexia
	Organ failure
	Nutritional support
	Failure-to-thrive
	Endocrine disturbances
Organ-specific studies	Biopsy studies: adipocytes
	muscle
	A–V differences: limbs
	fat pad
Wasting	Anorexia nervosa & bulimia
	'Institutional starvation'
	AIDS
Obesity	Energy-sparing defects
	Appetite control

major change in the way that recommendations for dietary energy are established. It recognised that estimates of energy expenditure provide a sounder basis for establishing requirements than estimates of intake. The concept of a Physical Activity Level (PAL, derived as total energy expenditure divided by BMR) was established and has now entered the energy vocabulary. The clear dissection and exposition of the principles of energy expenditure put forward in this document have created a greater level of knowledge among general nutritionists than ever before.

Reproduction

The late 1960s and early 1970s witnessed the seminal work by Hytten, Thompson, Lind and others, much of which was condensed into Hytten and Leitch's *The Physiology of Human Pregnancy* (1971): a tome so sought after that the Dunn's photocopied copy was kept under virtual lock and key for many years. The question as to whether Hytten's estimates of the energy cost of pregnancy were reasonable formed the basis of the five-country multi-centre studies coordinated by Professor Durnin and described in his chapter (p. 254). These broadly supported Hytten's estimates for most of the communities concerned, but revealed important energy-conserving adaptations in under-nourished Gambian women.

Lactation also came under renewed scrutiny with the resurgence of breast-feeding after a post-war period dominated by bottle-feeding. The major questions centred around establishing the efficiency of conversion of dietary-to-milk energy and hence the overall energetic stress of milk synthesis. The question of whether milk output is compromised at marginal energy intakes in developing countries also received considerable attention, and the consensus has swung from 'yes' to 'no' as improved methods of measuring milk production have yielded higher estimates in underprivileged women (Prentice *et al.*, 1986). It is concluded that the earlier literature reporting very low levels of milk output was largely generated from inappropriate measurement procedures which inhibited milk flow by ignoring the importance of demand feeding.

In all aspects of human reproductive energetics, there has been a very pronounced move away from the use of small experimental animals as models for human reproduction since 1966. This has occurred as the dangers of quantitative extrapolation from small animals to man have become apparent.

Nutrition in developing countries

Elsewhere in this volume (pp. 303, 314) Whitehead and Waterlow describe the work carried out at the Medical Research Council's Units in Uganda and Jamaica. To these must be added the many important contributions from the Department of Human Nutrition at the London School of Hygiene and Tropical Medicine through their collaborations with institutes overseas, and the research from the Dunn's fieldstation in Keneba, The Gambia.

Over the 25 years in question, there has been a marked change in emphasis from protein deficiency, through a period when the protein and energy components of PEM held equal sway, to the current situation where there is greater emphasis on energy. The post-colonial links with many developing countries, together with a formerly (but fast disappearing) enlightened view about the value of long-term scientific investment in such projects, has ensured that British science has held its head high.

Work and exercise

Once again the name of Durnin emerges as being highly influential, this time in conjunction with Passmore. They provided an inheritance for later researchers in the form of their book *Energy, Work and Leisure* (Durnin & Passmore, 1967), which summarised comprehensive studies of the energy costs of different occupational and recreational activities. Since its publication there has been little need to extend their database, and it might be said that there has been little progress. However, interest in the field has been rekindled by the development of the doubly labelled water method (see below) and by an awareness that we are experiencing important social changes away from work and towards leisure activity as the major determinant of people's energy requirements. The relationship between physical inactivity and coronary heart disease highlighted by the now-classic studies of civil servants (Morris *et al.*, 1980) has also renewed attention in this area.

Diet

There have been significant developments in the past quarter century in a number of areas linking diet and energy expenditure. A good example is the rapid increase in knowledge about 'unavailable' carbohydrate and the realisation that some of it is in fact available. It is now appreciated that an energy value must be ascribed to some of these substances since colonic fermentation renders their energy at least partly available to the host (Cummings and Englyst, p. 125 this volume). It is also appreciated that their influence in delaying and extending the release of energy across the gut lumen, and in providing some of the energy in the form of short-chain fatty acids may have significant effects on energy metabolism.

The ability of food companies to modify fats and carbohydrates in order to reduce their effective energy value has profound implications for research in this field which will be returned to in comments on future horizons.

The final area relating to diet and energy metabolism is one of very great interest. It relates to a recent awareness that the energy balance equation has been over-simplified. For many years, the scientific community in this field has tended to assume that it is not necessary to make a distinction between calories from fat, carbohydrate, protein or alcohol since, once they have been absorbed, they are mutually interconvertible. It is now believed that substrate inter-conversion is less favoured than hitherto assumed and that the dietary source of energy may be absolutely critical to the way in which the body maintains substrate balance. For instance, it now appears that *de novo* fat synthesis from carbohydrate is of minimal quantitative significance in people consuming a typical high-fat Western diet. The intake of dietary fat may therefore be the major determinant of fatness, and obesity may legitimately be described as an excessive *fat* balance rather than an excessive *energy* balance.

Clinical states

This has been an area of mixed fortunes. On the one hand, little progress arguably has been made in terms of identifying the underlying causes of the deteriorating nutritional status which often accompanies cancers, infections or injuries, and there remains significant controversy as to whether hypermetabolism or inanition is the primary cause. On the other hand, there has been remarkable progress in the fields of enteral and parenteral support. This has required an increasingly sophisticated knowledge of the patient's energy and substrate requirements. The strength of the Clinical Metabolism and Nutritional Support Group within the Nutrition Society bears witness to the progress occurring in this particular field.

Organ-specific studies

British nutritionists have not featured very strongly in the world literature on studies involving biopsy samples; perhaps because of a greater sensitivity concerning the acceptability of such procedures. However, this has not affected progress with arterio-venous (A–V) difference studies. In particular, the novel A–V studies across the abdominal fat pad developed by Frayn and colleagues in Oxford promise to yield exciting new insights in the near future.

Wasting syndromes

With the exception of the self-evident cause of weight loss in anorexia nervosa, there is also continuing controversy as to the primary causal defect in weight-losing syndromes such as infant malnutrition, wasting in the elderly and AIDS. The questions are similar to those posed for acute infections: Is failure to eat enough food or inanition the primary cause? Is there a failure in absorption or utilisation of nutrients? Or is energy expenditure raised? Very recently, significant progress does seem to have been made and a consensus that energy expenditure is not grossly abnormal in most cases seems to be emerging. This has the important effect of removing a metabolic excuse as to why such people have a deteriorating nutritional status, and of re-focusing attention on their nutritional support.

Obesity (see also Garrow p. 53)

There is no doubt that obesity has been the single most powerful stimulus to recent research on human energy metabolism. Figure 5.1, showing the results of a Medline search using human obesity and energy as key words, illustrates the massive increase in research effort in this direction. The search for an energy-sparing hypometabolic defect in obesity has almost exactly mirrored the search for energy-wasting hypermetabolic defects in wasting syndromes. Both seem to have arisen from an unwillingness to accept that food intake could be sufficiently perturbed to be the only, or even the major, cause of the displaced energy balance.

In the particular case of obesity, there have been three main threads of evidence supporting the view that food intake might be 'normal'. The first is the simple fact that the majority of overweight patients claim not to eat any more food than their lean friends. The second is that formal studies of energy intake using weighed diet records or recall methods tend to support this claim. The third is that, as described by Professor Stock (p. 3), genetically obese rodents certainly do exhibit energy-sparing alterations in brown adipose tissue (BAT) metabolism which cause them to become obese even when they are pair-fed to genotypically lean litter mates. This conviction that the defect was not on the intake side, together with the self-reinforcing excitement of brown fat research, dominated British studies of obesity for at least a decade from 1975 to 1985 and later. The polarisation of thinking is perhaps best illustrated by reference to the Royal College of Physicians' report on Obesity published in 1983, which contains numerous section or chapter headings referring to energy expenditure or thermogenesis, and only one referring to food intake (RCP, 1983).

The late Professor Derek Miller was one of the first to appreciate the potential elegance of a solution to obesity which revolved around a 'thrifty' defect, and his contagious enthusiasm helped to launch a massive research effort in this direction. The resultant studies in small animals by

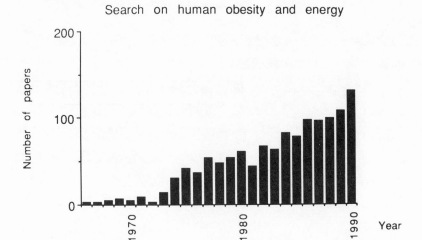

Fig. 5.1. Results of a Medline search using keywords 'human', 'obesity' and 'energy'.

Rothwell and Stock, Trayhurn, York and others have led to a more detailed understanding of uncoupling in BAT and its impairment in obese genotypes than is possessed for any other aspect of energy metabolism, and they stand as a model to be emulated by human orientated researchers. Unfortunately their past record has not been so good and the quality of human studies on obesity has been variable to say the least. None the less it is believed that a consensus is emerging against the likelihood of an energy-sparing defect as the primary cause of obesity. This new swing of the pendulum is encouraging new research on the physiological basis for appetite control and on the means by which the organism maintains macronutrient, as opposed to energy, balance. This realignment of research away from the earlier domination by studies of thermogenic defects is favoured, but at the same time with caution against a full swing of the pendulum and reverse polarisation. It is vital that an open and balanced stance is maintained which acknowledges that the etiology of obesity is likely to be multifactorial, with the different factors having a variable influence in different variants of obesity.

Twenty-five years of technological development

The past 25 years have witnessed two major technological developments which provide an excellent platform from which to launch the next 25 years

Whole-body calorimeters in Britain

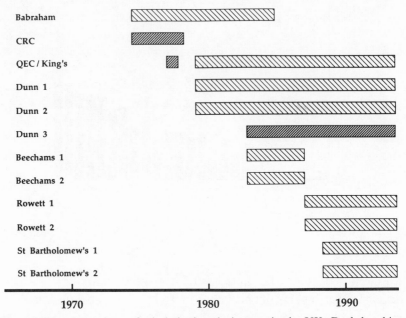

Fig. 5.2. The chronology of whole-body calorimeters in the UK. Dark hatching represents direct or direct/indirect chambers. Light hatching represents indirect chambers.

of research. These are the re-emergence of whole-body calorimetry and the doubly labelled water method.

The former was at least partly stimulated by a letter to *Nature* in 1973 entitled 'How much food does man require?'. The signatories were Durnin, Edholm, Miller and Waterlow, and they made a plea for serious support for high-tech methods in order to further the limited understanding of man's food needs (Durnin *et al.*, 1973). Figure 5.2, which summarises the subsequent history of whole-body calorimeters in Britain, shows that their pleas did not go unheeded. There are currently eight functional calorimeters in the UK, representing almost half of the world's capacity. Almost all of these, and at least four others elsewhere in the world, have benefited from the technical advice of an outstanding bio-engineer, Peter Murgatroyd, who has successfully harnessed the power of modern gas analysis, data-logging and computing equipment to create a new generation of whole-body calorimeters. Although these still function on the same basic principles of gas exchange employed by Atwater and Rosa's first chamber, commissioned at the turn of the century, they are

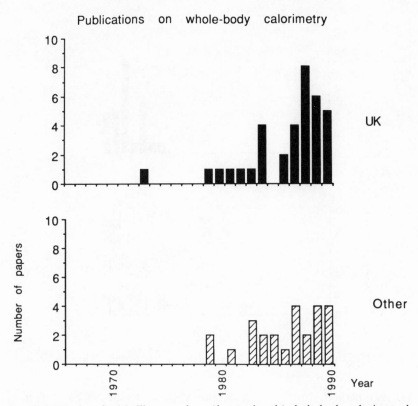

Fig. 5.3. Results of a Medline search on 'human' and 'whole-body calorimetry'.

unrecognisable in terms of acceptability to subjects, ease of use, response time, data-handling and many other features.

In spite of the technical advances which can now be capitalised upon, whole-body calorimeter studies will always have a rather slow throughput. For instance, in the authors' own unit a small study is currently being performed which requires six subjects to spend 7 days in a calorimeter on three occasions. The actual measurements themselves will therefore occupy a minimum of 186 days assuming no down-time. It is therefore not surprising that results are relatively slow to percolate through to the literature. However, Fig. 5.3 shows that their appearance is now accelerating, and that the UK currently contributes around half of the world literature in line with its share of instruments. The future for whole-body calorimetry looks increasingly promising as it is learnt how best to apply it in the study of the mechanisms controlling human energy balance.

The second major development has been the doubly labelled water

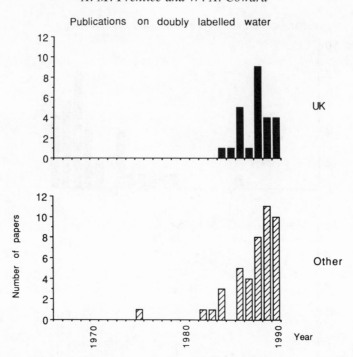

Fig. 5.4. Results of a Medline search on 'human' and 'doubly labelled water'.

(DLW) method. This was first developed by Professor Nathan Lifson at the University of Minnesota in the late 1940s, but was restricted to use in small animals for the next four decades owing to the prohibitive cost of ^{18}O at the dose levels required for human studies. It was only in the early 1980s that Dr Dale Schoeller from Chicago started to validate the method in man, having realised that improvements in the precision of mass spectrometers had made it possible to administer economically viable doses of isotope to humans. The Dunn Clinical Nutrition Centre took up the challenge a little later, encouraged by Roger Whitehead's enthusiasm for novel technology, his eye for an important breakthrough and his willingness to invest the necessary capital to obtain a suitable mass spectrometer. The first biological, as opposed to validation, results were published in 1985, and there has been a rapid expansion of the literature since then, with the UK contributing about one-third (see Fig. 5.4).

There still remains a number of sceptics who are not convinced that the doubly labelled water method (DLW) provides reliable data in spite of the extensive cross-validation studies which have been performed. Their caution is useful in stressing that the method should not be viewed as a golden arrow, and that it certainly can give misleading results in some circumstances or if incorrectly performed. In order to try to stimulate a high level of quality control, the International Dietary Energy Consultancy Group convened a workshop at which all human-orientated DLW research groups were represented. This working group considered all aspects of DLW and published a consensus document containing recommendations for human applications of the technique (IDECG/IAEA, 1990).

The authors share the view of many others that the DLW method represents an exceptional breakthrough in technology by providing us with the first ever non-invasive and accurate means of assessing energy expenditure in genuinely free-living people. They believe that Nathan Lifson certainly deserved the Rank Prize in Nutrition awarded to him some 40 years after his initial discovery.

Future horizons

The progress in establishing whole-body calorimetry and the doubly labelled water method provides an excellent launch-pad for future research, particularly as it is accompanied by parallel technical advances in related fields. For instance, the assessment of body composition is crucial to many studies of energy expenditure, either as the basis for expressing expenditure data or because changes in body composition are the end result of any discrepancies between energy intake and expenditure. The lack of accuracy and precision in currently available techniques has been a major handicap to progress. Novel methods for assessing composition are rapidly emerging and, whilst there are some unhelpful devices being marketed, others show great promise for the future. These include total body electrical conductivity (TOBEC), magnetic resonance imaging (MRI) and dual X-ray absorptiometry (DEXA). In addition to these, there are numerous potentially exciting tools for making non-invasive *in vivo* measurements of energy metabolism. Magnetic resonance spectroscopy of high-energy phosphate compounds probably leads the field at present.

Areas of great challenge lie ahead. Just a few are highlighted. There is a need to integrate research on energy expenditure with an understanding of the intrinsic factors such as cytokines which may modulate it during disease processes. There is a need to perform studies which simultaneously consider the regulation of energy intake as well as expenditure with a greater emphasis on appetite than has existed hitherto. A continuation of the research alluded to in the section on obesity and relating to the processes which control macronutrient, as opposed to energy, balance should prove fruitful. Other areas of immense potential are those of genetics and molecular biology. It is not a question of whether it will become possible to identify energy-related genetic lesions, but of when they will be identified. The possibilities of treatment and eventually of gene therapy will then unfold. But perhaps the most imminent challenge is posed by the rapid advances in food technology which are producing no-fat fats and modified starches in order to reduce the energy density of diets and allow 'overeating' without becoming obese. The possible beneficial or adverse effects of these covert manipulations which are bound to confuse cognitive satiety signals will need to be monitored.

References

Durnin, J. V. G. A., Edholm, O. G., Miller, D. S. & Waterlow, J. C. (1973). How much food does man require? *Nature*, **242**, 418.
Durnin, J. V. G. A. & Passmore, R. (1967). *Energy, Work and Leisure*. London: Heinemann.
Hytten, F. E. & Leitch, I. (1971). *The Physiology of Human Pregnancy*. Oxford: Blackwell Scientific Publications.
IDECG/IAEA. (1990). *The Doubly-Labelled Water Method for Measuring Energy Expenditure: Technical Recommendations for Use in Humans.* Prentice, A. M., ed., Vienna: International Atomic Energy Agency.
Morris, J. N., Everitt, M. G., Pollard, R. *et al.* (1980). Vigorous exercise in leisure time: protection against coronary heart disease. *Lancet*, **ii**, 1207–10.
Prentice, A. M., Paul, A. A., Prentice, A., Black, A. E., Cole, T. J. & Whitehead, R. G. (1986). Cross-cultural differences in lactational performance. In *Human Lactation 2: Maternal and Environmental Factors*. Hamosh, M. & Goldman, A. S., eds, pp. 13–44, New York: Plenum Publishers.
Royal College of Physicians (1983). Obesity: a report of the Royal College of Physicians. *Journal of the Royal College of Physicians*, **17**, 1–112.

6

Obesity in man

J. S. GARROW

Obesity is a more serious problem in man than in other mammalian species, for reasons which are social rather than metabolic. It is suspected that all mammals will become too fat if they live long enough, and have access to unlimited quantities of palatable food. However, farm animals are fed and slaughtered according to a regimen which produces the most commercially profitable carcass, while ageing predators in the wild become less adept at hunting and may themselves become prey before obesity overtakes them. Obesity is certainly a problem among animals kept in zoos, and among domestic pets, especially if the pet owner is also obese (Mason, 1970). Even the laboratory rat, fed on a semi-synthetic diet, will have reduced life expectancy if allowed to eat *ad libitum* (Ross, 1972). Therefore, it is not at all surprising that ageing human beings tend to become obese: the questions which have intrigued researchers over the last 50 years have been first: Why do some people become much more obese than others in the same environment? and second: Does it matter?

The experience of life insurance companies strongly suggests that it does matter: actuaries have long known that there is a range of desirable weight-for-height, below and above which mortality risks increase. Among normal-weight men the chief causes of death are cardiovascular disease and cancer. Among men who are more than 20% overweight these risks are increased by a factor of 1.48 between the age of 35 and 49 years, and by 1.36 between 50 and 74 years (Preston & Clarke, 1966). These observations have been confirmed many times, for both men and women, and among both insured and non-insured populations (Garrow, 1988).

Measurement of body fat in man

The scientific study of obesity in man became possible with the development of an adequate method for measuring the fat content of living
subjects. Pace and Rathbun (1945) showed that the fat-free carcass of
eviscerated guinea-pigs had a quite constant water content (about 73%),
and chemical analyses of six adult human cadavers by Mitchell *et al.*
(1945), Widdowson, McCance & Spray (1951), and Forbes, Cooper &
Mitchell (1953; Forbes, Mitchell & Cooper, 1956) showed this was also
true in man. This evidence that body weight was the sum of fat plus a fat-
free body of approximately constant composition was used by Behnke,
Feen & Welham (1942) who assumed that the fat-free body had a density
of 1.1 g/ml and fat a density of 0.9 g/ml. They measured the body volume
of athletes, using Archimedes' principle, and showed that, although they
were overweight for height, this could not be due to excess fat, but excess
lean tissue, because the total body density was high. Various tracers were
used to estimate the volume of water spaces in living subjects (Keys *et al.*,
1950) and hence to estimate the change in lean tissue compartments in
malnourished subjects (McCance & Widdowson, 1951).

A third independent method for estimating fat-free mass in man became
available when Burch and Spiers (1953) showed that it was possible to
detect the very weak gamma radiation which originated in the natural
isotope ^{40}K present in all potassium, including that in human tissue. Since
fat-free tissue has a fairly constant potassium concentration (66 mmol/kg
in men and 60 mmol/kg in women), but fat contains no potassium, a
measurement of total body potassium yielded an estimate of fat-free mass
in the subject. There are now improved techniques for measuring body
density, total body water and total body potassium, which are reviewed
elsewhere (Garrow, 1988), but these are still inconvenient and expensive
techniques. Measurement of skinfold thickness is probably the most
practical technique for field use, provided the subjects are not severely
obese. The equations of Durnin and Womersley (1974) permit a calculation
of percentage body fat from measurements of skinfold thickness at four
sites.

The essential changes in body composition which occur when a normal
adult becomes obese are illustrated in Table 6.1. It is assumed that the
initial fat content was about 17% by weight (12 kg in 70 kg), but, of
course, this fat represents 68% of the energy content of the body. During
the development of obesity, the additional tissue stored is about 75% fat
and 25% fat-free tissue (Garrow, 1988), so, with the addition of 12 kg fat,

Table 6.1. *Components of body weight and energy stores [A] in a hypothetical normal adult, and [B] in an obese adult with twice the normal fat stores*

Component	[A] Weight (kg)	[A] Energy (Mcal)	[A] Energy (MJ)	[B] Weight (kg)	[B] Energy (Mcal)	[B] Energy (MJ)
Water	42	0	0	45	0	0
Protein	12	48	200	13	52	217
Fat	12	108	451	24	216	903
Glycogen	0.5	2	8	0.5	2	8
Minerals, etc.	3.5	0	0	3.5	0	0
Total	70.0	158	659	86.0	270	1128

there is also a gain of about 1 kg protein and 3 kg water, to bring total body weight to 86 kg. (It is assumed for simplicity that there is no change in the glycogen or mineral content of the body, but this is not quite true. However, such changes will have a negligible effect on the energy stores of the body.)

Why fatness causes disease

One of the points on which there has been controversy concerns the extent to which the excess mortality observed in 'overweight' individuals can be ascribed to obesity: i.e. excessive fat stores. It has already been mentioned that athletes may be overweight by virtue of a large muscle mass, and old people who are of 'normal' weight in fact have less lean tissue and more fat than young adults of similar stature. Research in the last decade has shown that the primary metabolic defect in obesity concerns resistance to the action of insulin: this is seen in genetically determined or experimental obesity in laboratory rodents (Jeanrenaud, 1991) and also in experimentally overfed normal human volunteers (Sims *et al.*, 1973). Intra-abdominal fat has a greater effect in inducing metabolic abnormalities than an equivalent amount of subcutaneous fat, because intra-abdominal fat has higher rates of lipolysis, and can generate high fluxes of fatty acids in the portal circulation (Bjorntorp, 1985).

There is now a plausible explanation for the association between obesity and the diseases to which obese people are particularly prone: cardio-vascular diseases, non-insulin-dependent diabetes mellitus, certain cancers, osteoarthritis and gallstones. In the past the link between obesity and these diseases has been dismissed as coincidental: Keys *et al.* (1984) reported of the Seven Nations Study: 'The risk of all-causes or CHD death did not increase with increasing body weight in any of the regions of the study.' The significant risk factors for heart disease were thought to be age, cigarette smoking, blood pressure and serum cholesterol concentration: adding obesity as an additional variable to these did not improve the ability to predict the risk of death from heart disease. However, the risk factors are themselves related, and further analysis shows that obesity is an independent factor contributing to high blood pressure, diabetes and heart disease, although the effect is less strong in men over the age of 50 years (as studied by Keys) than in younger men or in women (Hubert, 1984).

The liability of obese people to form gall-stones is explained by the high concentration of cholesterol in their bile. The risk of some cancers is significantly greater in obese people: these are in colon, rectum and prostate in men; and endometrium, uterus, cervix, ovary, breast and gall-bladder in women. Apart from the gall-bladder (which is probably related to gall-stone formation and biliary obstruction) the other cancers are related to sex-hormone activity, so the conversion of androgens to oestrogens by aromatase in adipose tissue is probably at least part of the explanation. Osteoarthritis of weight-bearing joints is plausibly explained by the increased mechanical load attributable to the excess body fat (Garrow, 1988).

The changing prevalence of obesity

To discuss prevalence, it is necessary to agree a definition of obesity. There is now an international consensus that the most convenient measure of obesity is weight divided by height squared, since Quetelet (1869) observed that, among people of normal physique, weight was proportional to height squared. Keys *et al.* (1972) renamed this 'BMI', or body mass index, but in view of the long priority of Quetelet it will be here referred to as Quetelet's Index (QI): the units being kg/m^2. The mortality and morbidity associated with overweight begins to become evident in the range QI 25–30 (Garrow, 1988), so it is convenient to define obesity as QI > 30. If it is assumed that the hypothetical subject in Table 6.1 was 1.73 m tall, his QI initially would be $70/1.73 \times 1.73 = 23.4$, and, after becoming obese (assuming his height did not change), his QI would be 28.7. To reach QI = 30 he would have to increase in weight to 90 kg, so this usually represents a more than doubling of the normal fat stores. In 1980, in the UK 6% of men and 8 % of women between the ages of 16 and 64 years were obese by this criterion, and, in 1987, this prevalence had increased to 8 % and 12 % respectively (Gregory *et al.*, 1990). In every country for which there are reliable serial data, the prevalence is increasing.

Aetiology of obesity

There is not space in this short chapter to mention all the explanations which have been offered for the occurrence of obesity in man, but which have failed to receive experimental support. Astwood (1962) predicted that it would be shown to be due to a genetically determined enzyme defect, but, in view of the considerations of energy balance set out below, it is difficult to see what metabolic function this enzyme would have. Various fat-mobilising substances have been reported, but not a significant difference between lean and obese subjects in the production of these substances. Hirsch (1975) suggested that something – perhaps the level of nutrition in early life – fixed the number of fat cells in the body, and hence determined the risk of subsequent obesity, but recent studies show that fat cell number can change to accommodate differences in fat content even in adult life. The activity of energy-wasting brown adipose tissue has been shown to be crucial in the aetiology of obesity in some genetically-obese rodents (Stock & Rothwell, 1982), but there is little evidence for a defect in thermogenesis in obese human subjects. Obesity has been blamed on physical inactivity (Mayer, Roy & Mitra, 1956), but this hypothesis has not withstood experimental testing (Porikos & Pi-Sunyer, 1984).

It is obvious that the increased energy stores which characterise the obese state could not have been deposited unless energy intake had exceeded energy output. However, attempts to show that obese people have a higher energy intake than lean people have usually failed, so it has often been hypothesised that obese people must have (or have had, at some stage) an unusually low energy output. However, the study of human obesity has been greatly helped by the development of various devices for measuring daily energy expenditure by which this hypothesis can be experimentally tested. These are either chambers in which it is possible to measure heat loss or metabolic gas exchange, or a more or less portable apparatus for measuring gas exchange. The last decade has seen the application of a technique by which both the hydrogen and oxygen molecules in body water are isotopically labelled, and the difference in the rate of decrease in the two labels indicates carbon dioxide production and hence metabolic gas exchange (Garrow, 1988). Whichever technique has been used, the results have always indicated that obese people have a higher energy expenditure than lean controls measured by the same technique. The laws of thermodynamics therefore require that the energy intake of obese people is, on average, higher than that of lean controls in order to maintain body weight.

The possibilities remain either that obese people were 'energy thrifty' before becoming obese, or that they conserve energy more effectively than normal when on a low energy diet, and both these theories have been proposed. The difficulty of studying the 'pre-obese' state is obvious: there is some evidence that children of obese parents (who are liable to become obese) have a low metabolic rate, but this has not been confirmed in adult offspring of obese parents (Avons & James, 1986). The evidence concerning obese people who have lost weight is that their energy requirements, although less than in the obese state, are not different from controls of the same age and body composition (Dore *et al.*, 1982). Some people (who are usually lean) identify themselves as 'hard gainers': despite efforts to overeat their weight does not significantly change, while others (usually fat) say they very readily gain weight with the slightest increase in food intake. This phenomenon was investigated by Webb and Annis (1983), who overfed 'easy' and 'hard' gainers by 1000 kcal (4.2 MJ) daily for 30 days. The observed weight gain (2.5 v. 2.2 kg), and efficiency of weight gain (58 % v. 51 %) was similar for the two groups, the slight difference being in favour of greater weight gain in the 'hard' gainers. Current interest therefore centres on the factors which regulate energy intake in lean and obese subjects.

The classical work on the control of food intake was conducted on laboratory rodents fed on laboratory chow. In this simple model it can be shown that centres in the hypothalamus determine food intake and thus regulate energy balance. However, as Edholm (1973) observed: man is not a rat, and in any case when a rat is offered food more like that eaten by man regulation of energy balance is not so precise. In man, many factors affect food intake. If the energy density of food is covertly altered, or if energy expenditure is increased by exercise, there is incomplete compensation in *ad libitum* food intake (Porikos & Pi-Sunyer, 1984). It appears that long-term regulation of energy balance in man depends on cognitive control (Garrow, 1974). If this analysis is correct, it implies that cognitive control is defective in obese people, but this hypothesis is almost impossible to test experimentally.

Treatment of obesity

To remove excess fat stores it is necessary to generate a negative energy balance: that much is agreed. However, there is dispute about whether this should be done by increasing energy output (either by physical exercise or a thermogenic drug) or decreasing energy absorption from ingested food (by bowel-bypass surgery or by a drug which blocks some digestive enzyme) or by restricting food intake. The problems and dangers associated with the first two options have been reviewed elsewhere (Garrow, 1988), and, on balance, restriction of energy intake, or 'dieting', is the most promising option. The most extreme form of dieting, which achieves the most rapid weight loss, is total starvation, but this has proved unsatisfactory for several reasons: some patients unexpectedly died; too high a proportion of the weight lost was lean tissue rather than fat, and metabolic rate was therefore unnecessarily reduced; it did not provide the patient with experience useful as a basis for weight maintenance when the goal weight was reached; and in the long term it is difficult to avoid deficiencies of essential nutrients.

There is now keen commercial competition to find a dietary formulation which will retain the advantages of starvation (simplicity and rapid weight loss) while avoiding the above disadvantages (COMA, 1987). Conflicting schools of thought hold deeply entrenched positions, so it is unlikely that consensus will be reached. The author's view is that the best diet is one composed of ordinary food, which provides enough protein, vitamins, minerals and dietary fibre, but about 500–1000 kcal (1.7–3.4 MJ) less than requirements for weight maintenance, which will cause weight loss of 0.5–1.0 kg/week. The fundamental problem, however, is how best to help a severely overweight person to keep to such a diet for many months, and thereafter not to regain the weight which has been lost.

In this field, behavioural psychologists have made a major contribution over the last two decades. It has come to be realised that, in most people (not merely obese ones), eating is triggered by many non-nutritional stimuli, and that manipulation of these stimuli may make it much easier to keep to a diet. Behavioural methods have not quite fulfilled their early expectations of curing obesity (Stunkard, 1985), but they have certainly contributed to maintenance of weight loss. It is believed that, in the next few years, the focus of research will swing towards the *social* determinants of obesity, since these seem to provide clues for effective therapy. Table 6.2 shows some data from a large survey in Finland by Rissanen *et al.* (1991).

It is well established that, in many countries, there is an inverse

Table 6.2. *Relative risk*[a] *(and n) of gaining > 5 kg in 5 years related to parity and educational attainment in Finnish women aged 25–44 y*

Childbirths	Education		
	High	Medium	Low
0	1.0 (201)	1.5 (708)	1.4 (1860)
1	0.8 (48)	1.5 (126)	1.6 (265)
2+	0.6 (11)	2.8 (22)	3.3 (42)

[a] Corrected for age, BMI and interaction: parity × education.
Rissanen *et al.* (1991).

relationship between prevalence of obesity and socioeconomic status, for which there is no satisfactory explanation. A plausible idea is that discrimination against obese people results in those who are constitutionally predisposed to obesity being over-represented in the less affluent sections of society. The negative association between parity and socioeconomic status might also be part of the explanation if the metabolic changes during pregnancy predisposed to weight gain. However, Table 6.2 shows a complex interaction between parity and educational status in relation to 'significant weight gain', which is operationally defined as a gain of at least 5 kg in 5 years. Those of a higher educational status have a lower risk of weight gain at all parities, but increasing numbers of childbirths during the 5-year survey period *increases* the difference between the educational groups. This observation defies any metabolic explanation. The hypothesis which seems best to fit the data was advanced some time ago: that the long-term regulation of energy balance in man is achieved by cognitive control when fluctuations in body weight exceed acceptable limits (Garrow, 1974). It appears that highly educated Finnish women seldom permit themselves significant weight gain, and, if they have babies, they are still more vigilant that this should not happen.

Conclusion

It seems that the direction in which obesity research is leading us is a hopeful one. It is not true, as Astwood (1962) suggested, that fat people are born fat, and that nothing much can be done about it. Obesity is the natural consequence of affluence and longevity, but not the inevitable price that must be paid for those otherwise desirable circumstances. There is still much to be discovered about the causes of individual variations in energy requirements, and about the metabolic derangements which accompany excessive fat storage, but it seems that enough is known about the principles of energy balance in man for it to be asserted that virtually anyone can, if he or she so desires, achieve and maintain the body composition which is associated with health and long life.

References

Astwood, E. B. (1962). The heritage of corpulence. *Endocrinology*, **71**, 337–41.

Avons, P. & James, W. P. T. (1986). Energy expenditure of young men from obese and non-obese families. *Human Nutrition: Clinical Nutrition*, **40C**, 259–70.

Behnke, A. R., Feen, B. G., & Welham, W. C. (1942). The specific gravity of healthy men; body weight and volume as an index of obesity. *Journal of the American Medical Association*, **118**, 495–8.

Bjorntorp, P. (1985). Regional patterns of fat distribution. *Annals of Internal Medicine*, **103**, 994–5.

Burch, P. R. J. & Spiers, F. W. (1953). Measurement of the gamma radiation from the human body. *Nature (London)*, **172**, 519–21.

Committee on Medical Aspects of Food Policy. (1987). *The Use of Very-Low-Calorie Diets in Obesity*. London: HMSO, 32 pp.

Dore, C., Hesp, R., Wilkins, D. & Garrow, J. S. (1982). Prediction of energy requirements of obese patients after massive weight loss. *Human Nutrition: Clinical Nutrition*, **36C**, 41–8.

Durnin, J. V. G. A. & Womersley, J. (1974). Body fat assessed from body density and its estimation from skinfold thickness: measurement on 481 men and women from 16–72 years. *British Journal of Nutrition*, **32**, 77–97.

Edholm, O. G. (1973). *Energy Balance in Man*. Apfelbaum, M. ed., Paris: Masson.

Forbes, R. M., Cooper, A. R. & Mitchell, H. H. (1953). The composition of the adult human body as determined by chemical analysis. *Journal of Biological Chemistry*, **203**, 359–66.

Forbes, R. M., Mitchell, H. H. & Cooper, A. R. (1956). Further studies on the gross composition and mineral elements of the adult human body. *Journal of Biological Chemistry*, **223**, 969–75.

Garrow, J. S. (1974). *Energy Balance and Obesity in Man*. Amsterdam: Elsevier/North Holland.

Garrow, J. S. (1988). *Obesity and Related Diseases*. London: Churchill Livingstone, 329 pp.

Gregory, J., Foster, K., Tyler, H. & Wiseman, M. (1990). *The Dietary and Nutritional Survey of British Adults*. London: HMSO, 430 pp.

Hirsch, J. (1975). Cell number and size as a determinant of subsequent obesity. In *Childhood Obesity*. Winick, M., ed., pp. 15–21, New York: John Wiley.

Hubert, H. B. (1984). The nature of the relationship between obesity and cardiovascular disease. *International Journal of Cardiology*, **6**, 268–74.

Jeanrenaud, B. (1990). Neuroendocrinology and evolutionary aspects of experimental obesity. In *Progress in Obesity Research*. Oomura, Y., Tarve, S., Inoue, S. and Shimazu, T., eds, London: John Libbey, pp. 409–421.

Keys, A., Brozek, J., Henschel, A., Mickelsen, O. & Taylor, H. L. (1950). *The Biology of Human Starvation*. Minneapolis: University of Minnesota Press, 1385 pp.

Keys, A., Fidanza, F., Karvonen, M. J., Kimura, N. & Taylor, H. L. (1972). Indices of relative weight and obesity. *Journal of Chronic Diseases*, **25**, 329–43.

Keys, A., Menotti, A., Aravanis, C., Blackburn, H., Djordevic, B. S., Buzina, R., Dontas, A. S., Fidanza, F., Karvonen, M. J., Kimura, N., Mohacek, I., Nedeljkovic, S., Puddu, V., Punsar, S., Taylor, H. L., Conti, S., Kromhout, D. & Toshima, H. (1984). The seven countries study: 2289 deaths in 15 years. *Preventive Medicine*, **13**, 141–54.

McCance, R. A. & Widdowson, E. M. (1951). A method of breaking down the body weights of living persons into terms of extracellular fluid, cell mass and fat, and some applications of it to physiology and medicine. *Proceedings of the Royal Society, B*, **138**, 115–30.

Mason, E. (1970). Obesity in pet dogs. *Veterinary Record*, **86**, 612–16.

Mayer, J., Roy, P. & Mitra, K. P. (1956). Relation between caloric intake, body weight and physical work. *American Journal of Clinical Nutrition*, **4**, 169–75.

Mitchell, H. H., Hamilton, T. S., Steggerda, F. R. & Bean, H. W. (1945). The chemical composition of the adult human body and its bearing on the biochemistry of growth. *Journal of Biological Chemistry*, **158**, 625–37.

Pace, N., & Rathbun, E. N. (1945). Studies on body composition: water and chemically combined nitrogen content in relation to fat content. *Journal of Biological Chemistry*, **158**, 685–91.

Porikos, K. P. & Pi-Sunyer, F. X. (1984). Regulation of food intake in human obesity: studies with caloric dilution and exercise. *Clinical Endocrinology and Metabolism*, **13**, 547–61.

Preston, T. W. & Clarke, R. D. (1966). Mortality of impaired lives. *Transactions of the Faculty Actuaries*, **29**, 251–315.

Quetelet, L. A. J. (1869). *Physique Sociale*. Brussels, C. Muquardt, vol. 2, p. 92.

Rissanen, A. M., Heliovaara, M., Knekt, P., Reunamen, A. & Aromaa, A. (1991). Determinants of weight gain and overweight in adult Finns. *European Journal of Clinical Nutrition*, **45**, 419–30.

Ross, M. H. (1972). Length of life and calorie intake. *American Journal of Clinical Nutrition*, **25**, 834–8.

Sims, E. A. H., Danforth, E. Jr, Horton, E. S., Bray, G. A., Glennon, J. A. & Salans, L. B. (1973). Endocrine and metabolic effects of experimental obesity in man. *Recent Progress in Hormone Research*, **29**, 457–96.

Stock, M. & Rothwell, N. (1982). *Obesity and Leanness: Basic Aspects*. London: John Libbey. 98 pp.

Stunkard, A. J. (1985). Behavioural management of obesity. *Medical Journal of Australia*, **142**, suppl., S13–20.

Webb, P. & Annis, J. F. (1983). Adaptation to overeating in lean and overweight women. *Human Nutrition: Clinical Nutrition* **36C**, 117–31.

Widdowson, E. M., McCance, R. A. & Spray, C. M. (1951). The chemical composition of the human body. *Clinical Science*, **10**, 113–25.

Part two
Metabolism of the major nutrients

7

Digestive physiology of ruminant livestock: a review of recent developments

D. E. BEEVER

Introduction

Whilst the distinct anatomical features of the ruminant digestive tract have been known for more than a century, it is within the Society's lifetime that many of the mechanisms involved in the conversion of ingested feed to absorbed nutrients have been elucidated. In this respect, much is owed to Professor A. T. Phillipson and colleagues who set about resolving many issues which previous research had failed to elucidate. His initial interests involved the movements of various compartments of the ruminant stomach, but it was studies on the fate of odd and even carbon lower fatty acids that provided the focus for much of the research which has occurred subsequently. In this connection, Barcroft, McAnally & Phillipson (1944) demonstrated that volatile fatty acids (VFA) arising from microbial fermentation in the rumen were absorbed from the rumen whilst glucose was not a significant end product of digestion.

Phillipson was also aware of the importance of rumen microbial biomass synthesis (Phillipson, 1946), but inadequate techniques to determine quantitative yields limited progress until several papers (Hogan & Phillipson, 1960; Harris & Phillipson, 1962; Clarke, Ellinger & Phillipson, 1966) provided the focus for much of the subsequent research to examine nitrogen, carbohydrate and lipid digestion which has occurred. Subsequently, multi-disciplinary research involving physiologists, biochemists, microbiologists and nutritionists has confirmed often tentative qualitative descriptions of the digestive processes and provided quantitative data which have led to an improved understanding of the processes involved.

This chapter will highlight specific areas where there have been major advances, recognising the important contribution that improved techniques have made. Issues still requiring resolution will be identified whilst

65

topical issues such as the control of methanogenesis and the contribution of molecular biology will be discussed. The paper will aim to put current research knowledge into the context of ruminant animals being significant contributors of meat and milk by recognising that improvements in both the efficiency of production and composition of the product will only be achieved and sustained through an adequate knowledge of ruminant nutrition and metabolism.

Sites of nutrient digestion

Initial studies to partition nutrient digestion within the alimentary tract were restricted to the use of slaughter procedures in which animals were dosed with an indigestible marker prior to slaughter and, through subsequent reference of marker concentrations in specific digesta fractions, the relative contributions of various parts of the tract to whole tract digestion were assessed (Badaway *et al.*, 1958). Subsequently, these were replaced by surgical procedures in which total exteriorisation of digesta flow was effected (Ash, 1962) but, as marker techniques to quantify digesta flow were refined (Faichney, 1975), the use of simple T piece cannulae was established and has now become a routine technique for all classes of ruminant livestock. Early studies with sheep demonstrated that digestion of water soluble carbohydrates and starch occurred principally in the rumen, accounting for over 90 % of whole tract digestion which usually exceeded 95 % of total dietary intake (MacRae & Armstrong, 1969; Beever *et al.*, 1971). Similarly it was found that the digestion of hemicellulose and cellulose occurred principally in the rumen, with whole tract digestion varying according to the nature of the fibre source. In contrast, studies on diets containing ground maize indicated that, whilst whole tract starch digestion approached starch intake, ruminal contribution was often reduced, with significant quantities of starch entering the small intestine. Data presented in Table 7.1 (Karr, Little & Mitchell, 1966) for cattle receiving three levels of ground maize in the diet showed that whole tract digestion of starch exceeded 97 % of intake. However, the extent of starch digestion in the rumen was lower than that found by MacRae & Armstrong (1969) for rolled and whole barley fed to sheep, and as starch intake increased, the extent of ruminal digestion declined further, whilst limitations in the capacity of the small intestine to digest starch at high starch intakes were established. The origins of the extra starch entering the small intestine have never been fully elucidated, although it is assumed to be increased undegraded feed starch rather than microbial polysaccharide.

Table 7.1. *Partition of starch digestion on ground maize containing diets fed to cattle*

	Apparent digestibility (g/kg intake)			
			Intestines	
	Whole tract	Rumen	Small	Large
Ground maize + lucerne				
40 % ground maize	990	721	238	32
60 % ground maize	984	681	250	53
80 % ground maize	977	634	233	110

Karr *et al.* (1966).

Table 7.2. *Effect of concentrate type on carbohydrate digestion in the rumen of lactating dairy cows fed grass silage*

| | Sugar beet feed | | |
	Unmolassed	Molassed	Rolled barley
Starch (kg/d)			
Intake	0.19	0.27	5.22
Ruminally digested	–	–	3.79
Cellulose (kg/d)			
Intake	4.04	3.39	2.58
Duodenal flow	0.73	0.91	1.03
Ruminally digested (g/kg intake)	815	737	601

Similarly, Thomson *et al.* (1972) and Beever *et al.* (1972) found that reduction in the particle size of dried forage reduced the extent of fibre digestion in the rumen. They concluded that compensatory digestion of fibre in the large intestine was substantial, and only at high levels of intake was a depression in whole tract fibre digestibility observed.

In a study with dairy cows fed grass silage and three contrasting concentrates, Beever *et al.* (1988) showed substantial negative effects of both molasses and starch on fibre digestion. As expected, net ruminal digestion of starch was only observed on the barley based diet (Table 7.2). In contrast, unmolassed sugar beet feed provided the highest cellulose intake, and had the highest extent of cellulose digestion in the rumen.

Addition of molasses reduced cellulose intake, but ruminal digestion declined to 737 g/kg cellulose intake despite both diets being prepared from the same original crop. As expected, rolled barley provided the lowest cellulose intake but had the highest duodenal flow of cellulose, with the ruminal digestion of cellulose amounting to only 601 g/kg consumed. Such effects appear to be related to the increased digestion of starch and water-soluble carbohydrate on the barley and molassed sugar beet feeds respectively.

Hogan & Weston (1970) established the rumen as a principal site of digestion of nitrogenous compounds, involving the degradation of dietary protein and synthesis of microbial protein; they proposed an inverse relationship between dietary N concentration (g/kg digestible organic matter (DOM) content) and duodenal non-ammonia nitrogen (NAN) flow (g/g N intake), which showed that above 40 gN/kg DOM, NAN flow to the small intestine was less than N intake, indicative of protein wastage within the rumen. Despite the empiricism of this relationship, with no attempt to interpret the underlying mechanisms, its lasting value has been remarkable. Subsequently, McAllan, Siddons & Beever (1987) established important dietary differences with respect to concentrate and silage-based diets and those including substantial quantities of non-protein nitrogen such as urea. Hogan and Weston (1970) established that optimal rumen ammonia concentration should not exceed approximately 18 mg NH_3-N/100 ml if substantial ruminal losses of nitrogen were to be avoided. High rumen ammonia concentrations occur on diets which contain substantial quantities of readily digestible protein (e.g. forages, soluble protein supplements), particularly where energy and protein availability in the rumen are unbalanced. Such situations exist on ensiled forages, but, equally, high rumen ammonia concentrations have been found on fresh forages. Studies with dairy cows fed zero-grazed forage (Beever & Siddons, 1986) indicated rumen ammonia concentrations of 35–45 mg NH_3-N/100 ml with a net loss of ammonia from the alimentary tract equivalent to almost 30 % of N intake.

Microbial protein synthesis

By 1970 it was evident that further progress on elucidating the mechanisms of ruminal fermentation would only be achieved if reliable estimates of microbial biomass synthesis could be obtained. Diaminopimelic acid (DAPA) was identified as a potential marker of bacterial biomass but, despite refinements in the method of analysis (Hutton, Bailey & Annison,

1971), considerable doubt was expressed over the difficulty in obtaining samples of bacteria from duodenal digesta which were representative of bacteria leaving the rumen with respect to the concentration of DAPA. Ethylaminophosphonic acid was suggested as a protozoal marker, but similar criticisms and its possible occurrence in feed limited its application.

Quantitative identification of the microbial, undegraded feed and endogenous components of duodenal protein by mathematical reference to their individual amino acid profiles was undertaken by Evans, Axford & Offer (1975), but variability in the solutions obtained limited subsequent use of this technique. Smith & McAllan (1971) proposed the use of RNA as a microbial marker, and despite some problems with sample preservation, this technique has been adopted by many laboratories, especially those with no isotope facilities. Techniques using sulphur-35 (Roberts & Miller, 1969; Beever *et al.*, 1974) and nitrogen-15 (Nolan & Leng, 1972) were developed, and, more recently, labelled leucine has been proposed (Bruce, Marsden & Buttery, 1985). In a comparison of DAPA, ^{35}S, ^{15}N and amino acid profile methods Siddons, Beever & Nolan (1982) found substantial differences in marker concentrations of rumen and duodenal bacteria which were subsequently confirmed by Dawson *et al.* (1988). Thus estimates of microbial N synthesis by Siddons *et al.* (1982) ranged from 0.32 to 0.76 (grass silage) and 0.18 to 0.80 (dried grass) of total duodenal NAN, based on rumen microbes, whilst values were approximately 20% higher when duodenal microbes were used. Values based on DAPA were high (average 0.78), whilst those based on amino acid profiles were low (average 0.27). In contrast, values based on ^{35}S and ^{15}N were relatively similar within each diet comparison, and appeared to be more biologically acceptable. To date, however, this issue remains unresolved; the absence of an absolute standard prevents satisfactory validation of any of the methods proposed.

Despite such uncertainty, Thomas (1982) concluded that the efficiency of microbial synthesis was reduced on grass silage diets. Several reasons were advanced, but in a series of intraruminal infusions into cows fed grass silage, Rooke, Lee & Armstrong (1987) showed marked improvements in both the extent and efficiency of microbial N synthesis when energy supplements were supplied, with or without extra protein, whilst the response to urea or protein alone was marginal. There are other studies which suggest that the opportunity to manipulate microbial synthesis may be considerable. Pirt (1965) established the relationship between turnover rate of the microbial media and growth rate of the micro-organisms, and these were subsequently extended by Stouthamer & Bettenhausen (1973).

The concept of Y(ATP), expressed as grams of microbial biomass synthesised per mole ATP produced was advanced, and whilst an average value of 10.5 was initially proposed for the rumen ecosystem, it is now accepted that this will vary according to specific growth rate of the microbes, and in particular the partition of available hexose towards growth or fermentation (Black *et al.*, 1980/81). Harrison *et al.* (1975) found that doubling of rumen fluid outflow rate by infusion or dietary inclusion of buffer salts significantly increased the extent and efficiency of microbial protein synthesis despite no change in feed intake, and a marked increase in the ratio of acetate:propionate production.

Ammonia metabolism

Through the combined use of $(^{15}NH_4)_2 SO_4$, ^{14}C urea and ^{14}C bicarbonate, quantitative models of whole body metabolism have been proposed (Nolan, 1975, Nolan *et al.*, 1976, Mathison & Milligan, 1971), which identified the importance of ammonia and preformed amino acids as precursors of microbial N synthesis, and established the extent of nitrogen recycling between gut and body tissues. The full implications of such were developed by Siddons *et al.* (1985) for sheep fed grass silage in which rumen ammonia production equalled 75% of dietary N intake. Only one-third of ammonia production was incorporated into microbial protein and the remainder was absorbed across the rumen wall. Total microbial N synthesis was 35% of N intake, with one-third being derived from non-ammonia sources, presumably free amino acids and possibly peptides. Small intestinal NAN absorption was 38% of N intake, whilst 40% of body urea synthesis was recycled to the alimentary tract, with a greater proportion entering postruminal components.

Thus, on diets where energy and protein imbalances in the rumen have been suggested, the excessive production and absorption of ammonia will not only reduce amino acid supply to the animal, but increase hepatic ammonia levels. A key role of the liver is ammonia detoxification, but recent studies by Wilton, Gill & Lomax (1988), Fitch *et al.* (1989) and Maltby *et al.* (1991) have demonstrated increased hepatic amino acid utilisation under conditions of high portal ammonia supply, possibly impairing amino acid availability to peripheral tissues. In the study of Maltby *et al.* (1991) urea supplementation of maize silage enhanced both portal ammonia and amino acid supply. Hepatic ammonia removal was complete for both the control and supplemented diets, but hepatic amino acid utilisation increased substantially on the urea supplemented diet, such that total splanchnic output of amino acids was similar to that on the non-supplemented diet.

Protection of nutrients from ruminal degradation

Undoubtedly the rumen is the principal site of fibre digestion. However, the ruminal digestion of nutrients such as starch and protein is often in excess of microbial requirements. Attempts to protect starch from rumen digestion have been relatively unsuccessful, despite the benefits it may have of enhancing small intestinal glucose supply and reducing the negative effects of starch on fibre digestion in the rumen. In contrast, protection of dietary protein from rumen degradation has been more successful. The effect of heat treatment of forages was examined by Beever *et al.* (1976), but formaldehyde treatment of proteins has given more consistent results. Improvements in duodenal amino acid supply (Faichney, 1974) and animal productivity, measured in terms of wool growth (Ferguson, 1975), have been demonstrated provided the level of formaldehyde application was controlled in order to prevent the protein supplement from being rendered indigestible. In contrast, whilst formaldehyde-containing silage additives have shown increased duodenal flows of undegraded feed protein and hence total protein (Beever *et al.*, 1977; Thomson *et al.*, 1981), the effect of these on increased animal productivity has been inconsistent.

Technological advances in the production of pH sensitive polymers has led to the development of protected amino acid supplements. *In vitro* examination of such products revealed that the polymer coating of the amino acids was stable in rumen but sensitive to abomasal pH conditions. Beever *et al.* (1990*a, b*) examined such products in dairy cows and, whilst they could not establish a ruminal protection of more than 65%, substantial improvements in lysine and methionine concentrations of duodenal amino acids were observed. To date, however, the possible benefits of such products on animal productivity have not been adequately established.

Given the general desire to increase protein flow to the small intestine, whilst minimising excessive loss of nutrients during rumen fermentation, much interest has been shown in the nutritional value of fishmeal. Its low susceptibility to rumen fermentation is now established, and improvements in duodenal protein supply have been observed with such products. However, Beever *et al.* (1990*a, b*) reported that the response to increments of fishmeal may not be linear, whilst indicating significant changes in the relative yields of acetate and propionate.

Control of methanogenesis

Methane production is principally related to the extent of carbohydrate degradation in the rumen, but also the relative yields of the individual VFAs. The production of propionate requires hydrogen, and on diets that stimulate propionate production the net yield of fermentation hydrogen and hence methane is reduced. It was suggested that by enhancing propionate production, methane production would decline, and in this context some success has been achieved with the ionophores such as monensin and lasalocid (Chalupa, 1980). However, practical experience with such products is variable, and there are suggestions that the rumen environment may adapt to such manipulants, the overall effect being lost within 3–4 weeks of commencing the treatment.

If the current interest in reducing methane production is sustained, two approaches are worthy of consideration. Optimisation of animal productivity must be aimed for, as this will undoubtedly reduce methane production per unit of animal product. Further to this, attention should be focused on the ruminal disposal of monosaccharides. Both pentoses and hexoses arise from dietary carbohydrate degradation and, depending upon microbial growth rates, are used either in the synthesis of microbial biomass or fermented for the production of ATP which is required for microbial maintenance and growth. This partition of monosaccharide use will have a major bearing on the ultimate yield of methane, and could lead to much larger and sustainable reductions in methane production than have been achieved by manipulating the disposal of fermentation hydrogen.

Mathematical modelling

Through increased computing power improved mathematical procedures have been developed, and their application to the field of ruminant nutrition has greatly assisted the interpretation of research data. In this respect, compartmental analysis has been widely used in tracer studies to determine precursor–product relationships (Shipley & Clarke, 1972). Lactate in grass silage diets may comprise as much as 15 % of total dietary dry matter intake, but until recently its metabolic fate in the rumen was unclear. Chamberlain, Thomas & Anderson (1983) suggested that the major end product of lactate metabolism was propionate (and ultimately glucose), based on observing changes in the molar proportions of VFA following an intraruminal infusion of lactate. In contrast, using a 4-pool rumen model, Gill *et al.* (1985) found almost 60 % of ruminally produced lactate was converted to acetate, with only one-third converted to propionate, and showed that the approach of Chamberlain *et al.* (1983) was methodologically incorrect. Clearly, such findings have a major implication when assessing the glucose economy of silage-fed cattle.

Simulation modelling has been used to predict the outcome of rumen fermentation and to identify areas of inadequate knowledge, and it was Baldwin, Lucas & Cabrera (1970) who first proposed a mathematical model of nutrient digestion, microbial synthesis and VFA production. Further improvements to this model have been possible due to increased data availability (Baldwin, Koong & Ulyatt, 1977; Black *et al.*, 1980/81; France, Thornley & Beever, 1982), and recently Baldwin, Thornley & Beever (1987*a*) proposed a digestion model for lactating dairy cows which was subsequently combined with a nutrient metabolism model to create a full lactation model based on the utilisation of individual nutrients (Baldwin *et al.*, 1987*b*).

Behaviour of the model was generally satisfactory, but the need for further improvements was identified, as was the situation with the model recently proposed by Danfaer (1990). None the less, such developments represent major advances in the transfer of research information to the livestock industry. Current feed rationing systems practised in UK are based on metabolisable energy contents. For several reasons, these are rapidly becoming outdated (MacRae, Buttery & Beever, 1988), and suitable alternatives which adequately represent energy and protein interactions at both the gut and body tissue level and are capable of predicting both product yield and composition are urgently required.

Rumen fungi

Until the early 1970s bacteria and protozoa were considered the major components of the rumen microbial population, but in a series of papers, Orpin (1974*a, b*, 1975) and Bauchop (1979) identified obligate anaerobic fungi in rumen contents by demonstrating that certain motile cells, previously believed to be protozoan flagellates, were zoospores of Chytridiomycete fungi. Subsequently, the life cycle of rumen fungi was proposed (Lowe *et al.*, 1985), comprising a rhizoidal vegetative state followed by zoosporangia development and subsequent release of zoospores. Once released, the zoospores quickly colonise plant material where they germinate, and the resulting hyphae invade the fibrous components of rumen digesta. Turnover rates of the life cycle of between 8 and 30 h have been observed by Bauchop (1979) and Lowe *et al.* (1987). One function of rumen fungi may be primary invasion of plant material, thus enhancing bacterial penetration and digestion. However, Theodorou *et al.* (1989), using pure cultures of anaerobic rumen fungi, observed extensive degradation of forage cell walls, and cellulolytic, xylanolytic and glycolytic enzyme activities have been demonstrated (Mountfort & Asher, 1985). In co-culture, and particularly in the presence of methanogenic bacteria, the products of cellulose fermentation by rumen fungi are largely acetate and methane.

To date, the relative contribution of rumen fungi to total rumen fermentation has not been established, but recently Davies, Theodorou & Trinci (1990) isolated fungi in all parts of the digestive tract of forage-fed cattle, with the highest numbers of thallus-forming units being identified in rumen and omasal contents.

Genetic engineering of rumen microflora

With the recent advances in molecular biology, application of such techniques to manipulate the metabolic characteristics of the rumen microflora has been considered. Much of this interest has centred on attempting to insert genes into rumen bacteria in order to enhance the rate of fibre degradation and possibly to stimulate lignin degradation (Teather & Ohmiya, 1991). Equally, enhancement of microbial detoxification of anti-nutritional dietary factors by gene manipulation has been considered (Gregg & Sharp, 1990), and other claims to improve protein utilisation, modify microbial biomass composition and generate novel compounds have been made.

Despite considerable research investment, no significant and sustainable improvements have yet emerged, and problems associated with gene expression and survival of modified organisms in the rumen still remain. Whilst such initiatives must be encouraged, it is believed that inadequate attention was given to focusing such studies towards achievable targets, whilst the important ethical issue of releasing modified bacteria into the environment still remains to be addressed. By the time this Society enjoys its centennial celebrations such comments will be either fallacy or prophetic, but by then few of the present generation will have any further interests in the debate.

Conclusion

The lifetime of the Society has witnessed great advances in our quantitative understanding of rumen function, and the implications of such for ruminant livestock production. From an earlier position which provided sound generalisations (e.g. Annison & Lewis, 1959), the quantitative importance of energy and protein interactions in the rumen and their implications for metabolite availability to the whole animal have been established. For many years, however, research effort reflected the view that ruminal events were of sole importance in controlling ruminant animal productivity, and research to elucidate the control of nutrient metabolism in the whole body was limited. The last 10 years have seen a major reappraisal of this position. Improved techniques to measure protein and lipid metabolism in body tissues have become available and, with the improved understanding of the endocrinological control of metabolism, the research effort on ruminant nutrition is now more balanced. Sustainment of this approach is crucial if the UK ruminant livestock industry is to meet many of the challenges which it now faces with respect to environmental pollution, animal welfare and concern over quality of animal products for the human population.

Acknowledgements

Without the unfailing support of the staff of Ruminant Nutrition and Metabolism my contribution to this research area would not have been possible.

References

Annison, E. F. & Lewis, D. (1959). *Metabolism in the Rumen*. London: Methuen.

Ash, R. W. (1962). Gastro-intestinal re-entrant cannulae for studies of digestion in sheep. *Animal Production*, **4**, 309–12.

Badaway, A. M., Campbell, R. M., Cuthbertson, D. P., Fell, B. F. & MacKie, W. S. (1958). Further studies on the changing composition of the digesta along the alimentary tract of the sheep. 1. Total and non-protein nitrogen. *British Journal of Nutrition*, **12**, 367–83.

Baldwin, R. L., Lucas, H. L. & Cabrera, R. (1970). Energetic relationships in the formation and utilization of fermentation end-products. In *Physiology of Digestion and Metabolism in the Ruminant*, Phillipson, A. T., ed., pp. 319–34, Newcastle-upon-Tyne: Oriel Press.

Baldwin, R. L., Koong, L. J. & Ulyatt, M. J. (1977). A dynamic model of ruminant digestion for evaluation of factors affecting nutritive value. *Agricultural Systems*, **2**, 255–88.

Baldwin, R. L., Thornley, J. H. M. & Beever, D. E. (1987a). Metabolism of the lactating cow. II. Digestive elements of a mechanistic model. *Journal of Dairy Research*, **54**, 107–31.

Baldwin, R. L., France, J., Beever, D. E., Gill, M. & Thornley, J. H. M. (1987b). Metabolism of the lactating cow. III. Properties of mechanistic models suitable for evaluation of energetic relationships and factors involved in the partition of nutrients. *Journal of Dairy Research*, **54**, 133–45.

Barcroft, J., McAnally, R. A. & Phillipson, A. T. (1944). Absorption of volatile acids from the alimentary tract of sheep and other species. *Journal of Experimental Biology*, **20**, 120–9.

Bauchop, T. (1979). Rumen anaerobic fungi of cattle and sheep. *Applied Environmental Microbiology*, **38**, 148–58.

Beever, D. E., Thomson, D. J., Pfeffer, E. & Armstrong, D. G. (1971). The effect of drying and ensiling grass on its digestion in sheep. *British Journal of Nutrition*, **26**, 123–34.

Beever, D. E., Coehlo da Silva, J. F., Prescott, J. H. D. & Armstrong, D. G. (1972). The effect in sheep of physical form and stage of growth on the sites of digestion of a dried grass. *British Journal of Nutrition*, **28**, 347–56.

Beever, D. E., Harrison, D. G., Thomson, D. J., Cammell, S. B. & Osbourn, D. F. (1974). A method for the estimation of dietary and microbial protein in duodenal digesta of ruminants. *British Journal of Nutrition*, **32**, 99–112.

Beever, D. E., Thomson, D. J. & Cammell, S. B. (1976). The digestion of frozen and dried grass by sheep. *Journal of Agricultural Science, Cambridge*, **86**, 443–52.

Beever, D. E., Thomson, D. J., Cammell, S. B. & Harrison, D. G. (1977). The digestion by sheep of silages made with and without the addition of formaldehyde. *Journal of Agricultural Science, Cambridge*, **88**, 61–70.

Beever, D. E. & Siddons, R. C. (1986). Digestion and metabolism in the grazing ruminant. In *Control of Digestion and Metabolism in Ruminants*, Milligan, L. P., Grovum, W. L. & Dobson, A., eds, pp. 479–97, Englefield Cliffs, NJ: Prentice Hall.

Beever, D. E., Sutton, J. D., Thomson, D. J., Napper, D. J. & Gale, D. L. (1988). Comparison of molassed and unmolassed sugar beet pulp and barley as energy supplements on nutrient digestion and supply in silage fed cows. *Animal Production*, **46**, 490.

Beever, D. E., Gill, M., Dawson, J. M. & Buttery, P. J. (1990a). The effect of fishmeal on the digestion of grass silage by growing cattle. *British Journal of Nutrition*, **63**, 489–502.

Beever, D. E., Napper, D. J. & Sloan, B. (1990b). Use of protected amino acids to increase duodenal amino acid supply in lactating dairy cows. *Animal Production*, **50**, 550.

Black, J. L., Beever, D. E., Faichney, G. J., Howarth, B. R. & Graham, N. McC. (1980/81). Simulation of the effects of rumen function on the flow of nutrients from the stomach of sheep. Part 1. Description of a computer model. *Agricultural Systems*, **6**, 195–219.

Bruce, C. I., Marsden, M. & Buttery, P. J. (1985). Leucine metabolism by rumen bacteria *in vivo*. *Proceedings of the Nutrition Society*, **44**, 143A.

Chalupa, W. (1980). Chemical control of rumen microbial metabolism. In *Digestive Physiology and Metabolism in Ruminants*, Ruckebush, Y. & Thivend, P., eds, pp. 325–47, Lancaster: MTP Press.

Chamberlain, D. G., Thomas, P. C. & Anderson, F. J. (1983). Volatile fatty acid proportions and lactic acid metabolism in the rumen in sheep and cattle receiving silage diets. *Journal of Agricultural Science, Cambridge*, **101**, 47–58.

Clarke, E. M. W., Ellinger, G. E. & Phillipson, A. T. (1966). The influence of diet on the nitrogenous components passing to the duodenum and through the terminal ileum of sheep. *Proceedings of the Royal Society, B*, **166**, 63–79.

Danfaer, A. (1990). A dynamic model of nutrient digestion and metabolism in lactating dairy cows. *Beretning fra Statens Husdyrbrugsforsog*, **671**, National Institute of Animal Science, Denmark.

Davies, D., Theodorou, M. K. & Trinci, A. P. J. (1990). Anaerobic fungi in the digestive tract and faeces of growing steers: evidence for a third stage in their life cycle. *Abstract of 4th International Mycology Congress* (Reyensburg, Germany [FDR]) II E-226/3.

Dawson, J. M., Bruce, C. J., Buttery, P. J., Gill, M. & Beever, D. E. (1988). Protein metabolism in the rumen of silage-fed steers. *British Journal of Nutrition*, **60**, 339–53.

Evans, R. A., Axford, R. F. E. & Offer, N. W. (1975). A method for estimating the quantities of microbial and dietary proteins flowing in the duodenal digesta of ruminants. *Proceedings of the Nutrition Society*, **34**, 65A.

Faichney, G. J. (1974). Effects of formaldehyde treatment of casein and peanut meal supplements on amino acids in digesta and plasma of lambs and sheep. *Australian Journal of Agricultural Research*, **25**, 583–98.

Faichney, G. J. (1975). The use of markers to partition digestion within the gastro-intestinal tract of ruminants. In *Digestion and Metabolism in the Ruminant*, McDonald, I. W. & Warner, A. C. I., eds, pp. 277–91, Armidale, Australia: University of New England Publishing Unit.

Ferguson, K. A. (1975). The protection of dietary proteins and amino acids against microbial fermentation in the rumen. In *Digestion and Metabolism in the Ruminant*, McDonald, I. W. & Warner, A. C. I., eds, pp. 448–64, Armidale, Australia: University of New England Publishing Unit.

Fitch, N. A., Gill, M., Lomax, M. A. & Beever, D. E. (1989). Nitrogen and glucose metabolism by the liver of forage- and forage-concentrate-fed cattle. *Proceedings of the Nutrition Society*, **48**, 76A.

France, J., Thornley, J. H. M. & Beever, D. E. (1982). A mathematical model of the rumen. *Journal of Agricultural Science*, **99**, 343–53.

Gill, E. M., Siddons, R. C., Beever, D. E. & Rowe, J. B. (1985). Metabolism of lactic acid isomers in the rumen of silage fed sheep. *British Journal of Nutrition*, **55**, 399–407.

Gregg, K. & Sharp, H. (1991). Enhancement of rumen microbial detoxification by gene transfer. In *Physiological Aspects of Digestion and Metabolism in Ruminants*, Tsuda, T., Sasaki, Y. & Kawashima, R., eds, pp. 719–35, New York: Academic Press.

Harris, L. E. & Phillipson, A. T. (1962). The measurement of the flow of food to the duodenum of sheep. *Journal of Animal Production*, **4**, 97–116.

Harrison, D. G., Beever, D. E., Thomson, D. J. & Osbourn, D. F. (1975). Manipulation of rumen fermentation in sheep by increasing the rate of flow of water from the rumen. *Journal of Agricultural Science, Cambridge*, **85**, 93–101.

Hogan, J. P. & Phillipson, A. T. (1960). The rate of transport of food along the digestive tract of sheep. *British Journal of Nutrition*, **14**, 147–55.

Hogan, J. P. & Weston, R. H. (1970). Quantitative aspects of microbial protein synthesis in the rumen. In *Physiology of Digestion and Metabolism in the Ruminant*, Phillipson, A. T., ed., pp. 474–85, Newcastle-upon-Tyne: Oriel Press.

Hutton, K., Bailey, J. F. & Annison, E. F. (1971). Measurement of the bacterial nitrogen entering the duodenum of the ruminant using diaminopimelic acid as a marker. *British Journal of Nutrition*, **25**, 165–73.

Karr, M. R., Little, C. O. & Mitchell, G. E. Jr. (1966). Starch disappearance from different segments of the digestive tract of steers. *Journal of Animal Science*, **25**, 652–4.

Lowe, S. E., Griffith, G. G., Milne, A., Theodorou, M. K. & Trinci, A. P. J.

(1987). The life cycle and growth kinetics of an anaerobic rumen fungus. *Journal of General Microbiology*, **133**, 1815–27.

Lowe, S. E., Theodorou, M. K., Trinci, A. P. J. & Hespell, R. B. (1985). Growth of anaerobic rumen fungi on defined and semi-defined media lacking rumen fluid. *Journal of General Microbiology*, **131**, 2225–9.

MacRae, J. C. & Armstrong, D. G. (1969). Studies on intestinal digestion in sheep. 2. Digestion of some carbohydrate constituents in hay, cereal and hay-cereal rations. *British Journal of Nutrition*, **23**, 377–87.

MacRae, J. C., Buttery, P. J. & Beever, D. E. (1988). Nutrient interactions in the dairy cow. In *Nutrition and Lactation in the Dairy Cow*, Garnsworthy, P. C., ed., pp. 55–75, London: Butterworths.

Maltby, S. A., Lomax, M. A., Beever, D. E. & Pippard, C. J. (1991). The effect of increased ammonia and amino acid supply on post-prandial portal and hepatic nitrogen and energy metabolism in growing steers fed maize silage. *European Association of Animal Production, Zurich*, Publication No. 58. Wenk, C. & Boessinger, M. eds.

Mathison, G. W. & Milligan, L. P. (1971). Nitrogen metabolism in sheep. *British Journal of Nutrition*, **25**, 351–66.

McAllan, A. B., Siddons, R. C. & Beever, D. E. (1987). The efficiency of conversion of degraded nitrogen to microbial nitrogen in the rumen of sheep and cattle. In *Feed Evaluation and Protein Requirement Systems for Ruminants*, Jarrige, R. & Alderman, G., eds, pp. 111–28, Luxembourg: CEC.

Mountfort, D. O. & Asher, R. A. (1985). Production and regulation of cellulase by two strains of the rumen anaerobic fungus *Neocallimastix frontalis*. *Applied and Environmental Microbiology*, **49**, 1314–22.

Nolan, J. V. (1975). Quantitative models of nitrogen metabolism in sheep. In *Digestion and Metabolism in the Ruminant*, McDonald, I. W. & Warner, A. C. I., eds, pp. 416–31, Armidale, Australia: University of New England Publishing Unit.

Nolan, J. V. & Leng, R. A. (1972). Dynamic aspects of ammonia and urea metabolism in sheep. *British Journal of Nutrition*, **27**, 177–94.

Nolan, J. V., Norton, B. W. & Leng, R. A. (1976). Further studies of the dynamics of nitrogen metabolism in sheep. *British Journal of Nutrition*, **35**, 127–47.

Orpin, C. G. (1974a). The rumen flagellates *Callimastix frontalis* and *Monas communis*-zoospores of Phycomycete fungi. *Journal of Applied Bacteriology*, **37**, ix–x.

Orpin, C. G. (1974b). The rumen flagellate *Callimastix frontalis*: does sequestration occur. *Journal of General Microbiology*, **84**, 395–8.

Orpin, C. G. (1975). Studies on the rumen flagellate *Neocallimastix frontalis*. *Journal of General Microbiology*, **91**, 249–62.

Phillipson, A. T. (1946). The physiology of digestion in the ruminant. *Veterinary Record*, **58**, 82–5.

Pirt, S. J. (1965). *Principles of Microbe and Cell Cultivation*. Oxford: Blackwell.

Roberts, S. A. & Miller, E. L. (1969). An estimate of bacterial protein synthesis in sheep on a constant feeding regime. *Proceedings of the Nutrition Society*, **28**, 32A.

Rooke, J. A., Lee, N. H. & Armstrong, D. G. (1987). The effects of intraruminal infusions of urea, casein, glucose syrup and a mixture of casein and glucose syrup on nitrogen digestion in the rumen of cattle receiving grass-silage diets. *British Journal of Nutrition*, **57**, 89–98.

Shipley, R. A. & Clarke, R. E. (1972). *Tracer Methods for* In vivo *Kinetics.* New York: Academic Press.

Siddons, R. C., Beever, D. E. & Nolan, J. V. (1982). A comparison of methods for the estimation of microbial nitrogen in duodenal digesta of sheep. *British Journal of Nutrition*, **48**, 377–89.

Siddons, R. C., Nolan, J. V., Beever, D. E. & MacRae, J. C. (1985). Nitrogen digestion and metabolism in sheep consuming diets containing contrasting forms and levels of N. *British Journal of Nutrition*, **54**, 175–87.

Smith, R. H. & McAllan, A. B. (1971). Nucleic acid metabolism in the ruminant. 3. Amounts of nucleic acids and total and ammonia nitrogen in digesta from the rumen, duodenum and ileum of calves. *British Journal of Nutrition*, **25**, 181–90.

Stouthamer, A. H. & Bettenhausen, C. W. (1973). Utilisation of energy for growth and maintenance in continuous and batch cultures of micro-organisms. A re-evaluation of the method for the determination of ATP production by measuring molar growth yields. *Biochimica et Biophysica Acta*, **301**, 53–70.

Teather, R. M. & Ohmiya, K. (1991). Molecular genetics of rumen cellulase systems. In *Physiological Aspects of Digestion and Metabolism in Ruminants*, Tsuda, T., Sasaki, Y. & Kawashima, R., eds, pp. 701–17, New York: Academic Press.

Theodorou, M. K., Longland, A. C., Dhanoa, M. S., Lowe, S. E. & Trinci, A. P. J. (1989). Growth of *Neocallimastix sp.* strain R. 1 on Italian ryegrass hay: removal of neutral sugars from plant cell walls. *Applied and Environmental Microbiology*, **55**, 1363–7.

Thomas, P. C. (1982). Utilisation of conserved forages. In *Forage Production in Ruminant Animal Production, British Society of Animal Production Occasional Publication No. 6*, Thomson, D. J., Beever, D. E. & Gunn, R. G., eds, pp. 67–76, Thames Ditton: BSAP.

Thomson, D. J., Beever, D. E. Coehlo da Silva, J. F. & Armstrong, D. G. (1972). The effect in sheep of physical form on the sites of digestion of a dried lucerne diet. *British Journal of Nutrition*, **28**, 31–41.

Thomson, D. J., Beever, D. E., Lonsdale, C. R., Haines, M. J., Cammell, S. B. & Austin, A. R. (1981). The digestion by cattle of grass silage made with formic acid and formic acid-formaldehyde. *British Journal of Nutrition*, **46**, 193–207.

Wilton, J. C., Gill, M. & Lomax, M. A. (1988). Uptake of ammonia across the liver of forage-fed cattle. *Proceedings of the Nutrition Society*, **47**, 153A.

8

Nitrogen metabolism in the ruminant

PETER J. BUTTERY

The 50 years that the Society has been in existence have seen the discovery of virtually all current knowledge on ruminant nitrogen metabolism, although the contributions made by several individuals during the late nineteenth and the first part of the twentieth century must not be forgotten (see Chalmers, 1961). Space prevents a comprehensive review of the subject, and it has been necessary to concentrate on a few topics which partially reflect the author's current and past interests and also to restrict the numbers of citations to published work.

Metabolism in the rumen

The 1940s saw not only the birth of the Society but also the discovery of most of the major features of nitrogen metabolism in the rumen. As recently as 1938 it was suggested that the rumen was merely a storage reservoir of food awaiting mastication and that it took little or no part in digestion (see Chalmers, 1961). Even though these views were common in the late 1930s there are several reports which indicate clearly that their authors were far from convinced that the rumen was only a food reservoir. As early as the 1890s, Zuntz (1891) postulated that the microorganisms in the rumen might synthesise their protein from simple nitrogenous components and so reduce the dietary protein needs of the animal. Pearson & Smith (1943) appreciated that protein was broken down to simple nitrogenous compounds in the rumen and that these materials were then used for microbial protein synthesis, but it was the work of McDonald (1948) that highlighted the importance of the large quantities of ammonia produced in the rumen. His work established three main features of rumen nitrogen metabolism, namely that the amount of ammonia in the rumen is dependent upon the type of dietary protein and carbohydrate, that a

80

considerable amount of ammonia passes through the rumen wall and hence reaches the liver and thirdly, that absorbed ammonia re-enters the rumen in the form of urea via the saliva. These concepts were subsequently developed and now form the basis of our current knowledge. Several reviews were published at the end of the 1950s, perhaps most notable being the monograph by Annison & Lewis (1959). The schematic representation they gave for nitrogen metabolism is almost identical to that which would depict today's knowledge; they even appreciated that the microorganisms could use peptides. The main achievements since then have been to quantify many of the transactions they postulated.

The central role played by ammonia in nitrogen metabolism in the rumen was emphasised by McDonald (1948) and this, coupled with the work of Virtanen (Land & Virtanen, 1959), formed the background to numerous studies in which a wide variety of non-protein nitrogenous compounds were fed to ruminants in attempts to reduce the animals' requirements for dietary protein. The responses obtained were very variable, but at the time the importance of balancing nitrogen supply to that of energy was not appreciated by many workers. The need to maintain a sufficiently high ammonia concentration to saturate the demands of the rumen bacteria but not high enough to induce ammonia toxicity in the animal was also not considered by most workers. Controversy raged as to what was the required concentration, some groups maintaining that less than 5×10^{-3} M was sufficient (Satter & Slyter, 1974; Pisulewski *et al.*, 1981), while others recommended much higher values. In a study in which sheep were fed low nitrogen/high energy diets supplemented with varying amounts of urea, abomasal non-protein nitrogen flow did not increase when ammonia concentrations exceeded 11.4×10^{-3} M (Allen & Miller, 1970). Mehrez, Ørskov & McDonald (1977) determined the rumen ammonia concentration required to give maximal digestion of dry matter confined in a Dracon bag suspended in the rumen, and suggested that ammonia concentrations needed to be in the order of 14×10^{-3} M to obtain maximal digestion of the fibre components of the diet. Studies with rumen microorganisms in culture threw some light on the subject when it was discovered that some species of rumen microorganisms had two pathways for fixing ammonia, one operating at low ammonia concentrations and another operating at higher concentrations (see, for example, Jenkinson, Buttery & Lewis, 1979; Scheifer, Davis & Bryant, 1980). In addition to interest in ammonia metabolism in the rumen, the impact of excess ammonia on the metabolism of the animal itself occupied many groups, and several attempts were made to find out the exact biochemical and physiological basis of ammonia toxicity both in ruminants (see, for example, Chalmers, Jeffray & White, 1971) and non-ruminants (for example, Visek, 1972). While it was relatively easy to study the effects of high concentrations of ammonia on metabolism, it was much more difficult to demonstrate that the ammonia challenges likely to be obtained when conventional feedstuffs are fed were of any great significance (see, for example, the study by Leonard, Buttery & Lewis, 1977). The possibility that ammonia resulting from the digestion of some forages and silages may have a deleterious effect cannot, however, be excluded.

The need to quantify the extent of microbial protein production in the rumen set a considerable challenge. It was necessary to be able to measure the amount of microbial protein in duodenal or abomasal digesta. (Protein chemists were not really interested in working with such smelly mixtures!) The methods developed all relied on the measurement of a metabolic marker in the digesta and in a sample of bacteria isolated either from the rumen or the digesta from the abomusum or the duodenum. Some of the techniques available at the end of the 1970s are presented in Table 8.1. There have been few developments in this area since. Several experiments were conducted to determine which method was the best, but no one had an absolute standard against which to evaluate accuracy of any techniques (see, for example, Ling & Buttery, 1978). It is of interest that the method which relies on determining RNA in the digesta and in bacteria (see McAllan & Smith, 1969) arose from studies to determine the significance of the binding of magnesium to the nucleic acid from rumen microorganisms and not from a programme specifically designed to measure microbial protein synthesis (McAllan, personal communication).

This ability to give an indication of the extent of microbial protein synthesis in the rumen enabled quantitative measures of the energetic efficiency of microbial protein synthesis *in vivo* to be made and a wide variety of values were obtained. Some of this variation obviously reflected genuine variability in the efficiency of the process, but some of it must have reflected the methods used (see Buttery & Lewis, 1982). Many of the experiments designed to investigate the control of microbial protein production in the rumen yielded inconclusive results largely because too few animals were used to gain any statistical significance in the data.

Perhaps the biggest contribution to quantitative knowledge on the rates of nitrogen metabolism came from studies using ^{15}N as a tracer and the pioneering work of Nolan and Leng (1972) at Armidale, Australia, Pilgrim *et al.* (1970) at Adelaide, Australia and in Canada by Mathison & Milligan (1971). These studies were applicable to the rumen in steady state, but

Table 8.1. *Some methods for determining the fraction of undegraded feed in duodenal digesta in ruminants*

	Method	Principle of operation
(i)	$^{35}SO_4$ incorporation	Bacterial and protozoal sulphur amino acids labelled; requires separation of microbial fraction and assay of radio-activity in (a) methionine, (b) cysteine or (c) organic sulphur of microbial fraction and duodenal digesta
(ii)	$^{32}PO_4$ incorporation	Bacterial and protozoal nucleic acids labelled; requires assay of activity in digesta and microbial nucleic acids; activity of ^{32}P prevents widespread use
(iii)	^{15}N incorporation	Bacterial and protozoal nitrogen labelled; need to isolate a microbial fraction from the digesta; ^{15}N difficult to assay
(iv)	Diaminopimelic acid (DAPA)	This amino acid occurs in the cell walls of some bacteria; does not occur in feed; requires assay of DAPA in microbial fraction and digesta
(v)	Aminoethylphosphonic acid	This amino acid occurs in the lipid fraction of some protozoa; this may occur in some feeds; can be difficult to assay; occurs in bacteria
(vi)	Constrained optimization of amino acid profile	Requires amino acid analysis of feed, microbial and digesta fractions
(vii)	RNA	RNA content of digesta compared with concentration in microbial fraction; analytical and storage problems can be encountered

For references to techniques see:
Ling & Buttery (1978).
Stern & Hoover (1979).

unfortunately under most feeding conditions the rumen is rarely in a steady state. Truly dynamic models to describe rumen metabolism in non-steady state conditions are now being developed (see, for example, Gill, Beever & France, 1989).

The need to predict the extent of the breakdown of dietary constituents in the rumen is crucial to virtually all decisions associated with feeding ruminants. While very useful data can be obtained from sophisticated experimentation with animals fitted with abomasal or duodenal cannulae, such procedures require elaborate laboratories, and much simpler techniques have many attractions. A wealth of information on the degradation of feedstuffs and rumen function in general has been obtained by the exploitation of the relatively simple *in situ* Dacron bag technique for which Ørskov must take considerable credit (Ørskov & McDonald, 1979).

The ability to consider nitrogen metabolism in the rumen in quantitative terms led to the development of schemes for predicting the response of ruminants to dietary nitrogen supply. The basic concepts of the scheme promoted by the Agricultural Research Council (1980) were that by initially calculating from the rumen fermentable energy in the diet, the supply of simple nitrogenous compounds required for maximal activity of the rumen microorganisms could be determined. The protein production from the microorganisms could then be compared with the expected protein requirements of the tissues of the animal. Any shortfall could then be made up by ensuring that the diet had sufficient dietary protein which escapes ruminal degradation. The foundations for this scheme were laid in a most stimulating paper by Miller (1973), presented at a meeting of the Nutrition Society, and the scheme itself was unveiled in 1977 (Roy *et al.*, 1977). Even in 1991 the scheme continues to be refined, but the main stumbling blocks seem to be the difficulty in describing rumen activity in truly dynamic rather than static terms, particularly allowing for asynchrony in the metabolism of the nitrogenous and the energy-yielding components of the diet, ascribing values to the energetic efficiency of microbial protein synthesis and in accurately predicting the efficiency of utilisation of the protein leaving the duodenum by the animal's tissues.

Metabolism in the tissues of the animal

The technical difficulties associated with working with large animals resulted in the development of knowledge of protein metabolism in the ruminant lagging behind that of the small laboratory animals. During the late 1960s and early 1970s techniques were developed to quantify the extent of protein synthesis and to a limited extent protein degradation in the tissues of intact animals. Initial studies concentrated on laboratory animals, but when the techniques were applied to sheep and cattle it was clear that there was nothing peculiar about the rates of protein metabolism in ruminants (see the stimulating review presented to the Society by Reeds & Lobley, 1980, Table 8.2). It is now universally accepted that protein and amino acid metabolism in ruminant tissues is similar to that in other mammals.

The concept that the requirements of ruminant tissues for essential amino acids were similar to those of non-ruminants was difficult to

Table 8.2. *Protein synthesis in animals of different body size*

Species	Bodyweight (kg)	Protein synthesised[a] ($g/kg\ BW^{0.75}\ per\ d$)
Rat (growing)	0.35	16.7
Rabbit (adult)	3.6	15.0
Pig (growing)	30	18.9
Sheep (adult)	63	15.7
Man (adult)	62	12.5
Cattle (adult)	500	16.1

[a] Data calculated from plasma flux measurements of $[1-^{14}C]$-leucine corrected for catabolism of leucine and taken from Reeds & Lobley (1980).

establish, but studies with isotopically labelled compounds eventually yielded the necessary data (see, for example, Downes, 1961; Black *et al.*, 1957). Comparison of the amino acid profile of microbial protein with the expected requirements of growing, lactating and wool-producing ruminants indicated that production might be increased by increasing the supply of certain amino acids, especially methionine and cysteine, to the duodenum. A particularly novel approach to this area were the experiments of Storm & Ørskov (1984), who isolated large quantities of rumen microorganisms and then infused them into the abomasum of sheep maintained by intragastric infusion. For amino acids to act as effective supplements for ruminant diets they need to be protected from rumen degradation but still become available to the tissues on leaving the rumen. Numerous preparations and derivatives of several amino acids, especially of methionine, were developed which meet these criteria (see Ferguson, 1975). The commercial exploitation of these materials was thwarted by an inability to predict the response of the animal when they were added to conventional diets. Part of the problem is that, in many cases, two or more amino acids rapidly become co-limiting. Despite the numerous studies, especially in the 1970s, protected amino acids are now rarely used commercially.

The importance of ruminants as meat-producing animals resulted in many attempts to increase their rate of protein deposition by manipulation of their endocrine status, initially by the use of implants of steroid hormones or their analogues. This practice is still used in many countries of the world, including the United States, but relatively recently was banned in the European Economic Community despite scientific evidence which clearly indicates that if the preparations based upon natural steroids are used according to the manufacturer's instructions they present no hazard to the consumer of the meat, the animal or indeed those caring for the animal (Lamming *et al.*, 1987). Studies on the mode of action of the growth promoters principally designed for use with cattle have yielded some interesting observations on the control of lean deposition. The anabolic agent trenbolone was shown to increase muscle mass by decreasing the rate of muscle protein degradation, which at the time was a very surprising finding (Vernon & Buttery, 1976). Protein degradation rate was shown to be a major factor in the myogenic response seen to treatment of mammals with beta agonists (see MacRae & Lobley, 1991). Not all growth enhancers work this way, for example growth hormone stimulates muscle protein synthesis (MacRae & Lobley, 1991). Response of ruminants to growth promoters is usually only apparent when the animals are fed good quality diets (Breier *et al.*, 1986).

Although the size of most domesticated ruminants has created problems for many metabolic studies, it has for some studies been a distinct advantage. The elegant work of Bergman and his colleagues (see, for example, Bergman & Pell, 1984) quantified the uptake and release of amino acids by the organs of the sheep, and made a significant contribution to knowledge of interorgan transport of amino acids. Studies by Linzell and co-workers (see Linzell & Annison, 1975) contributed significantly to knowledge of protein metabolism in the mammary gland.

The future

Knowledge of the transactions of nitrogen in the rumen is still at a level where it is difficult to predict with any precision the supply of amino acids reaching the duodenum. This is particularly so when ammonia and amino acid production is not synchronised with the availability of energy. If ruminant feeding schemes are to gain the precision needed for intensive livestock production then they must be able to predict the supply of amino acids to the tissues. Attention needs to be given to methods of defining precisely the biochemical composition of feeds and how this influences the proportions of individual species of rumen microorganisms and hence the supply of amino acids to the animal's tissues. Manipulation of the microbial population of the rumen is an attractive idea and has been achieved by the use of antibiotic-feed additives, e.g. rumensin.

An alternative approach in the future is the use of genetically manipulated organisms. Genetic manipulation of rumen microorganisms has been achieved (see, for example, Thompson & Flint, 1989), but the difficulty of maintaining a modified organism in the rumen should not be underestimated. Some encouragement comes from the successful intro-duction of rumen microorganisms from Hawaiian goats which have the ability to catabolize dihydroxypyridine (a metabolite of mimosine, a toxic non-protein amino acid found in the *Leucaena* bush) into Australian cattle and hence give them the ability to detoxify mimosine (Jones & Megarrity, 1986).

Developments in nitrogen metabolism of the tissues of the ruminant are likely to follow those of mammals in general. Of particular interest to the nutritionist will be studies on the control of gene expression and hormonal activity by nutrient supply (see Pell & Bates, 1990).

Manipulation of ruminants to enhance protein deposition at the expense of fat without the use of exogenously applied hormones is now a reality. The use of the immune response has many attractions. Although the binding of hormones by antibodies usually decreases their activity, certain monoclonal antibodies to growth hormone have been shown to potentiate its somatogenic activity (Aston *et al.*, 1986; Wallis *et al.*, 1987). More recently, immunological enhancement of the galactopoietic response to exogenous growth hormone has been demonstrated in lactating sheep (Pell & Bates, 1990). The diabetogenic activity of endogenous, as well as exogenous applied, growth hormone was also shown to be potentiated in young lambs given monoclonal antibodies against growth hormone (Pell & Bates, 1990). This suggests that a similar immunological approach could be used to enhance the effect of other bioactive peptides which control nitrogen deposition. An alternative approach is the use of anti-idiotypic antibodies, for example, anti-idiotypic antisera produced in sheep to rat growth hormone antibodies have been shown to stimulate body weight gain in hypophysectomised rats (Gardner *et al.*, 1990). Interestingly, however, no increases in circulating IGF-1 levels were detected. Develop-ments in the use of the immune response are currently being constrained by difficulties in controlling the immune response and by the need to develop adjuvants which do not cause abscesses in treated animals.

Now that transgenic animals are a reality there is little doubt that eventually ruminant animals with enhanced protein deposition will be routinely produced. One of the main requirements is to advance knowledge of the control of protein deposition. Increasing the copies of growth hormone genes in pigs and sheep has only met with limited success; although some animals have shown increased growth and enhanced lean deposition most also exhibited several detrimental abnormalities. Transgenic animals (e.g. mice) containing extra copies of insulin-like growth factor 1 genes have been produced and, although these animals were larger and did not show the same deleterious features associated with the growth hormone transgenic animals, many of the desirable features associated with enhanced circulating growth hormone were lost (Matthews *et al.*, 1988). The future probably lies in manipulating genes whose products only influence a limited number of metabolic processes. The recent report of the introduction of the *c-ski* gene from chicken into mice is interesting (Sutrave, Kelly & Hughes, 1990). These animals had enhanced growth of muscles containing type 2 fibres. Improvement of the supply of amino acids to the tissues of ruminants could potentially be achieved in two ways, first by manipulation of the rumen micro-organisms (see above), and secondly by manipulation of the animal itself, for example by production of transgenic sheep which express the cysteine synthesising enzymes (Rogers, 1990). Such animals should have an enhanced wool growth. One of the major constraints in the production of transgenic ruminants is the time taken to obtain lines of transgenic animals suitable for breeding. Brenig & Brem (1991) calculated that this would take 4–5 or 8–9 years after the appropriate gene constructs have been produced to establish transgenic lines of sheep or cattle respectively. The use of these potential methods of enhancing lean deposition in ruminants can only become a commercial reality when, and if, the general public accepts that they are safe and ethical.

Protection of the environment is now a major concern, and nitrogen pollution from ruminant livestock often presents serious problems. Research into factors which regulate the efficiency of capture of amino acids by the tissues and ammonia and other nitrogenous materials by the rumen micro-organisms is likely to pay considerable dividends besides being a very interesting scientific challenge.

Acknowledgement

The author wishes to thank Professors Frank Annison and Dyfed Lewis for introducing him to the fascinations of ruminant nutrition and biochemistry. Attempting to understand the complexities of nitrogen transactions in the ruminant has been and still is a most stimulating challenge.

References

Agricultural Research Council (1980). *Nutrient Requirements of Ruminant Livestock*. Farnham royal: Commonwealth Agricultural Bureaux.

Allen, S. A. & Miller, E. L. (1970). Determination of nitrogen requirements for microbial growth from the effect of urea supplementation of low-N diets on abomasal N flow and N recycling in wethers and lambs. *British Journal of Nutrition*, **36**, 353–68.

Annison, E. F. & Lewis, D. (1959). *Metabolism in the Rumen*. London: Methuen.

Aston, R., Holder, A. T., Preece, M. A. & Ivanyi, J. (1986). Potentiation of the somatogenic and lactogenic activity of human growth hormone with monoclonal antibodies. *Journal of Endocrinology*, **110**, 381–8.

Bergman, E. N. & Pell, J. M. (1984). Integration of amino acid metabolism in the ruminant. In *Herbivore Nutrition*, Gilchrist, F. M. C. & Mackie, R. I., eds, pp. 613–30, Craighill: Science Press.

Black, A. L., Klieber, M., Smith, A. H. & Stewart, D. N. (1957). Acetate as a precursor of amino acids of casein in the intact dairy cow. *Biochimica et Biophysica Acta*, **23**, 54–9.

Breier, B. H., Bass, J. J., Butler, J. H. & Gluckman, P. D. (1986). The somatotrophic axis in young steers, influence of nutritional status on pulsatile release of growth hormone and circulating concentration of insulin-like growth factor-1. *Journal of Endocrinology*, **116**, 169–77.

Brenig, B. & Brem, G. (1991). Principles of genetic manipulation of livestock. In *Animal Biotechnology and the Quality of Meat Production*, Fiems, L. O., Cottyn, B. G. & Demeyer, D. I., eds, pp. 31–49. Amsterdam: Elsevier.

Buttery, P. J. & Lewis, D. (1982). Nitrogen metabolism in the rumen. In *Forage Protein in Ruminant Animal Production*, Thomson, D. J., Beever, D. E. & Gunn, R. G., eds, pp. 1–11. Thames Ditton: British Society of Animal Production.

Chalmers, M. I. (1961). Protein synthesis in the rumen. In *Digestive Physiology and Nutrition of the Ruminant*, Lewis, D., ed., pp. 205–26. London: Butterworths.

Chalmers, M. I., Jeffray, A. E. & White, F. (1971). Movements of ammonia following intraruminal administration of urea or casein. *Proceedings of the Nutrition Society*, **30**, 7–17.

Downes, A. M. (1961). On the amino acids essential for the tissues of the sheep. *Australian Journal of Biological Science*, **14**, 254–9.

Ferguson, K. A. (1975). The protection of dietary proteins and amino acids against microbial fermentation in the rumen. In *Digestion and Metabolism in the Ruminant*, McDonald, I. W. & Warner, A. C. I., eds, pp. 448–64. Armidale: The University of New England Publishing Unit.

Gardner, M. J., Morrison, C. A., Stevenson, L. Q. & Flint, D. J. (1990). Production of anti-idiotypic antisera to rat growth hormone antibodies capable of binding to growth hormone receptors and increasing body weight gain in hypophysectomized rats. *Journal of Endocrinology*, **125**, 53–9.

Gill, M., Beever, D. E. & France, J. (1989). Biochemical bases needed for the mathematical representation of whole animal metabolism. *Nutrition Research Reviews*, **2**, 181–200.

Jenkinson, H., Buttery, P. J. & Lewis, D. (1979). Assimilation of ammonia by *Bacteroides amylophilus* in chemical cultures. *Journal of General Microbiology*, **113**, 305–13.

Jones, R. J. & Megarrity, R. G. (1986). Successful transfer of DHP degrading bacteria from Hawaiian goats to Australian ruminants to overcome the toxicity of *Leucaena*. *Australian Veterinary Journal*, **63**, 259–62.

Lamming, G. E., Ballarini, G., Baulieu, E. E., Brookes, P., Elias, P. S.,
    Ferrando, R., Gallic, C. L., Heitzman, R. J., Hoffman, B., Karg, H.,
    Meyer, H. H. D., Michel, G., Poulsen, E., Rico, A., Van Leewen, F. X. R.
    & White, D. S. (1987). Scientific report on anabolic agents in animal
    production. Veterinary Record, 121, 389–92.
Land, H. & Virtanen, A. I. (1959). Ammonia salts as nitrogen source in the
    synthesis of protein by the ruminant. Acta Chemica Scandinavica, 13,
    489–96.
Leonard, M. C., Buttery, P. J. & Lewis, D. (1977). The effects on glucose
    metabolism of feeding high urea diets to sheep. British Journal of Nutrition,
    38, 455–62.
Ling, J. R. & Buttery, P. J. (1978). The simultaneous use of ribonucleic acid, ^{35}S,
    2, 6-diaminopimelic acid and 2-aminoethylphosphoric acid as markers of
    microbial nitrogen entering the duodenum of sheep. British Journal of
    Nutrition, 39, 165–79.
Linzell, J. L. & Annison, E. F. (1975). Methods of measuring the utilization of
    metabolites absorbed from the alimentary tract. In Digestion and
    Metabolism in the Ruminant, McDonald, I. W. & Warner, A. C. T., eds, pp.
    306–19, Armidale: The University of New England Publishing Unit.
McAllan, A. B. & Smith, R. H. (1969). Nucleic acid metabolism in the
    ruminant. Determination of Nucleic acids in Digesta, British Journal of
    Nutrition, 23, 671–82.
McDonald, I. W. (1948). The absorption of ammonia from the rumen of
    sheep. Biochemical Journal, 42, 548–57.
MacRae, J. C. & Lobley, G. E. (1991). Physiological and metabolic implications
    of conventional and novel methods for the manipulation of growth and
    production. Livestock Production Science, 27, 43–68.
Mathison, G. W. & Milligan, L. P. (1971). Nitrogen Metabolism in Sheep,
    British Journal of Nutrition, 25, 351–66.
Matthews, L. S., Hammer, R. E., Behringer, R. R., D'Ercole, A. J., Bell, G. I.,
    Brinster, R. L. & Palmiter, R. D. (1988). Growth enhancement of
    transgenic mice expressing human insulin-like growth factor I.
    Endocrinology, 123, 2827–33.
Mehrez, A. Z., Ørskov, E. R. & McDonald, I. (1977). Rates of ruminal
    fermentation in relation to ammonia concentration. British Journal of
    Nutrition, 38, 437–43.
Miller, E. L. (1973). Evaluation of foods as sources of nitrogen and amino
    acids. Proceedings of the Nutrition Society, 32, 79–84.
Nolan, J. V. & Leng, R. A. (1972). Dynamic aspects of ammonia and urea
    metabolism in sheep. British Journal of Nutrition, 35, 177–94.
Ørskov, E. R. & McDonald, I. (1979). The estimation of protein degradability
    in the rumen from incubation measurements weighted according to rates of
    passage. Journal of Agricultural Science, Cambridge, 92, 499–503.
Pearson, R. M. & Smith, J. A. B. (1943). The utilization of urea in the bovine
    rumen. 1. Methods of analysis of the rumen ingesta and preliminary
    experiments in vivo. Biochemical Journal, 37, 142–8.
Pell, J. M. & Bates, P. C. (1990). The nutritional regulation of growth hormone
    action. Nutrition Research Reviews, 3, 169–92.
Pilgrim, A. F., Gray, F. V., Weller, R. A. & Bellin, C. B. (1970). Synthesis of
    microbial protein from ammonia in the sheep's rumen and the proportion
    of dietary nitrogen converted into microbial protein. British Journal of
    Nutrition, 24, 589–98.

Pisulewski, P. M., Okorie, A., Buttery, P. J., Haresign, W. & Lewis, D. (1981). Ammonia concentrations and protein synthesis in the rumen. *Journal of the Science of Food and Agriculture*, **32**, 759–66.

Reeds, P. J. & Lobley, G. E. (1980). Protein synthesis: are there real species differences? *Proceedings of the Nutrition Society*, **39**, 43–52.

Rogers, G. E. (1990). Improvement of wool production through genetic engineering. *Trends in Biotechnology*, **8**, 6–11.

Roy, J. H. B., Balch, C. C., Miller, E. L., Ørskov, E. R. & Smith, R. H. (1977). Calculation of the N-requirement for ruminants from nitrogen metabolism studies. *Proceedings of the Second International Symposium on Protein Metabolism and Nutrition*, Taminga, S., ed., pp. 126–9. Wageningen: Centre for Agricultural Publishing and Documentation.

Satter, L. D. & Slyter, L. L. (1974). Effect of ammonia concentration on rumen microbial protein production *in vivo*. *British Journal of Nutrition*, **32**, 199–208.

Scheifer, D. M., Davis, G. L. & Bryant, M. P. (1980). Ammonia saturation constants for predominant species of rumen bacteria. *Journal of Dairy Science*, **63**, 1248–63.

Stern, M. D. & Hoover, W. J. (1979). Methods for determining factors affecting microbial protein synthesis: a review. *Journal of Animal Science*, **49**, 1590–603.

Storm, E. & Ørskov, E. R. (1984). The nutritive value of rumen micro-organisms in ruminants. The limiting amino acids of microbial protein in growing sheep determined by a new approach. *British Journal of Nutrition*, **52**, 613–20.

Sutrave, P., Kelly, A. M. & Hughes, S. (1990). *Ski* can cause selective growth of skeletal muscle in transgenic mice. *Genes and Development*, **4**, 1462–72.

Thompson, A. M. & Flint, H. J. (1989). Electroporation induced transformation of *Bacteroides ruminocola* and *Bacteroides uniformis* by plasmid DNA. *FEMS Microbiology Letters*, **61**, 101–4.

Vernon, B. G. & Buttery, P. J. (1976). Protein turnover in rats treated with trenbolone acetate. *British Journal of Nutrition*, **36**, 575–9.

Visek, W. J. (1972). Effects of urea hydrolysis on cell lifespan and metabolism. *Federation Proceedings*, **31**, 1178–93.

Wallis, M., Daniels, M., Ray, K. P., Cottingham, J. D. & Aston, R. (1987). Monoclonal antibodies to bovine growth hormone to potentiate effects of the hormone on somatomedin C levels and growth of hypophysectomized rats. *Biochemical and Biophysical Research Communications*, **149**, 187–93.

Zuntz, N. (1891). Remarks on the digestion and the nutritional value of cellulose. *Pfluger's Archiv fur die gesamte Physiologie des Menschen und die Tiere*, **49**, 477–84.

9

Protein metabolism in man

ALAN A. JACKSON

Introduction

The Nutrition Society was formed at a time when two advances were being made of fundamental importance to the understanding of protein nutrition: the refinement of the concept of protein quality (Rose, 1938) and the concept of the dynamic state of the body constituents (Schoenheimer, 1942). During the past 50 years the concepts of protein quality have been applied to the human and there has been a greater exploration of the metabolic interrelations of amino acids. A new area, the measurement and exploration of aspects of protein turnover at the level of the whole body and individual tissues, represents the major conceptual and practical development of recent time (Waterlow, 1984).

Recent data have caused the detailed application of some of the principles developed during the earlier years to be reassessed critically. For many of the classical studies, the investigators were much more cautious in the interpretation of their own experimental results than those who later adopted the principles they expounded. The original scientists took care to express their conclusions in guarded terms, with due allowance for conceptual modification as understanding advanced. However, the conceptual modification did not always take place and there has been a tendency towards ossification of thought. A good example of this is the tortuous route to the present understanding of the absorption of protein and amino acids (Matthews, 1991).

Classical perceptions

Amino acids: indispensable or essential?

The identification of mechanisms which explained the processes through which nitrogen balance could be maintained, such as urea synthesis, gave

92

a rational basis to the determination of the amount of protein required in the diet. The identification of amino acids as the functionally active components of protein made it possible to determine quality chemically in rational terms. By 1914, Osborne and Mendel had enunciated a most important principle which embodied the concept of limiting nutrients (Rose, 1938):

That the tissues either form a typical protoplasmic product or none at all, now seems to be axiomatic in physiology.

The principle is implicit to the methods used extensively in nutrition, whereby nitrogen balance is used as a marker for adequacy of a diet or a range of nutrients. During the early part of the century the individual amino acids were identified and isolated. By feeding diets of purified amino acids the effect of a deficiency of a single amino acid could be determined. This was the basis of the experimental approach adopted by Rose, in which he used the ability of a diet to maintain an acceptable rate of weight gain as the outcome variable for amino acids adequacy.

By 1938 it was clear that under the experimental conditions adopted rats required ten amino acids to support the rate of weight gain seen on the full diet (Rose, 1938). Eight of the ten were subsequently found to be necessary for the maintenance of weight and nitrogen balance in adult humans. In rats, the omission of histidine was associated with weight loss. More recent studies in humans show that the ability to maintain weight and nitrogen balance in the short term on a diet deficient in histidine might be accounted for by progressive depletion of the histidine contained within the pool of carnosine in muscle (FAO/WHO/UNU, 1985). In the rat, a diet deficient in arginine was associated with a reduced rate of weight gain. The requirement for dietary arginine is being reassessed for humans.

The results of Rose gave rise to the classification of amino acids into two broad groups, indispensable (essential) and dispensable (non-essential). '...we define an indispensable dietary component as one which cannot be synthesised by the animal organism, out of the materials *ordinarily available* at a speed commensurate with the demands for *normal* growth' (Rose, 1938). The classification has become widely accepted, but has been used in a much more rigid way than was implied by the experimental results obtained. The identification of amino acids as indispensable gave rise to the idea that they could not be formed at all in the body. Conversely, the idea that some amino acids were dispensable was taken by many to mean that they did not have to be present in the diet under any circumstances. It is interesting that the two amino acids accepted as being conditionally indispensable, arginine and histidine, were seen as being the exceptions to

the general rule, whereas they probably represent the rule, with indispensable and dispensable amino acids representing the two extremes
(Jackson, 1989).

Metabolic activity of amino acids

The second great conceptual advance depended upon technological
innovations in the separation and measurements of stable isotopes. By
1942, Schoenheimer and his colleagues had demonstrated unequivocally
that, when labelled amino acids were added to the diet, a substantial
proportion of the label could be retained in the body. The label was
identified as an integral component of the proteins in all of the tissues
examined. These studies gave rise to the principle that the materials which
comprised the substance of the body were engaged in a constant turnover,
and that the material from the diet was an integral part of the exchange.
The identification of enzyme systems which allowed for the movement of
amino groups between carbon skeletons encouraged the view that the
movement of amino groups between carbon skeletons was limitless
(Jackson & Golden, 1981).

In 1950, Aqvist showed that, although there was exchange of ^{15}N-
labelled amino groups between the carbon skeletons, the exchange was
channelled and in some situations restricted. The limited use of nitrogen
tracers for the study of intermediary metabolism has meant that this area
of investigation has not been greatly advanced over the last 40 years
(Jahoor, Jackson & Golden, 1988). It is clear from the limited data
provided by these studies that the metabolic channelling of nitrogen
represents a most important area of enquiry for the future (Fig. 9.1).

Protein turnover

One consequence of the demonstration that proteins exist in a dynamic
state was the attempts to measure the intensity of the rate at which proteins
turned over. Early explorations of the theoretical and practical issues
involved did not lead to any widespread use of the methods until they were
developed as a tool to address specific problems such as the failure of the
mechanisms for protein synthesis in childhood malnutrition (Waterlow,
1984). The history and development of these ideas and approaches by
Waterlow and his colleagues (Waterlow, Garlick & Millward, 1978a) has
become a citation classic for the decade, demonstrating the enormous
influence the work has had upon metabolic study. The most useful
development of all by Waterlow appears to have been overlooked: the

atoms % excess × 1000

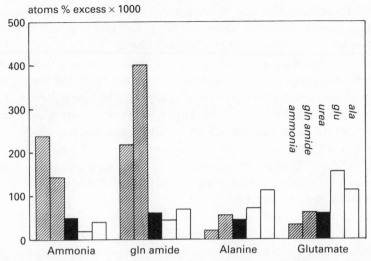

Fig. 9.1. Rats were given a constant intravenous infusion of one of four ^{15}N-labelled compounds, ammonia, glutamine amide, alanine and glutamate. The level of enrichment of ammonia, glutamine amide, urea, glutamate and alanine were measured in the free hepatic pool after 6 hours' infusion (Jahoor *et al.*, 1988). Similar levels of enrichment were found in urea (solid square) with the infusion of each label, but the distribution of label amongst the precursors, transaminators (shaded square) and deaminators (open square) (Jackson & Golden, 1981) varied with the origin of the label.

single dose/end product method (Waterlow, Golden & Garlick, 1978*b*; Fern *et al.*, 1981). It is non-invasive and simple to use in practice, therefore it can be used for field studies. The isotope is presented orally and follows the natural fate of dietary protein. By using nitrogen as a tracer the fate of amino acids is followed in terms of the nitrogen pool, rather than the carbon pool. The results of studies on protein turnover have contributed greatly to advancing understanding and conceptual development by demonstrating that the external exchange represented by balance is only a pale shadow of the intensity of the internal exchange.

Human requirements

Assessment of protein status

Central to all considerations of protein nutriture is the assessment of protein status. There has been confusion as to how this might best be achieved, which to an extent relates to insufficient care in differentiating state from function. Measurements of state such as body weight, body composition, plasma concentrations of amino acids and proteins are in general measures of amounts. Measurements of function such as nitrogen balance, enzyme activities, measures of tissue function and protein turnover are in general measures of rates of change.

The indicators used by earlier workers in the definition of amino acid and protein requirements were a normal rate of weight gain and acceptable nitrogen balance in growing animals. This approach has the limitation that it is not applicable to adults. Adult requirements have been based upon approaches which require the definition of nitrogen balance, which as a method is difficult, laborious and lacks precision (FAO/WHO/UNU, 1985). Similar difficulties are experienced in attempting to assess amino acid or protein requirements in unusual or pathological states. Increasingly it seems that the classification introduced by Rose lacks flexibility, and alternative systems of classification have been proposed (Jackson, 1982; Laidlaw & Kopple, 1987). These classifications recognise that, although the body may seek to match the endogenous synthesis of amino acids to its metabolic demands, the demands might not always be met. More and more situations can be identified in which individual amino acids have been shown to be 'conditionally essential' (Jackson, 1989).

Dispensable amino acids and non-essential nitrogen

For many years the attention given to the metabolic role played by the indispensable amino acids appeared to outweigh in importance any consideration of the metabolic activity of the dispensable amino acids. The perception was that the dispensable amino acids were unlikely to be limiting for metabolic processes.

In adulthood, the requirement for indispensable amino acids might only be 19% of total nitrogen intake (Munro, 1985). It has never been adequately explained why there should be such a high requirement, 81%, for dispensable amino acids and/or non-essential nitrogen. Indispensable amino acids have been shown to be a relatively poor source of non-essential nitrogen and the evidence indicates that the most efficient source of non-essential nitrogen is glutamic acid or an ammonium salt with glycine (Kies, 1972). When the protein intake of infants is progressively reduced to a point where nitrogen balance and growth can no longer be maintained, then growth and positive balance can be restored by the addition of either glycine or urea to the diet. The nitrogen from these sources is actively incorporated into body protein (Snyderman *et al.*, 1962). In adults, nitrogen balance could not be maintained on an intake of 0.57 g protein/kg/d and a generous intake of energy, but the addition of dispensable amino acids promoted positive nitrogen balance and enabled the energy intake to be reduced by 10 to 15% (Garza, Scrimshaw & Young, 1978). Therefore, the data show that there is a component of 'non-essential nitrogen' which is 'essential': an obvious contradiction in terms.

One example of the importance of this apparent contradiction is the demonstration that populations taking traditional diets appear to be able to exist on intakes of protein below the level considered to be compatible with life (Ooman, 1970). This practical observation cannot easily be explained by prevailing concepts of the requirements for protein and amino acids. The suggestion that it might be possible for man to fix atmospheric nitrogen through the metabolic activity of the colonic flora has not been supported by the experimental evidence.

Metabolic activity of individual dispensable amino acids

There has been an expansion of work on the specific metabolic functions of individual amino acids and the cooperativity between different tissues. The flux of glutamine in the body is far greater than required simply for acid base balance (Golden, Jahoor & Jackson, 1982), and glutamine has a complex metabolic role of wider significance (Newsholme, Crabtree & Ardawi, 1985). Glutamine released from muscle passes to the intestine where it acts as a source of energy for the bowel mucosa and gives rise to citrulline (Windmueller & Spaeth, 1980). The citrulline leaves the bowel, passes to the kidney to be formed into arginine (Windmueller & Spaeth, 1981), which is available for the rest of the body. Both arginine and glutamine are required for cellular proliferation, and may be involved in the activity of the immune system, wound healing and gastro-intestinal function (Barbul, 1986). Arginine as the immediate precursor of nitrous oxide may be involved in the maintenance of vascular tone, as a neurotransmitter and as an integral part of the inflammatory response (Moncada & Higgs, 1991). The sulphur amino acids, cysteine and taurine, have a complex metabolism, playing an important role in maintaining the integrity of cell function, acting as a membrane stabiliser, as well as having well defined roles as anti-oxidants. Glycine, like glutamine and arginine, is required for cell proliferation as a building block for DNA and RNA; like cysteine and taurine it plays a role in cell communication and membrane function (Jackson, 1991).

Protein, amino acids and growth

Children who are unwell lose their appetite, fail to grow and their development stops or regresses. Children who become stunted have a delay in mental development (Grantham-McGregor, 1988). It had been believed that normal growth and development required an adequate intake of good quality protein, and in illness protein was diverted towards dealing with the disease rather than for normal development. It has been difficult to obtain support for this general impression, as supplements of essential amino acids provided little clear benefit.

Linear growth takes place in a collagen matrix. The demands for glycine for linear growth are high, as one third of the amino acid residues in collagen are glycine. During periods of rapid growth, during pregnancy, in neonates or during recovery from malnutrition the requirements for glycine are barely satisfied (Jackson, 1991). The intracellular tripeptide glutathione (glutamate, cysteine and glycine) has a metabolic function central to the maintenance of cellular integrity (Kosower & Kosower, 1978). Reduced cellular levels of glutathione increase sensitivity to the damaging effects of a range of physical, chemical and therapeutic agents (Reed & Fariss, 1984). The intracellular concentration of glutathione is influenced by the dietary availability of cysteine and possibly of glycine also (Jackson, 1991). An inflammatory response, necessary for effective recovery from a wide range of insults, is a complex response mediated by cytokines. Nutritional factors influence the ability to produce cytokines, and patients unable to produce satisfactory levels of cytokines are at increased risk (Grimble, 1990). An increase in the amount and alteration in the pattern of proteins synthesised in the liver is an integral part of the acute phase response. Three amino acids in particular are required in unusually large amounts for the synthesis of these proteins, glycine, serine and cysteine (Grimble, 1990). The acute phase response in rats can be modulated by varying the availability of amino acids from the diet. Attempts to prevent wasting by the provision of extra protein may not be particularly successful if the pattern of amino acids in the proteins provided is not optimally suited to the pattern being synthesised. These metabolic relationships may help to explain some of the apparent conflict of ideas that have persisted over the years.

Adaptation and nitrogen balance

Central to Waterlow's ideas about protein metabolism was the concept of adaptation (Waterlow, 1968). What is the minimum intake which can be accommodated to allow for survival of some specified level of functional capability? It is clear that nitrogen balance might be defended in the face of a marginal reduction in energy intake (Kennedy et al., 1990) even though different levels of energy intake exert an influence upon nitrogen balance (Munro, 1985). An understanding of the processes whereby individuals can accommodate to changes in protein intake and the metabolic demand for protein are central to our definition of protein, amino acid and nitrogen requirements in health and disease.

Adults are capable of accommodating to a wide range of protein intakes without any obvious untoward effect. Nitrogen balance is maintained by a shift in the rate at which nitrogen is lost from the body as urea in urine. There has been a tendency to equate the rate of urinary urea excretion with urea production. However widespread, this presumption is incorrect. Although urea is appropriately considered to be an end product of mammalian metabolism, it has been known since 1946 that urea can be hydrolysed in the body to release nitrogen which is potentially available for further metabolic interaction. Several studies show that overall 75 % of urea production is excreted and 25 % salvaged, following hydrolysis by the microflora of the lower bowel, for further interaction (Hibbert & Jackson, 1991).

Urea kinetics

Urea salvaging appears to have all the characteristics of a controlled process, but the nature and details of the control still have to be resolved. It would appear that the most important influence upon the rate of salvage is the dietary intake of nitrogen or protein (Langran *et al.*, 1992; Danielsen & Jackson, 1991). In normal adults (Fig. 9.2), as protein intake falls, there is a decrease in the rate of urea excretion to maintain nitrogen balance. At intakes below the physiological minimal requirement for protein, urea excretion no longer falls, and may even rise, with the result that nitrogen balance can no longer be sustained. Biochemical studies in animals and some studies in man have shown that the activity of the urea cycle enzymes is sensitive to the dietary protein. Most of these studies have explored extremes of dietary intake and have not considered subtle changes around the physiological minimal requirement for protein. Figure 9.2 shows that, *in vivo*, the rate of urea production is relatively unresponsive to the intake of protein above the minimal requirement. Below this level, there is a sharp reduction in the rate of urea production. Therefore, as the dietary protein falls there is an increase in the rate of urea salvage. In individuals taking the physiological minimal protein intake the rate of salvage is greater than the intake of nitrogen. Below this level, salvage fails, in association with a reduction in urea production, an increase in urea excretion and an inability to maintain nitrogen balance.

The implication of these data is that the minimal requirement for protein

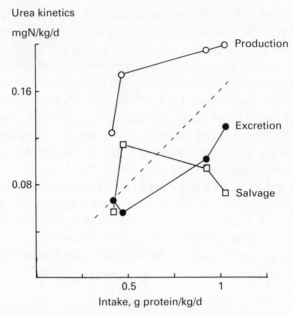

Fig. 9.2. Urea kinetics were measured in normal adult men (Langran *et al.*, 1992; Danielsen & Jackson, 1991) who were on abundant or marginal intakes of protein: urea production (open circle), urea excretion in urine (closed circle) and the salvage of urea through the lower bowel (open square). The dotted line represents the line of concordance i.e. protein intake expressed as g/kg/d and as mgN/kg/d.

requires an intact and functional system for the salvage of urea nitrogen, and the salvage of urea nitrogen is an intrinsic part of the mechanism of adaptation to a low protein diet. Philosophically, the minimal protein requirement presumes effective salvaging and we have no knowledge of the protein requirements without a salvage system. Therefore, the effective nitrogen intake of the body is represented by the dietary intake, plus a contribution of nitrogen derived from urea salvaging.

Functional metabolic demand

Protein requirements are not absolute, but have to be related to the metabolic demand. There are physiological and pathological situations where the demand increases. Demand increases during periods of growth in infancy or during catch up growth during recovery from some insult. In both situations the rate of urea salvaging is enhanced. In infants on a milk formula 80% of the urea produced was salvaged for further metabolic interaction (Wheeler, Jackson & Griffiths, 1991). During rapid catch up weight gain there was an increase in urea salvaging which related to the relative balance between the metabolic demand and the ability of the dietary intake to satisfy that demand (Jackson *et al.*, 1990).

The form in which the nitrogen from urea is made available represents an outstanding question of considerable importance. Non-essential nitrogen may be limiting for growth, and it is tempting to assume that the urea-N simply contributes to the synthesis of indispensable amino acids. However, some have found difficulties with ready acceptance of this simple solution. In the newborn period, and during catch up growth the contribution of salvaged nitrogen to total nitrogen availability might be as high as 40–50 %. The data from the Japanese workers which show that urea-N might be incorporated into dispensable amino acids, indispensable amino acids, and most particularly into lysine, has not been widely accepted (Tanaka *et al.*, 1980). There is a need for this work to be repeated. Millward *et al.* (1991) have obtained indirect evidence in adults on low protein diets that dispensable amino acids may be formed from urea salvaging. The proposals put forward by Pellet & Young (1988) that the requirements for indispensable amino acids in adults is greater than generally recognised might be explained by salvaged urea nitrogen.

Conclusions

It should be recognised that protein, amino acid and nitrogen requirements are not synonymous terms, and there is a need to explore the interrelationships in greater detail. The FAO/WHO/UNU (1985) expert consultation were not sympathetic to the view that non-essential nitrogen and salvaged urea nitrogen might play an important role in the nitrogen economy of the body. This viewpoint needs to be reassessed.

For the future the questions for which answers are required are:

1. Minimal protein requirements in the absence of urea salvaging.
2. Protein requirements with altered demand, growth, exercise and training, infection and trauma, in the absence of urea salvaging.
3. The quantitative and qualitative importance of urea salvaging to nitrogen economy.
4. Limits of *de novo* synthesis of non-essential amino acids; how do these relate to demand?
5. Conditions under which the rates of *de novo* synthesis may be increased or decreased.

6. How the pattern of amino acids required changes with demand and functional state.
7. The quantitative production of amino acids (non-essential and essential) from the lower bowel.

References

Aqvist, S. E. G. (1951). Metabolic relationships among amino acids studied with isotopic nitrogen. *Acta Chemica Scandanavica*, **5**, 1046–64.

Barbul, A. (1986). Arginine: biochemistry, physiology and therapeutic implications. *Journal of Parenteral and Enteral Nutrition*, **10**, 227–37.

Danielsen, M. & Jackson, A. A. (1992). Limits of adaptation to a low protein diet in normal adults: urea kinetics. *Proceedings of the Nutrition Society*, in press.

FAO/WHO/UNU (1985). Energy and protein requirements: *Report of a Joint Expert Consultation. Technical Report Series 724*. Geneva: World Health Organization.

Fern, E. B., Garlick, P. J., McNurlan, M. A. & Waterlow, J. C. (1981). The excretion of isotope in urea and ammonia for estimating protein turnover in man with ^{15}N-glycine. *Clinical Science*, **61**, 217–28.

Garza, C., Scrimshaw, N. S. & Young, V. R. (1978). Human protein requirements: interrelationships between energy intake and nitrogen balance in young men consuming the 1973 FAO/WHO safe level of egg protein with added non-essential amino acids. *Journal of Nutrition*, **108**, 90–6.

Golden, M. H. N., Jahoor, P. & Jackson, A. A. (1982). Glutamine production and its contribution to urinary ammonia in normal man. *Clinical Science*, **62**, 299–305.

Grantham-McGregor, S. (1988). Studies in behaviour and malnutrition in Jamaica. *Transactions of the Royal Society of Tropical Medicine and Hygiene*, **82**, 7–9.

Grimble, R. F. (1990). Nutrition and cytokine action. *Nutrition Research Reviews*, **3**, 193–210.

Hibbert, J. M. & Jackson, A. A. (1991). Variation in measures of urea kinetics over four years in a single adult. *European Journal of Clinical Nutrition*, **45**, 347–51.

Jackson, A. A. (1982). Amino acids: essential and non-essential? *Lancet*, **i**, 1034–7.

Jackson, A. A. (1989). Optimizing amino acid and protein supply and utilization in the newborn. *Proceedings of the Nutrition Society*, **48**, 293–301.

Jackson, A. A. (1991). The glycine story. *European Journal of Clinical Nutrition*, **45**, 59–65.

Jackson, A. A., Doherty, J., deBenoist, M-H., Hibbert, J. & Persaud, C. (1990). The effect of the level of dietary protein, carbohydrate and fat on urea kinetics in young children during rapid catch-up weight gain. *British Journal of Nutrition*, **64**, 371–85.

Jackson, A. A. & Golden, M. H. N. (1981). Deamination versus transamination. In *Nitrogen Metabolism in Man*, Waterlow, J. C. & Stephen, J. M. L., eds, pp. 203–213, London: Applied Science Publishers.

Jahoor, F., Jackson, A. A. & Golden, M. H. N. (1988). *In vivo* metabolism of nitrogen precursors for urea synthesis in the postprandial rat. *Annals of Nutrition and Metabolism*, **32**, 240–4.

Kennedy, N., Badaloo, V. & Jackson, A. A. (1990). Metabolic adaptation to marginal intakes of energy in young children. *British Journal of Nutrition*, **63**, 145–54.

Kies, C. (1972). Nonspecific nitrogen in the nutrition of human beings. *Federation Proceedings*, **31**, 1172–7.

Kosower, N. S. & Kosower, E. (1978). Glutathione status of cells. *International Review of Cytology*, **54**, 109–60;

Laidlaw, S. A. & Kopple, J. D (1987). Newer concepts of the indispensable amino acids. *American Journal of Clinical Nutrition*, **46**, 593–605.

Langran, M., Moran, B. J., Murphy, J. L. & Jackson, A. A. (1992). Adaptation to a diet low in protein: the effect of complex carbohydrate upon urea kinetics in normal man. *Clinical Science*, **82**, 191–5.

Matthews, D. M. (1991). *Protein Absorption: Development and Present State of the Subject*. New York: Wiley-Liss.

Millward, D. J., Price, G. M., Pacy, P. J. H. & Halliday, D. (1991). Whole-body protein and amino acid turnover in man: what can we measure with confidence? *Proceedings of the Nutrition Society*, **50**, 195–214.

Moncada, S. & Higgs, E. A. (1991). Endogenous nitrous oxide: physiology, pathology and clinical relevance. *European Journal of Clinical Investigation*, **21**, 361–74.

Munro, H. N. (1985). Historical perspective on protein requirements: objectives for the future. In *Nutritional Adaptation in Man*, Blaxter, K. & Waterlow, J. C., eds, pp. 155–168, London: John Libbey.

Newsholme E. A., Crabtree, B. & Ardawi, M. S. M. (1985). Glutamine metabolism in lymphocytes: its biological, physiological and clinical importance. *Quarterly Journal of Experimental Physiology*, **70**, 473–89.

Ooman, H. A. P. C. (1970). Interrelationship of the human intestinal flora and protein utilization. *Proceedings of the Nutrition Society*, **29**, 197–205.

Pellet, P. L. & Young, V. R. (1988). Protein and amino acid needs for adults. *Ecology of Food and Nutrition*, **21**, 321–30.

Reed, D. J. & Fariss, M. W. (1984). Glutathione depletion and susceptibility. *Pharmacological Reviews*, **36**, 25S–33S

Rose, W. C. (1938). The nutritive significance of the amino acids. *Physiological Reviews*, **18**, 109–36.

Schoenheimer, R. (1942). *The Dynamic State of the Body Constituents*. Cambridge, Mass.: Harvard University Press.

Snyderman, S. E., Holt, L. E., Dancis, J., Roitman, E., Boyer, A. & Baylis, M. E. (1962). 'Unessential' nitrogen: a limiting factor for human growth. *Journal of Nutrition*, **78**, 57–72.

Tanaka, N., Kubo, K., Siraki, K., Hoishi, H. & Yoshimura, H. (1980). A pilot study on protein metabolism in Papua New Guinea Highlanders. *Journal of Nutritional Science and Vitaminology*, **26**, 247–59.

Waterlow, J. C. (1968). Observations on the mechanism of adaptation to low protein intakes. *Lancet*, **ii**, 1091–7.

Waterlow, J. C. (1984). Protein turnover with special reference to man. *Quarterly Journal of Experimental Physiology*, **69**, 409–38.

Waterlow, J. C., Garlick, P. J. & Millward, D. J. (1978). *Protein Turnover in Mammalian Tissues and the Whole Body*. Amsterdam: North Holland Publishing Company.

Waterlow, J. C., Golden, M. H. N. & Garlick, P. J. (1978b). Protein turnover in man measured with ^{15}N: comparison of end products and dose regimes. *American Journal of Physiology*, **235**, E165–74.

Wheeler, R. A., Jackson, A. A. & Griffiths, D. M. (1991). Urea production and recycling in neonates. *Journal of Pediatric Surgery*, **26**, 575–7.

Windmueller, H. G. & Spaeth, A. E. (1980). Respiratory fuels and nitrogen metabolism *in vivo* in small intestine of fed rats: quantitative importance of glutamine, glutamate and aspartate. *Journal of Biological Chemistry*, **255**, 107–12.

Windmueller, H. G. & Spaeth, A. E. (1981) Source and fate of circulating citrulline. *American Journal of Physiology*, **241**, E473–80.

10

The metabolism of fat

M. I. GURR

Historical survey

Table 10.1 gives a survey of some milestones in research in lipid metabolism. What follows is a rather personal account of the development of specific areas of lipid research with particular regard to their nutritional relevance, and some thoughts about key areas for future research.

Digestion, absorption and transport of lipids

Details of the amino acid sequences of pancreatic lipase, co-lipase and phospholipase are now well known, as are the molecular architecture of the mixed micelles formed by the products of fat digestion and the re-assembly of the absorbed products once they have entered the enterocytes (Tso, 1985). What is still surprisingly obscure is the precise mechanism by which the components of the mixed micelles cross the brush border and enter the enterocytes.

Almost certainly the most exciting and far-reaching advances have been in probing the composition and structure of the plasma lipoproteins and especially the way in which these particles deliver their lipids to target cells (Gurr & Harwood, 1991). The amino acid sequences of many of the apolipoproteins have been determined and specific metabolic functions assigned to them. Thus, apoprotein C_2 on the surface of chylomicrons and very low density lipoproteins (VLDL) are absolutely essential for the activity of lipoprotein lipase, the enzyme responsible for hydrolysing their triacylglycerols prior to the uptake of fatty acids into cells. Apoprotein A_1 in high density lipoproteins (HDL) activates the enzyme that converts unesterified cholesterol into cholesteryl esters as part of a process now thought to be responsible for scavenging excess cholesterol in tissues,

105

Table 10.1. *Historical milestones*

1814, 16	Chevreul: characterisation of fats (triacylglycerols), cholesterol[1]
1880s	Thudicum: brain phospholipids[1]
	Lawes & Gilbert: biosynthesis of fat from carbohydrates[2]
1900	Pfluger: fat absorption[2]
1929	Burr & Burr: essential fatty acids[2]
1930s	Rittenberg, Schoenheimer, Hevesy: tracers for lipid metabolism[1]
	Davson, Danielli: lipids in membranes[2]
	Kurzrok & Lieb, Von Euler: prostaglandins[3]
	Frazer: reassessment of fat absorption[2]
1940s	Tiselius, Gurd: lipoprotein separation, characterisation[1]
	Hilditch: separation and analysis of glycerides[5]
	Tswett: adsorption chromatography
1950s	James & Martin: GLC[2]
	Ahrens, Groen, Kinsell, Keys and others: dietary fatty acids and blood cholesterol[4]
	Sinclair: relative deficiency of EFA and arterial disease[2]
	Wakil, Vagelos, Lynen, Bloch, Brenner: fatty acid synthesis, desaturation[5]
1960s	Van Deenen & de Haas: stereospecific synthesis of lipids[2]. TLC becomes widely used.
	Van Dorp, Bergstrom: labelled arachidonic acid conversion into prostaglandin[2]
1970s	Brown & Goldstein: LDL receptors[2]
	Singer & Nicholson: fluid-mosaic membrane[2]
	Strittmatter: desaturase purification[2]
1980s	HPLC becomes widely used
	Brown & Goldstein, Steinberg: scavenger receptors; origins of foam cells[5]
	Hawthorn, Michell, Berridge: phosphoinositides and second messengers[5]

[1] Cited by Lovern (1955).
[2] Full reference in reference list.
[3] Cited by Van Dorp *et al.* (1964).
[4] Cited by Gurr, Borlak & Ganatra (1989).
[5] Cited by Gurr & Harwood (1991).

membranes and lipoproteins and transporting it to the liver for further processing. Apoproteins B and E on the surface of several classes of lipoproteins recognize and interact with receptors on cell surfaces (Brown & Goldstein, 1986).

The number of LDL receptors on the cell surface is subject to feedback regulation such that, if cholesterol accumulates in cells faster than it is needed for membrane synthesis (or, in the adrenal cell, the synthesis of steroid hormones as well), the cell stops making new receptors (Brown & Goldstein, 1986). Cholesterol entering the cell from the plasma also reduces the activity of hydroxymethylglutaryl-CoA reductase, thereby reducing the cell's own cholesterol synthesis. In this way, if the diet contains a particularly large amount of cholesterol, endogenous synthesis is reduced and body stores are maintained more or less constant. In one study, about two-thirds of the subjects were able precisely to regulate their cholesterol synthesis in this way (McNamara *et al.*, 1987).

Triacylglycerols as energy reserves: regulation of synthesis, storage and utilisation

The 1960s saw the dissecting of the intermediate steps in the biosynthesis of fatty acids. Fatty acid synthetase has the novel structure of a 'multicatalytic polypeptide chain', i.e. a single polypeptide on which reside all seven enzymic activities needed for the production of long chain fatty acids from acetate (e.g. see Gurr & Harwood, 1991). This cytoplasmic enzyme is 'soluble', which has been a great help in both elucidating its structure and, more important from a nutritionist's point of view, understanding how its activity is regulated by diet via the secretion of specific hormones.

Availability of dietary energy from carbohydrate for fat synthesis is important, and up to 20-fold differences have been observed in the concentrations of fatty acid synthetase in the liver between starved and re-fed animals. Insulin is probably the most important mediator but other hormones, oestradiol, hydrocortisone and growth hormone are probably involved at the level of gene transcription. Important nutritional effects that are recognised in broad outline, but whose detailed mechanisms are still obscure, are in the inhibition of fatty acid synthesis by dietary fatty acids, particularly the inhibitory potency of linoleic acid (Jeffcoat, 1979). These effects are of nutritional significance, since one of the consequences of the high fat consumption in industrialised countries is that endogenous fatty acid synthesis is largely suppressed. Equally important are the mechanisms by which dietary and hormonal factors have different effects on different tissues. While the liver is highly subject to the regulatory constraints just described, the fatty acid synthetase of brain is unaffected by day-to-day dietary fluctuations, which is just as well!

Adipose tissue lipoprotein lipase is activated by insulin when fuel is plentiful, while at the same time the enzyme in muscle is inhibited. During fasting or starvation the reverse is true. Mammary gland lipoprotein lipase is regulated by prolactin so that lipid in circulating lipoproteins can be used for milk fat synthesis.

Progress in understanding the regulation of pathways of fatty acid desaturation has been slow because, whereas fatty acid synthetase is a 'soluble' cytoplasmic enzyme, the desaturases are bound firmly to membranes and have been difficult to solubilise and purify. However, the gene for the rat liver 9-desaturase has now been cloned (Strittmatter *et al.*, 1988) but not that for the 6-desaturase. There are considerable differences in the biochemistry of unsaturated fatty acids between different species and even between tissues within a species, so that over-enthusiastic extrapolations from as yet limited data are not acceptable. The immediate fate of ingested long chain saturated fatty acids in man is obscure but it seems likely that many are rapidly desaturated and this needs further research.

Triacylglycerol and phosphoglyceride metabolism are interrelated despite the very different roles and cellular locations of these two types of lipids. Diacylglycerols are key intermediates in the biosynthesis of both triacylglycerols (for storage tissues) and phospholipids (for membranes) (Fig. 10.1). The characteristic combinations of fatty acids in phosphoglycerides (e.g. the very striking pairing of stearic and arachidonic acids in phosphatidylinositol) are achieved mainly by exchange of fatty acids after the basic phospholipid molecule has been built. However, some selectivity may also occur in the choice of diacylglycerol species that enter the pathways of triacylglycerol or phosphoglyceride biosynthesis (Fig. 10.1, Gurr & Harwood, 1991).

Phosphatidate phosphohydrolase stands at the branch-point of triacylglycerol and phospholipid biosynthesis and plays a regulatory role. It occurs in an inactive form in the cytoplasm as a reservoir of potential activity and in its active form on the endoplasmic reticulum membranes. Nutritional state influences the translocation from cytoplasm to membrane through changes in intracellular concentrations of non-esterified fatty acids and insulin. Such '*ambiquitous enzymes*' promise exciting new insights into metabolic regulation with some nutritional relevance.

When the body needs to consume fuel reserves, low ratios of circulating insulin/glucagon 'switch off' pathways of biosynthesis and storage, and release the inhibition of triacylglycerol lipase within the fat cells. This is achieved through regulation of the activity of adenylate cyclase in the fat cell membrane, thus controlling production of cyclic-AMP, which in turn regulates the degree of phosphorylation of the lipase by a protein kinase, converting inactive into active lipase. Fatty acids thereby released from the

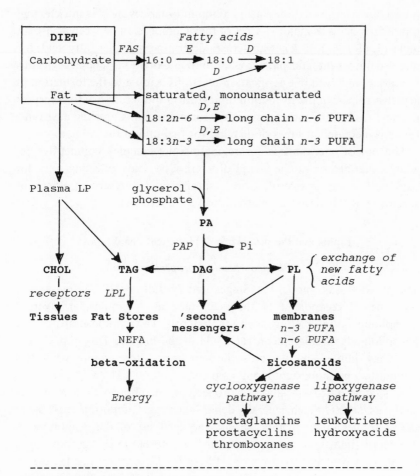

CHOL Cholesterol
DAG   Diacylglycerol
D   Desaturation
E   Elongation
FAS   Fatty acid synthetase
LP   Lipoprotein
LPL   Lipoprotein lipase
NEFA Non-esterified fatty acids
PA   Phosphatidate
PAP   Phosphatidate phosphohydrolase
Pi   Inorganic phosphate
PL   Phospholipid
PUFA Polyunsaturated fatty acids
16:0, 18:0, 18:1, 18:2, 18:3. - Palmitic, stearic,
oleic, linoleic, *alpha*-linolenic acids

Fig. 10.1 Origins and fates of body lipids.

fat cell are transported on plasma albumin to tissues such as muscle, that utilise fatty acids as major sources of fuel. Competition between acyl-CoA molecules for various acyltransferases determines whether fatty acids are directed into synthetic pathways or into β-oxidation. These acyltransferases are involved in esterification reactions leading to the formation of acylglycerols or in the formation of acyl-carnitines necessary to transport the acyl-CoAs into the mitochondria for oxidation. Carnitine acyltransferase is increased at times of demand for fuel utilisation.

The precise mechanisms for regulating the complex competitive reactions that determine the fate of different fatty acids, selecting some for oxidation, some for esterification in specific lipids, preserving others for specific vital functions, are matters for future research.

Lipids and the properties of biological membranes

Physico-chemical properties

The 'fluid-mosaic model' of Singer and Nicholson (1972) envisages a fundamental component of the membrane as a bimolecular layer of phospholipids interacting with cholesterol. The composition of the phospholipids is different on each side of the bilayer. This implies that lipids have limited ability to cross the membrane, although they may travel around to a certain extent along its plane.

It is common to talk about a property of membranes known (imprecisely) as *fluidity*, which generally depicts the degree of motion available to the molecules in the membrane and the flexibility of the membrane. A degree of fluidity is necessary for membrane enzymes, receptors and transporter proteins to function efficiently. Lipids are key factors in determining the fluidity of membranes as a result of the properties of the fatty acyl chains and interactions between acyl chains and cholesterol, and between polar headgroups of phospholipids and membrane proteins. Cholesterol is vital to the function of mammalian membranes in ways that are still not precisely understood: virtually no other steroid will substitute for it. In general, the shorter the chain length and the higher the degree of unsaturation of the fatty acids, the more fluid the membrane. However, beyond a certain degree of unsaturation, the fluidity properties of acyl chains reverse. Very highly unsaturated fatty acids adopt helical structures that are able to pack together more closely than the kinked structures of mono- and diunsaturated fatty acids (Stubbs & Smith, 1990). While dietary fat composition may markedly influence membrane fluidity and therefore function, the degree to which this is so is difficult to predict because, as the degree of unsaturation increases initially, tending to increase fluidity, compensation may be brought about by increases in the cholesterol/phospholipid ratio. Other homeostatic controls may also be operating.

Eicosanoids

Aside from their 'structural' role, membrane polyunsaturated fatty acids (PUFA) constitute a store of substrates for their biologically active metabolites, the *eicosanoids*. Among the first actions of an 'agonist' or stimulator molecule (e.g. neurotransmitters, hormones, growth factors) on the cell membrane is to stimulate the activity of a specific phospholipase that releases a fatty acid, normally arachidonic acid (20:4 *n*-6), from position 2 of a membrane phospholipid. The fatty acid may become a substrate for enzymes that catalyse its oxidation along two alternative pathways (Fig. 10.1, Sanders, 1988). The *cyclo-oxygenase pathway* produces prostaglandins, prostacyclins and thromboxanes, while the *lipo-oxygenase pathway* generates leukotrienes, named from the cells in which they were first identified. These oxygenated metabolites have been implicated in the regulation of many physiological processes including reproduction, haemostasis, inflammation, cell-mediated immunity, insulin release, bone calcification and the function of the kidney and the eye.

   In so far as changes in dietary lipids may influence the composition of fatty acids in membranes, they have the potential to influence the spectrum of eicosanoids produced and hence modify the numerous physiological functions enumerated above. For example, high dietary inclusions of *n*-3 polyunsaturated fatty acids characteristic of certain fatty fish, result in the replacement of membrane arachidonic acid by *n*-3 fatty acids that give rise to eicosanoids with different activities. Thus, platelets produce a thromboxane from arachidonic acid that is a powerful vasoconstrictor and strongly promotes aggregation. That produced from eicosapentaenoic acid (20:5 *n*-3) has these activities to a much weaker degree. Potential for thrombus formation is thereby much reduced (Sanders, 1988). Precisely how the appropriate balance of eicosanoids with their often opposing activities is regulated, and the extent to which diet plays a part, remain a major challenge for research.

Lipid peroxidation

Polyunsaturated fatty acids are susceptible to oxidation by the oxygen which all cells need (Halliwell & Gutteridge, 1989). Free radical reactions generate oxygenated fatty acid products. The cyclo-oxygenase and lipoxygenase reactions described above are examples of carefully regulated, enzymically catalysed free-radical peroxidation processes. Unregulated chemically catalysed peroxidation, however, leads to the formation of lipid and lipid peroxide free radicals and their low molecular weight breakdown products in chain reactions that can exact enormous damage on surrounding tissue and lead to disease processes. Such unwanted oxidation is normally curbed by the presence of antioxidants, mainly α-tocopherol. The presence of a highly organised membrane structure that incorporates the antioxidant molecules, closely packed with the fatty acid chains, is a major factor in preventing peroxidation *in vivo*. The presence of adequate vitamin E and other antioxidants in the diet that act synergistically, such as vitamin C and selenium, are now thought to be important for maintaining membrane lipid integrity.

Membrane lipids in cell signalling

Binding of an agonist to its receptor results in a rapid hydrolysis of phosphatidylinositol bisphosphate by a specific phospholipase C producing inositol,1,2,5-triphosphate (IP_3) and diacylglycerol (DAG), both of which have 'second messenger' functions (Gurr & Harwood, 1991). Thus, IP_3 and DAG are involved in the regulation of phosphorylase kinase and glycogen synthetase respectively through their actions on protein kinases, while DAG is degraded by a lipase, releasing arachidonic acid and initiating the production of eicosanoids. Nutrition may turn out to be important if it influences the properties of membranes sufficiently to modulate the activity of these second messenger sequences.

Specific lipid requirements for early development

From conception, the cells of the growing fetus need to incorporate lipids into their rapidly proliferating membranes. The fetus is totally dependent on the placental transfer of substrates from the mother's circulation. Glucose is the major substrate from which the fetus is able to elaborate the glycerol moiety of its lipids and the non-essential fatty acid components. A crucial question in developmental biology is how the essential fatty acids, linoleic (18:2 *n*-6) and α-linolenic acid (18:3 *n*-3) are acquired as they cannot be synthesised by mammalian tissues. A common finding is a higher concentration of arachidonic acid in fetal than in maternal plasma. Arachidonic acid appears to be selectively trapped into placental phospholipids for export to the fetal circulation. The process by which the proportion of long chain PUFA increases in phospholipids, progressing from maternal blood to cord blood, fetal liver and fetal brain has been termed '*biomagnification*' (Crawford *et al.*, 1976). Ruminants have adopted similar mechanisms to conserve EFA with supreme efficiency because dietary EFA are extensively destroyed by hydrogenation in the rumen (Gurr, 1988).

A large proportion of long chain PUFA synthesised or accumulated during the perinatal period is destined for the growth of the brain, 50 % of whose acyl groups comprise 20:4 *n*-6, 22:4 *n*-6, 22:5 *n*-6 and 22:6 *n*-3. Amounts of the precursor EFA are very low. In piglets, used as models because the temporal development of brain is similar to man's, brain and liver are able to synthesise long chain PUFA from linoleic and linolenic acids in the period immediately before and after birth (Purvis, Clandinin & Hacker, 1983). Such studies are important because premature babies may be born well before brain development has reached its peak. It is crucial, therefore, that the lipids in the infant's food are able to contribute to the brain growth that would have occurred in the fetus. Any long chain EFA that the fetus could not elaborate for itself and had to be supplied by the mother's circulation or the placenta will now have to be contributed by the milk. Human milk contains a high proportion of long chain fatty acids in comparison with cow's milk, but these may not be sufficient for some premature infants. Appropriate feeding strategies will require greater knowledge of the relative abilities of the placenta and other maternal tissues, the fetus and new-born's own tissues to supply long chain PUFA.

Current controversies and future directions

Needs for PUFA

Most practical diets should satisfy requirements for the two EFA to avoid overt EFA deficiency. There is uncertainty, however, about requirements for their elongation products in certain conditions and about additional needs in conditions such as pregnancy and lactation or for inducing 'optimal' plasma lipoprotein profiles, haemostasis and immune function or the body's capacity for adaptation. The importance of diet as a determinant of plasma lipoprotein concentrations is contentious, many believing that dietary lipids are major determinants of plasma lipoprotein composition and an essential means of controlling what they regard as an important 'risk factor' for CHD. Others point to the failure of many community studies to demonstrate a strong, or even any, relationship between dietary fats and blood lipids, despite clear indications that plasma lipids are amenable to dietary change under carefully controlled experimental conditions. The 1980s have also seen renewed interest in the different activities of specific saturated, monounsaturated and polyunsaturated fatty acids with respect to plasma lipoprotein profiles (Gurr *et al.*, 1989).

Defence against lipid peroxidation

Lipid peroxidation can modify the properties of membranes and of lipoprotein particles and their interaction with receptors. LDL modified by peroxidation are not taken up by apoB,E receptors but by macrophage 'scavenger' receptors. The lipid-filled macrophages may go on to become the foam cells of atherosclerotic plaques (Gurr & Harwood, 1991). These findings are tending to put more emphasis on the dietary roles of both lipid-soluble and water-soluble antioxidant vitamins. The relative importance of lipid peroxidation *in vivo* is a matter of hot dispute that will be important to resolve in the 1990s.

Overnutrition

There is keen interest now in abdominal fat distribution because it has particular association with hypertriglyceridaemia, hyperinsulinaemia, increased 'insulin resistance', hypertension and type II diabetes (Anon, 1991). A preoccupation of the last decade or so has been the reduction of dietary energy, particularly fat, and the food industry has provided a bewildering range of modified fat products as dietary aids. An important question is: do they work? The recent studies of Foltin *et al.* (1990) suggest that many people compensate their energy intake after consumption of low-fat products and that the success of substituting low fat for high fat foods may be limited. These are issues of vital importance for fat nutrition and need further exploration.

Lipid research techniques

There is a need to develop minimally invasive techniques for metabolic studies. These may include: adipose tissue compositional analysis for assessment of the intake of dietary fatty acids and their impact on metabolism (e.g. see Hudgins, Hirsch & Emken, 1991); the use of certain cells as surrogates for less accessible tissues (e.g. mononuclear leukocytes to study the regulation of cholesterol biosynthesis in response to diet: McNamara *et al.*, 1987); perfused placenta and umbilical artery for insights into fetal–maternal relationships (Crawford *et al.*, 1990); physical techniques for information on lipids in membranes (Stubbs & Smith, 1990), and stable isotopes to trace lipid metabolic pathways (Emken *et al.*, 1990). Advances in methodology are needed in the study of haemostatic phenomena, where there is some question about the relevance of currently used preparations *in vitro* and *in vivo* to haemostasis in the living blood.

Concepts

The idea that lipids are an inert cellular grease has long since been abandoned. It is now time to discard ideas that lipids can be considered in isolation from other cellular components and that their roles can be separated into entirely 'structural' or 'metabolic' roles. The 'structural' lipids of membranes provide a vast store of substrates for the production of compounds involved in cell signalling. Too much emphasis has been placed on a single plasma lipid profile, which is, after all, only a snapshot of lipids on their way from one part of the body to another. Studies must be integrated to combine observations of both plasma and tissue lipids over a period of time, and the period immediately following a meal is now being recognised as extremely important. The over-emphasis on fatty acids, especially, the tendency to speak in broad categories of 'saturated' or 'polyunsaturated' fatty acids, when they comprise a multitude of structures with different nutritional and physiological properties, must be abandoned. Dietary fats contain many components which, although present in small quantities, may exert important physiological effects.

This paper has been concerned with *fat metabolism*. While dietary lipids clearly have important influences on lipid metabolism in the body, nutritionists should be cautious about ascribing too much importance to diet in general and dietary lipids in particular. The body has an enormous capacity to adapt to external circumstances, to borrow from body stores and to pay back later. This is not to say that nutrition is not important, but it needs to be seen in perspective with the whole of life.

References

Anon. (1991). The metabolic basis for the 'apple' and 'pear' body habitus. *Nutrition Reviews*, **49**, 84–6.

Bergstrom, S., Danielsson, H. & Samuelsson, B. (1964). The enzymic formation of prostaglandin E_2 from arachidonic acid: prostaglandins and related factors. *Biochimica et Biophysica Acta*, **90**, 207–10.

Brown, M. S. & Goldstein, J. L. (1986). A receptor-mediated pathway for cholesterol homeostasis. *Science*, **232**, 34–47.

Burr, G. O. & Burr, M. M. (1929). A new deficiency disease produced by the rigid exclusion of fat from the diet. *Journal of Biological Chemistry*, **82**, 345–67.

Crawford, M. A., Costeloe, K., Doyle, W., Leighfield, M. J., Lennon, E. A. & Meadows, N. (1990). Potential diagnostic value of the umbilical artery as a definition of neural fatty acid status of the fetus during its growth: the umbilical artery as a diagnostic tool. *Biochemical Society Transactions*, **18**, 761–6.

Crawford, M. A., Hassam, A. G., Williams, G. & Whitehouse, W. L. (1976). Essential fatty acids and fetal brain growth. *Lancet*, **i**, 452–3.

Davson, H. & Danielli, J. F. (1943). *The Permeability of Natural Membranes*. Cambridge: Cambridge University Press.

Emken, E. A., Adlof, R. O., Rakoff, H., Rohwedder, W. K. & Gulley, R. M. (1990). Metabolism *in vivo* of deuterium-labelled linolenic and linoleic acids in humans. *Biochemical Society Transactions*, **18**, 766–9.

Foltin, R. W., Fischman, M. W., Moran, T. H., Rolls, B. J. & Kelly, T. H. (1990). Caloric compensation for lunches varying in fat and carbohydrate content by humans in a residential laboratory. *American Journal of Clinical Nutrition*, **52**, 969–80.

Frazer, A. C. (1946). The absorption of triglyceride fat from the intestine. *Physiological Reviews*, **26**, 103–19.

Gurr, M. I. (1988). Comparative aspects of nutrient metabolism: lipid metabolism. In *Comparative Nutrition*, Blaxter, K. & Macdonald, I. eds, pp. 73–89. London: John Libbey.

Gurr, M. I., Borlak, N. & Ganatra, S. (1989). Dietary fat and plasma lipids. *Nutrition Research Reviews*, **2**, 63–86.

Gurr, M. I. & Harwood, J. L. (1991). *Lipid Biochemistry: An Introduction*. London: Chapman & Hall.

Halliwell, B. & Gutteridge, J. M. C. (1989). *Free Radicals in Biology and Medicine*. 2nd edn. Oxford: Clarendon Press.

Hudgins, L. C., Hirsch, J. & Emken, E. A. (1991). Correlation of isomeric fatty acids in human adipose tissue with clinical risk factors for cardiovascular disease. *American Journal of Clinical Nutrition*, **53**, 474–82.

James, A. T. & Martin, A. J. P. (1952). Gas–liquid partition chromatography: the separation and micro-estimation of volatile fatty acids from formic to dodecanoic acid. *Biochemical Journal*, **50**, 679–90.

Jeffcoat, R. (1979). The biosynthesis of unsaturated fatty acids and its control in mammalian liver. *Essays in Biochemistry*, **15**, 1–36.

Lawes, J. B. & Gilbert, J. H. (1877). On the formation of fat in the animal body. *Journal of Anatomy and Physiology*, **11**, 577–88.

Lovern, J. A. (1955). *The Chemistry of Lipids of Biochemical Significance*. London: Methuen.

McNamara, D. J., Kolb, R., Parker, T. S., Batwin, H., Samuel, P., Brown, C. D. & Ahrens, E. H.(1987). Heterogeneity of cholesterol homeostasis in man. Responses to changes in dietary fat quality and cholesterol quantity. *Journal of Clinical Investigation*, **79**, 1729–39.

Pfluger, E. (1900). Über die Gesundheitsschudigungen welche durch den Genuss von Pferdelfleisch verursacht werden. (Nebst einem Beitrag über die Resorption der Fette). *Archiv für die gesammte Physiologie* (Pfluger's), **80**, 111–38.

Purvis, J. M., Clandinin, M. T. & Hacker, R. R. (1983). Chain elongation-desaturation of linoleic acid during the development of the pig.

Implications for the supply of polyenoic acids to the developing brain. *Comparative Biochemistry and Physiology*, **75B**, 199–204.

Sanders, T. A. B. (1988). Essential and trans fatty acids in nutrition. *Nutrition Research Reviews*, **1**, 57–78.

Sinclair, H. M. (1957). Food and Health. *British Medical Journal*, **2**, 1424–6.

Singer, S. J. & Nicholson, G. L. (1972). The fluid mosaic model of the structure of cell membranes. *Science*, **175**, 720–31.

Strittmatter, P., Thiede, M. A., Hackett, C. S. & Ozols, J. (1988). Bacterial synthesis of active rat stearoyl-coA desaturase lacking the 26-residue amino terminal amino acid sequence. *Journal of Biological Chemistry*, **263**, 2532–5.

Stubbs, C. D. & Smith, A. D. (1990). Essential fatty acids in membranes: physical properties and function. *Biochemical Society Transactions*, **18**, 779–81.

Tso, P. (1985) Gastrointestinal digestion and absorption of lipid. *Advances in Lipid Research*, **21**, 143–86.

Van Deenen, L. L. M. & de Haas, G. H. (1964). The synthesis of phosphoglycerides and some biochemical applications. *Advances in Lipid Research*, **2**, 167–234.

Van Dorp, D. A., Beerthuis, R. K., Nugteren, D. H. & Vonkeman, H. (1964). The biosynthesis of prostaglandins. *Biochimica et Biophysica Acta*, **90**, 204–7.

11

Sugars – still the Cinderella of nutrients?

IAN MACDONALD

Fifty years ago the teaching in one London medical school was that all absorbed carbohydrates were converted in the body to glucose and this incorrect information did not suggest to the future doctor that carbohydrates in the diet were other than cheap, common, and inconsequential, sources of energy for the body. This error had not, apparently, reached the USA Academy of Sciences by 1989 where, in their volume on *Diet and Health*, the following sentence appears 'After absorbtion [*sic*], fructose and galactose are converted in the liver to glucose, the blood sugar'!

A textbook of medical physiology published a year after the formation of the Nutrition Society (Bard, 1942) quoted the classical work of Cori, published in 1925, to tell its readers that galactose was absorbed from the intestine of the rat slightly more rapidly than glucose and that fructose absorption was approximately half as slow again and reported that when the monosaccharides were given intra-peritoneally there was no difference in their rate of uptake into the blood. The fact that this textbook was quoting findings reported 17 years earlier would suggest that even before the birth of the Nutrition Society it must have been felt that there was little further to learn about sugars. However, in 1953, an attempt was made to find out the reason why different monosaccharides were absorbed from the gut at different rates, and it was suggested that the process involved phosphorylation in the intestinal mucosa and subsequent liberation in the blood stream, a mechanism analogous to the formation of urine in the renal tubules (Darlington & Quastel, 1953). It was not until the early 1960s that the bioenergetics of monosaccharide absorption were understood and that it did not involve phosphorylation, but Na^+ (Crane, 1960).

At the time of the inauguration of the Nutrition Society, knowledge of the maximum tolerance of various sugars by man relied on work published in 1915 (Woodyatt, Sansun & Wilder) when a continuous intravenous infusion was given to volunteers until glycosuria occurred. Though the findings are probably reliable, it is unlikely that these experiments would be considered ethical today.

Turning to the Nutrition Society in its early days, it seems that the metabolism of sugars was not a subject that interested members or others in experimental research, but then, perhaps this was not surprising with the total involvement of the country at war. The consequences that this had on providing food for the population was of overwhelming importance. The niceties of metabolic research in carbohydrates or any other nutrient could wait for calmer times. In fact the first five volumes of the *Proceedings* contained no mention of sugars, and in the first six volumes of the *British Journal of Nutrition* there were only two references to sugars, except in large animals which were obviously important in the food supply, and indeed food shortages lasted for some time after the end of the war.

It is perhaps not surprising, therefore, that the first mention of sugar in the *British Journal of Nutrition* was in connection with the dietary intake of the UK population. In Volume 1 there was an article describing an 'estimate of the amounts of foods required to meet the needs of calories, protein and calcium of the population of the UK'. For those over 15 years of age they suggested an intake of total sugar of 27 oz/week, which was approximately 13% of the dietary energy for men and 17% for women (Bransbury *et al.*, 1947). In the discussion in this paper, the statement is made that 'excessive consumption of sugar is not looked on with favour because it displaces more nutritious foods from the diet, tends to pervert the taste and blunt the appetite of children and seems to play a part in causing dental caries' and the authors hoped that their recommended consumption level 'would meet the tastes of the majority, with a minimum of dissent from nutritional experts'. So what is new?

In the next volume of the *British Journal of Nutrition*, Bransbury, Daubney & King (1948) analysed the composition of the food intake of 33 adults 'enlisted because of their scientific training and ability to carry out the work satisfactorily' and it is perhaps of interest to note that they reported that the mean energy intake per day was 2022 Cals, with 17% of this provided by sugar.

Methodology

Another reason for the seeming lack of interest in the metabolism of sugars could lie in the methods available at the time for *in vivo* studies. In 1941 the method for estimating blood glucose was based on a colorimetric method (Folin & Malmros, 1929) using ferricyanide or a volumetric method involving the reduction of cupric to cuprous ions (Schaffer & Hartmann, 1921). Both these methods are tedious and only specific for reducing substances in the blood, not for individual monosaccharides. The discovery of the glucose oxidase method for measuring blood or serum glucose levels was of considerable importance (Keston, 1956), and a little later a reliable and relatively simple method became available for the estimation of serum insulin (Hales & Randle, 1963). These two techniques led to a greater understanding of the metabolism of dietary sugars in man, and the use of isotopically labelled ^{14}C and ^{13}C in the sugar molecule has enabled the molecular handling of these compounds, both in their absorption in the gut (Semenza, 1981) and their biochemistry in the liver (Hers & Hue, 1983) to be studied.

Fifty years ago biochemistry did not exist as such and was practised under the name of chemical physiology, and much of the research in this area was into metabolic processes The need and desire to study the chemistry of the cell led to a huge expansion of biochemical knowledge and information. By no means the least among the contributors at that time was Krebs, whose 'cycle' encouraged understanding of the metabolism of sugars. In passing, it is of interest to observe that studies at the cellular level are becoming even more precise, and it will be interesting to watch the impact of molecular biology on nutrition in general and sugars in particular.

Sugars and metabolism in man

Though in the past 50 years the rate of new knowledge of the metabolism of sugars in man has not been as rapid as that seen in protein and lipids, in fact much of what is known today about glucose metabolism in man was known at the time the Society was formed. It is in the control of glucose metabolism that advances have been made in the past 50 years. The recognition of glucagon and the discovery that hormones released from the wall of the intestine, due to the presence of sugars in the gut lumen, increased and will continue to increase our understanding of factors controlling the metabolism of sugars.

Metabolism of fructose and lipids

It is now known that fructose is not almost entirely converted to glucose in the intestinal wall and liver, as was taught at the time of the birth of the Nutrition Society, and perhaps because of this there has been an increase in our understanding of the metabolism of fructose in man.

It is largely the role of fructose in lipid metabolism where most has been learnt. Fructose produces a much greater hepatic lipogenesis than does glucose (Macdonald, 1968), probably due to the much greater capacity of the enzyme fructokinase to phosphorylate fructose than the combined activities of glucokinase and hexokinase the phosphorylate glucose in the liver (Heinz, Lamprecht & Kirsch, 1968; Zakim, Herman & Gordon, 1969). Later work showed that after intravenous infusion in man the incorporation of ^{14}C fructose into plasma VLDL is consistently higher than that of ^{14}C glucose (Wolfe & Ahuja, 1977), and this further supported the view that fructose is more lipogenic than glucose.

Many of the studies on the effects of fructose on plasma lipids have used sucrose as the source of fructose, and a high intake of sucrose does raise the triglyceride level in the blood. Furthermore, the extent of this elevation depends on the age and sex of the consumer (Macdonald, 1966), with pre-menopausal women apparently exempt from this lipogenic effect. This response is probably not marked in normal persons consuming usual levels of fructose, but those with raised fasting serum triglyceride concentrations show a marked increased in the lipogenic response to fructose (Kaufmann, Poznanski & Blondheim, 1966). There is some experimental evidence to suggest that, compared with glucose, dietary fructose is associated with much more triglyceride accumulating in the liver (Macdonald, 1962), though it seems clear that the fatty liver in kwashiorkor is due to a relative excess of dietary carbohydrate, usually as starch, which is a glucose polymer. Waterlow (p. 314) concludes that a deficiency of amino acids reduces the ability to synthesise the apo-proteins necessary to transport triglycerides from the liver to peripheral tissues.

Uric acid metabolism

When blood fructose levels are raised acutely, as after the ingestion of a relatively large amount of sucrose, blood uric acid levels are also raised (Macdonald, Keyser & Pacy, 1978) and, though the significance of this is questionable in most persons, a large intake can provoke, in those with raised blood uric acid levels, an attack of gout.

Galactose

It was in 1951 that the major route of the catabolism of galactose in man was first described, known as the Leloir pathway after the person who first described it (Leloir, 1951). All the enzymes of this pathway are located in the soluble fraction of the cell, and show the highest activity in the liver, hence the practice at one time of giving galactose by mouth as a measure of liver function.

Sugars and disease

Inborn errors of metabolism

In the past 50 years, advances in the techniques of assessing enzyme activity have led to an identification of the enzymes responsible for several inborn errors of metabolism. Those that relate to dietary sugars include:

Lactose intolerance (Holzel, Schwarz & Sutcliffe, 1959)
Sucrose intolerance (Burgess et al., 1964)
Galactosaemia (Isselbacher et al., 1956)
Benign fructosaemia (Schapira, Schapira & Dreyfus, 1962)
Fructose intolerance (Froesch *et al.*, 1959)
Pentosuria (Wang & van Eys, 1970)

Sugars as a cause of disease

A standard textbook of Clinical Medicine published in 1950, 9 years after the foundation of the Nutrition Society, stated that soft, pulpy, sweet and farinaceous foods encourage caries (Warner, 1950). Other comparable textbooks of medicine at that time make no reference to monosaccharides as such, and the word 'sugar' seemed to be synonymous with what we now call glucose, so it is perhaps not surprising that dietary sugars as we know them seemed then to play no part in the aetiology or prevention of disease in man. Has the situation, in this respect, changed all that much? Sugars have a major role in the cause of dental caries, and some sugars, notably sucrose, are thought by some to be a factor in the causation of overweight and obesity, possibly as a result of their organoleptic properties. The cause of many other diseases of the developed world has been laid at the door of sugars, and sucrose seems to have been singled out as the most disreputable in this respect.

Much of the apparent role of sucrose in the aetiology of disease in man needs the support of scientific evidence so, perhaps, when the Society celebrates its centenary more precise knowledge of the contribution of dietary sugars in the aetiology of disease in man will be known. Perhaps clinical medicine will be the Prince Charming for the metabolism of sugars.

References

Bard, P. (1942). In *Macleod's Physiology in Modern Medicine*, 9th edn, pp. 785–786. London: Kimpton.

Bransbury, E. R. Daubney, C. G. & King, J. (1948). Comparison of nutrient values of individual diets found by calculation from food tables and by chemical analysis. *British Journal of Nutrition*, **2**, 232–6.

Bransbury, E. R., Magee, H. E., Bowley, M. C. & Stanton, B. R. (1947). The food needs of the United Kingdom. *British Journal of Nutrition*, **1**, 275–83.

Burgess, E. A., Levin, B., Mahalanabis, D. & Tonge, R. E. (1964). Hereditary sucrose intolerance: levels of sucrose activity in the jejunal mucosa. *Archives in Diseases of Childhood*, **39**, 431–3.

Crane, R. K. (1960). Intestinal absorption of sugars. *Physiology Reviews*, **40**, 789–825.

Darlington, W. A. & Quastel, J. H. (1953). Absorption of sugars from isolated surviving intestine. *Archives in Biochemistry and Biophysics*, **43**, 194–207.

Cori, C. F. (1925). The rate of absorption of hexoses and pentoses from the intestinal tract. *Journal of Biological Chemistry*, **66**, 691–715.

Folin, O. & Malmros, H. (1929). An improved form of Folin's method for blood glucose determination. *Journal of Biological Chemistry*, **83**, 115–20.

Froesch, E. R., Prader, A., Wolf, H. P. & Labhart, A. (1959). Die hereditare Fructose intoleranz. *Helvetica Paediatrica Acta*, **14**, 99–112.

Hales, C. N. & Randle, P. J. (1963). Immunoassay of insulin with insulin–antibody precipitate. *Biochemical Journal*, **88**, 137–46.

Heinz, F., Lamprecht, W. & Kirsch, J. (1968). Enzymes of fructose metabolism in human liver. *Journal of Clinical Investigation*, **47**, 1826–932.

Hers, H. G. & Hue, L. (1983). Gluconeogenesis and related aspects of glycolysis. *Annual Reviews in Biochemistry*, **52**, 617–53.

Hers, H. G. & Joassin, G. (1961). Anomalie de l'aldolase dans l'intolerance au fructose. *Enzyme Biology Clinics*, **1**, 4–14.

Holzel, A., Schwarz, V. & Sutcliffe, K. W. (1959). Defective latose absorption causing malnutrition in infancy. *Lancet*, **i**, 1126–8.

Isselbacher, K., Anderson, E. P., Kurahashi, K. & Kalchar, H. M. (1956). Congenital galactosemia, a single enzymatic block in galactose metabolism. *Science*, **123**, 635–6.

Kaufmann, N. A., Poznanski, R. & Blondheim, S. H. (1966). Effect of fructose, glucose, sucrose and starch on serum lipids in carbohydrate induced hypertriglyceridemia and in normal subjects. *Israel Journal of Medical Science*, **2**, 715–26.

Keston, A. S. (1956). Specific colorimetric enzymatic analytical reagents for glucose. *Abstract of the 129th Meeting of the American Chemical Society*, Dallas, Texas. p. 310.

Leloir, L. F. (1951). Enzymatic transformation of uridine diphosphate glucose into galactose derivative. *Archives in Biochemistry and Biophysics*, **33**, 186–90.

Macdonald, I. (1962). Some effects of carbohydrate in experimental low protein diet. *Journal of Physiology* (London), **160**, 306–16.

Macdonald, I. (1966). Influence of fructose and glucose on serum lipid levels in men and pre- and post-menopausal women. *American Journal of Clinical Nutrition*, **18**, 369–72.

Macdonald, I. (1968). Ingested glucose and fructose in serum lipids in healthy men and after myocardial infarction. *American Journal of Clinical Nutrition*, **21**, 1366–73.

Macdonald, I., Keyser, A. & Pacy, D. (1978). Some effects, in men, of varying the load of glucose, sucrose, fructose, or sorbitol on various metabolites in blood. *American Journal of Clinical Nutrition*, **31**, 1305–11.

Schaffer, P. A. & Hartmann, A. F. (1921). The iodometric determination of copper and its use in sugar analysis. *Journal of Biological Chemistry*, **45**, 349–90;

Schapira, F., Schapira, G. & Dreyfus, J. C. (1962). La lesion enzymatique de la fructosurie benigne. *Enzyme Biology Clinics*, **1**, 170–5.

Semenza, G. (1981). Intestinal oligo- and di-saccharidases. In *Carbohydrate Metabolism and its Disorders*. Randle, P. J., Steiner, D. F. & Whelan, W. J., eds, pp. 425–79, Academic Press.

Wang, Y. W. & van Eys, J. (1970). The enzymatic defect in essential pentosuria. *New England Journal of Medicine* **282**, 892–6.

Warner, E. C. (1950). In *Savill's System of Clinical Medicine*. London: E. Arnold. 264 pp.

Wolfe, R. R. & Ahuja, S. P. (1977). Effects of intravenously administered fructose and glucose on splanchnic secretion of plasma triglycerides in hypertriglyceridemic men. *Metabolism*, **26**, 963–78.

Woodyatt, R. T., Sansun, W. D. & Wilder, R. M. (1915). Prolonged and accurately timed intravenous injection of sugar. *Journal of the American Medical Association*, **65**, 2067–9.

Zakim, D., Herman, R. H. & Gordon, W. C. (1969). The conversion of glucose and fructose to fatty acids in the human liver. *Biochemical Medicine*, **2**, 427–37.

12

Complex carbohydrates

J. H. CUMMINGS and H. N. ENGLYST

The dietary complex carbohydrates comprise starch and non-starch polysaccharides (NSP) (British Nutrition Foundation, 1990). Conventionally, dietary carbohydrate is divided into monosaccharides and disaccharides which are referred to as sugars whilst starch and NSP are clearly polysaccharides. In between these two groups are a number of carbohydrates which have largely been neglected both analytically and physiologically, yet may well have important properties relevant to health (Hidaka et al., 1986). They are carbohydrates with three or more sugar molecules and include raffinose, stachyose, fructo-oligosaccharides and some dextrins.

Neither the chemical nor physiological boundary between the oligosaccharides and complex carbohydrates is clear. In dividing oligosaccharides from polysaccharides the US Food and Drug Administration (FDA) has recently suggested that carbohydrates with a DP (degree of polymerisation) of 10 or more should be classified as polysaccharides (Federal Register, 1990). This cut-off point (DP 10) has the convenient advantage that it represents the approximate boundary between carbohydrates that are precipitated by an 80 % ethanol solution and those that remain in solution, although this is by no means an exact division.

Chemistry

Starch

Starches are the major storage polysaccharide in most higher plants. Other storage polysaccharides include fructans such as inulin (artichokes, chicory), mannans (konjac) and galactomannans (guar, locust bean gum). Starches are α-glucans. Two types exist: amylopectin, which is 70–80 % of total starch, and amylose, which usually comprises 20–30 %. Amylopectins are large molecules made up of more than 10000 glucose residues held together by $\alpha1$–4 and $\alpha1$–6 linkages in a branched tree-like structure. Amylose is a smaller linear molecule with only $\alpha1$–4 linkages. Starch is stored in plants as partially crystalline granules, in which amylopectin has clusters of interchain branching points and domains of short DP chains. These short chains exist as double helices and give rise to an alternating pattern of crystalline (arrays of double-stranded helices) and amorphous (zones of dense branching) regions (Biliaderis, 1991). This partially crystalline structure has distinct patterns on X-ray diffraction. Three main types exist: A, B and C. Type A is thermodynamically the most stable form, and is found in cereal starches. The B form is characteristic of banana, potatoes and other tubers, and the C pattern is found in legumes. The size and crystalline nature of starch granules influences their susceptibility to pancreatic enzymes. In general, starch granules showing X-ray diffraction patterns B and C tend to be more resistant to pancreatic amylase.

Starches are insoluble in cold water, but on heating they swell and eventually their molecular organisation breaks down and loses its crystallinity (Fig. 12.1). The granule is totally disrupted and at this stage the starch is readily attacked by enzymes. The whole process of disruption and swelling is known as gelatinisation (Biliaderis, 1991) and is the essence of cooking starchy foods. On cooling, gelatinised starch recrystallises, a change known as retrogradation. Retrograded starch, particularly amylose, is resistant to enzymic attack. The physical determinants of starch gelatinisation and recrystallisation are complex (Morris, 1990; Biliaderis, 1991), but are of vital importance for starch digestion because even simple food processes such as can occur during the preparation of a meal, like heating and cooling, will affect the nutritional quality of starchy foods.

NSP

Non-starch polysaccharides are principally the polysaccharides of the plant cell wall and are non-α-glucans. They include cellulose and the non-cellulosic polysaccharides, pectin and hemicellulose. They are a very diverse group of molecules with varying degrees of water solubility, size and structure (Selvendran & Robertson, 1990). A number of other non-α-glucan polysaccharides exist which are neither storage nor cell wall constituents. These include plant gums and exudates (gum arabic), seed mucilages (ispaghula), bacterial polysaccharides (xanthan), chemically modified starches and synthetic compounds such as polydextrose.

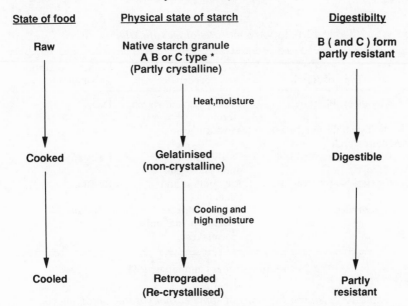

Fig. 12.1. The effects of cooking and cooling on the physical state of starch and its digestibility *in vivo*.

Measurement

Starch

In view of the importance to health of starch, there is a need to have good laboratory methods for its measurement both for research purposes and also for food tables and labelling. A single value for total starch is of limited use because of the widely varying digestibility of different starch types. This variability depends primarily on intrinsic factors such as crystalline state, although such knowledge alone does not entirely predict digestibility by individuals. This is because starchy foods are exposed to highly variable external influences during digestion in the gut. However, any measurement of the digestibility of starchy foods must be based on the intrinsic factors as only this will give reproducible values to compare different foods. A classification of starchy foods for nutritional purposes has been proposed based on these intrinsic factors (Table 12.1).

These categories of starch may be determined in the laboratory by controlled enzymic hydrolysis and measurement of the released glucose using glucose oxidase. Total starch (TS) is measured as the glucose released by complete enzymic hydrolysis of starch following gelatinisation in boiling water and treatment with potassium hydroxide to disperse

Table 12.1. In vitro *nutritional classification of starch*

Type of starch	Example of occurrence	Probable digestion in small intestine
Rapidly digestible starch	Freshly cooked starchy food	Rapid
Slowly digestible starch	Most raw cereals	Slow but complete
Resistant starch		
1. Physically inaccessible starch	Partly milled grain and seeds	Resistant
2. Resistant starch granules	Raw potato and banana	Resistant
3. Retrograded starch	Cooled, cooked potato, bread and cornflakes	Resistant

From Englyst & Cummings, 1990.

Table 12.2. *Starch fractions of some carbohydrate containing foods*

Sample	Dry matter (%)	g/100 g dry matter				
		RDS	SDS	RS	TS	SDI^a
White bread	54.5	69	7	1	77	90
Shredded Wheat	91.3	66	4	—	71	94
Lincoln biscuit	95.6	23	23	—	46	50
Potato starch (raw)	81.8	6	19	75	99	6
Banana flour	99.1	3	15	57	75	4
Spaghetti (freshly cooked)	28.3	41	33	5	79	52
Peas (frozen)	18.3	12	2	5	20	60
Haricot beans	41.4	8	19	18	45	18

^{a} Starch digestibility index $\left(\dfrac{RDS}{TS} \times 100\right)$.

retrograded amylose. Rapidly digestible starch (RDS) and slowly digestible starch (SDS) are measured after incubation with pancreatic amylase and amyloglucosidase at 37 °C. A value for RDS is obtained as the glucose released after 20 minutes and SDS as the glucose released after a further 100 minutes incubation. Resistant starch (RS) is calculated as the starch not hydrolysed after 120 minutes incubation. If required, separate values may be obtained for physically inaccessible starch (RS_1), resistant starch granules (RS_2) and retrograded amylose (RS_3). Some values for these starch fractions in food are given in Table 12.2 (Englyst, Kingman & Cummings, 1992).

Non-starch polysaccharides

NSP can be measured by the Englyst method which has been well documented elsewhere (Englyst & Cummings, 1988; Englyst & Hudson, 1987).

Other methods for the determination of 'dietary fibre' have been published, including the enzymatic–gravimetric method of Prosky (Prosky *et al.*, 1988). This method measures a residue on a filter after the food has been sequentially treated with various enzymes. A correction has to be made for residual minerals and protein. Values obtained by the gravimetric procedure are generally, but not always, higher than the values obtained by the Englyst NSP procedure, especially for processed foods. The main reasons are that the gravimetric technique includes some retrograded starch and lignin-measuring substances formed during food processing.

In a recent international collaborative study of dietary fibre methods (Wood *et al.*, 1992) the Prosky procedure was tested against the Englyst colorimetric and GLC procedures. For the 12 test samples the mean total value obtained by the Prosky technique was 21 % higher than the mean by the Englyst GLC procedure. Despite this, considerably higher amounts of soluble fibre were measured by the Englyst technique. The mean value for the 12 samples measured by the Prosky technique was only two-thirds of that measured as soluble NSP by the Englyst procedures. In the Englyst procedure soluble fibre represents 43 % of total, but in the Prosky procedure only 23 %. This is because more of the cell-wall polysaccharides are extracted at the physiological pH 7 used in the Englyst procedure than at pH 5 used in the Prosky technique. For all three methods the between laboratory variation was considerably higher than the within laboratory variation. The Englyst NSP procedure is technically easier, quicker and cheaper to perform than the Prosky gravimetric procedure.

Digestion

Whilst it is relatively straightforward to categorise and measure complex carbohydrate, it is much more difficult to classify it according to its digestibility. The old notion that starch is broken down by pancreatic amylase and absorbed from the small bowel as glucose, whilst NSP simply provides bulk and passes through into faeces, is now known to be incorrect. Figure 12.2 summarises what is known of the site of carbo-

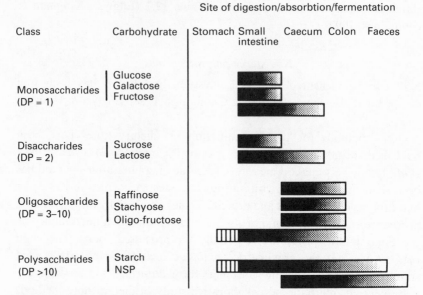

Fig. 12.2. Sites of carbohydrate digestion, absorption and fermentation in the human gut. Hatched bar represents digestion only; shaded bars represent digestion, absorption and fermentation. Intensity of shading reflects the amount of digestion/absorption/fermentation; darker shading indicates areas where the greater part of digestion/absorption/fermentation occurs (from Cummings & Englyst, 1991a).

hydrate digestion and absorption in the human gut in relation to its chemical type. Whilst most mono- and disaccharides are absorbed in the small bowel, it is known that large doses of fructose, normally absorbed by facilitated diffusion, can cause diarrhoea, whilst the majority of the world's population do not digest lactose. The oligosaccharides (raffinose, stachyose and oligo-fructose, DP 3–10) mostly escape digestion in the small bowel, although few good studies have been done in man on this point.

NSP consistently escape digestion in the small bowel (Englyst & Cummings 1985, 1986, 1987). This information is derived principally from the use of ileostomy patients as a model. Despite the ileostomist having many more bacteria in the terminal ileum than people with an intact gut, it is still possible to show, provided proper carbohydrate methodology is used, that all the ingested NSP is recoverable as NSP in the ileal contents. Measuring carbohydrate in ileal contents is technically quite difficult and it is here that gravimetric methods show up their limitations. NSP are largely but not always completely fermented in the large intestine (Cummings, 1981).

Starch

The realisation that starches are broken down at different rates and to differing extents in the human small bowel has been one of the major findings in nutrition in recent years. Understanding of starch hydrolysis in the gut is as yet incomplete and poses a number of methodological problems. Evidence for the site, rate and extent of starch breakdown may be obtained from *in vitro* studies, studies of blood glucose and insulin responses to starchy meals, breath hydrogen, ileostomy digestion, intubation of the ileum, the effects of starch on bowel habit, and study of colonic bacterial glycosidase activity (Cummings & Englyst, 1991*b*). None of these techniques alone gives the complete picture of the factors controlling starch digestibility, but together they allow some overall conclusions to be drawn.

Starch digestion primarily depends on its physical form, crystallinity, and the effect of any processing or cooking which affects gelatinisation and retrogradation. In addition a great range of starch digestibilities can be found within individuals which are the result of chewing, bowel transit time, presence of enzyme inhibitors, and overall composition of the meal. Starch which escapes digestion in the small bowel is broken down in the large intestine but not always completely so. Many people have observed whole grains and seeds in their own faeces which contain starch made resistant to any form of amylase attack by virtue of being physically enclosed in tough seed cases or cell walls. Moreover, some forms of resistant starch, especially retrograded amylose, are not digested by everyone. In feeding studies of healthy humans with retrograded amylose from maize we have observed that two out of five subjects were completely unable to break down the resistant starch whilst the other three fermented more than 80 % (Cummings & Englyst, unpublished observations). Such observations make it difficult to provide a universely applicable energy value for complex carbohydrate which is fermented rather than absorbed in the small bowel.

Physiology and metabolism

The physiological effects of complex carbohydrate and their implications for health is a burgeoning field which can only be summarised in the briefest way here. For further information see Kritchevsky, Bonfield & Anderson, 1990; Southgate *et al.*, 1990; BNF, 1990; Stephen, 1991. There is as yet no substantial book devoted to modern ideas concerning starch in human nutrition. 'Fibre' is still perceived as the key despite the fact that many of the effects ascribed to it are probably mediated through changes in starch digestion.

There are wide-ranging consequences of the digestion and metabolism of complex carbohydrates in the gut. Often it is difficult to separate the role of NSP and starch, but a number of important differences can be seen (Table 12.3). Chemically NSP and starch are very different and NSP have important physical properties which starch lacks. Ten times more starch than NSP is present in the diet, but starch exerts little effect on small bowel function whereas NSP, through its physical properties, may affect chewing, and lipid and carbohydrate absorption. Both NSP and RS are fermented in the colon, although RS may be fermented more to butyrate and lactate in addition to acetate and propionate.

Satiety

Current opinion is that NSP does have an effect on satiety and therefore indirectly may be important in obesity (Burley & Blundell, 1990). Satiety itself is a complex and poorly understood compendium of physiological events, to which NSP may contribute by a number of mechanisms including the provision of a physical barrier to nutrients which affects chewing, gastric emptying and nutrient release in the small intestine. Slowing of transit time in the upper bowel may also contribute through the ileal break. Post-absorptive effects of NSP, mediated through short chain fatty acids, are not currently thought to affect satiety, although salivary flow and appetite are both modulated in this way in the ruminant.

Convincing evidence that obesity can be either prevented or treated with complex carbohydrates alone is lacking. However, current advice for the obese is to increase their intake of complex carbohydrate if only to displace fat and sugar (Department of Health, 1991). Studies of the obese are in essence long term and difficult to make. High NSP intakes are associated with increased faecal energy losses, but compensatory reductions in urine output usually mean no change in energy balance.

Small bowel

The rate and extent of starch breakdown in the small bowel is important for the control of glucose and insulin metabolism. This phenomenon has been known for about 20 years (Crapo, Reaven & Olefsky, 1976) and led to the concept of the glycaemic index of foods (Jenkins *et al.*, 1981) and major changes in the management of diabetes. NSP also contributes to this

Table 12.3. *Contrasts between NSP and starch*

NSP	Starch
Not α-glucan	α-glucan
Wide variety of homo and hetero polysaccharides	Either amylose or amylopectin
Diet contains 10–30 g/day	Diet contains 100–300 g/day
Physical properties	No clear physical effects on
– plant cell wall	digestion
– water holding	
– surface binding	
Partly soluble (gels)	Gel formation unlikely in gut. RS insoluble
Not digested in small bowel	Partly digested
Cholesterol lowering	No effect detected as yet
Fermented to acetate/propionate/butyrate	RS possibly better source of butyrate and lactate

effect (Wolever & Jenkins, 1986) through its physical properties. Starch appears to have little influence on digestion and absorption of other nutrients in the small bowel. Resistant starch is by definition insoluble and lacks both the gel-forming or surface effects of NSP. By contrast NSP have clear effects on cholesterol absorption (Anderson, Deakins & Bridges, 1990), and through their ability to increase bile acid excretion and reduce deoxycholate formation may help prevent gallstones (Marcus & Heaton, 1986).

Large bowel

The large bowel exists primarily to salvage energy from NSP and resistant starch through fermentation. The microbiology of fermentation is reasonably well worked out, drawing on earlier studies of the rumen. However, the large bowel is a much more energy-depleted environment than the rumen and so does not model itself entirely on the foregut system. Much more proteolysis and amino acid fermentation probably takes place in the hind gut, which has implications for the pathogenesis of colonic and other disorders (Cummings & Macfarlane, 1991). Furthermore, hydrogen disposal, a major problem in anaerobic systems, may be different in man than in other species, with inorganic sulphate acting as a terminal electron acceptor in many people (Gibson *et al.*, 1990). Again, there are implications for the health of the colonic epithelium.

Short chain fatty acids are small molecules with diverse and fascinating properties (Roche, 1991). Whilst acetate serves primarily as a fuel for muscle, propionate has been implicated in the control of both cholesterol and carbohydrate metabolism in the liver. Butyric acid has important effects on epithelial cell growth and differentiation and SCFA in general may control cell turnover in the gut. It is an area of research one can safely expect to grow in the next decade.

Recommended intake of complex carbohydrate and food labelling

The recommendation for countries with Western-style diets to increase their intake of complex carbohydrate has become universal since it was first suggested by the US Senate Select Committee on Nutrition and Human Needs (1977) – the McGovern Report. Table 12.4 shows quantitative recommendations for starch and NSP intakes derived from the WHO (1990) and the UK (Department of Health, 1991) reports.

Starch

Limits for starch intake have usually been set by default, that is starch is considered to be an energy filler in the diet once limits have been set for fat and protein. The WHO report is typical in this respect, saying that the 'recommendations account for 25–45 % of the total energy intake as fat and protein. Since the Group does not recommend that alcohol be ingested, it follows that the remaining energy intake will be provided by carbohydrate, for which the lower and upper limits for the population nutrient goals are therefore set at 55 % and 75 %. The Group saw specific advantages associated with the intake of complex carbohydrates and has proposed a lower limit for this class (50 % of energy)'.

The UK Dietary Reference Values report took a similar approach, although in discussion the possible 'specific advantages' of starch were debated extensively: 'The Panel therefore proposed that starches and intrinsic and milk sugars should provide the balance of dietary energy not provided by alcohol, protein, fat and non-milk extrinsic sugars, that is on average 37 % of total dietary energy for the population.' The marked differences in recommendations for starch intakes between the two reports should be noted (Table 12.4).

What might be the specific advantages of consuming starch?

1. Starch as a substitute for saturated fat will lead to lower blood cholesterol.
2. Starch rather than sugar should lower the risk of dental caries.

Table 12.4. *Recommended intakes of dietary complex carbohydrate*

	WHO	UK DRV
Total % energy[a]	50–70	24 (population average)[b]
NSP	16–24	12–24 (average 18 g/day)

[a] % food energy only – excludes alcohol.
[b] assume intrinsic and milk sugar contribute 20 % food energy.

3. Starchy foods, namely cereals, pulses and vegetables, contain a wide variety of micronutrients which sugar and fatty foods usually do not.
4. Starchy foods are preferable to alcohol as a source of energy.
5. Starchy foods rather than fatty and sugary foods might limit the risk of obesity.
6. Some starch is resistant to digestion by pancreatic amylase and may contribute to the prevention of bowel cancer.
7. The type of starchy food is a major controlling factor for blood glucose and insulin levels.

The evidence for these statements is contained in the reference lists of the recent reports on this topic. Whilst none of it is unequivocal, few people interested in public health policy would not agree that this is prudent advice to the general population.

Non-starch polysaccharides

NSP are something of a newcomer to the dietary recommendations story. A number of national bodies have now made quantitative recommendations for increases in 'dietary fibre' intake, but because of the lack of an agreed definition of fibre and of a method for measuring it, these recommendations do not cross international boundaries very well. Therefore the BNF, WHO and the UK Department of Health have opted for NSP as the best index of fibre. Dietary NSP have been shown to have a wide variety of physiological effects, particularly on digestion, and are implicated in the aetiology of diseases such as bowel cancer, diverticular disease, diabetes, obesity, coronary heart disease and gallstones. It is clear, however, that the evidence in relation to most of these conditions is not sufficient to allow a quantitative estimate of need for the population to be made. Rather, it points to the goal of a diet characterised by high NSP (and starch) intakes.

When it comes to bowel habit, however, the role of NSP is much clearer and defined. The arguments for a recommended dietary amount therefore run as follows:

1. NSP increase stool output in a dose-related fashion up to about 32 g/day.
2. No other dietary component so affects bowel habit, although resistant starch is laxative and may contribute to faecal bulking in high starch/high NSP diets.
3. Constipation is a frequent problem in the UK, with almost half the population having stool weights below 100 g/day.
4. In epidemiological studies stool weights below 150 g/day are associated with increased risk of bowel cancer, diverticular disease and high deoxycholate levels in bile.
5. Therefore NSP intakes should be increased in order to increase average stool weight by about 25% in the UK. This means NSP intakes should rise from 13 to 18 g/day.

Labelling

What would be the most useful information the consumer should have to make informed decisions about complex carbohydrates in food? Clearly total starch and NSP should be given, but is there a case for further information? Starch may be divided in the laboratory into digestible and resistant starch and each fraction further sub-divided (Table 12.1). Whilst these further divisions give useful information on the way starch behaves in the gut and affects the glycaemic index, the finer points would probably be lost on the consumer. A 'digestibility index' (Table 12.2), which incorporates these fractions in a single figure, would probably be ideal.

Similarly for NSP a great deal of further information can be given, but the most widely recognised division is one on the basis of physical properties, namely solubility at pH 7. This correlates well with a number of physiological changes such as cholesterol-lowering and faecal bulking. For NSP therefore the best division is into total and soluble for the present.

References

Anderson. J. W., Deakins, D. A. & Bridges, S. R. (1990). Soluble fiber: hypocholesterolemic effects and proposed mechanisms. In *Dietary Fiber: Chemistry, Physiology and Health Effects*, Kritchevsky, D., Bonfield, C. & Anderson, J. W., eds, pp. 339–63, New York: Plenum.

Biliaderis, C. G. (1991). The structure and interactions of starch with food constituents. *Canadian Journal of Physiology and Pharmacology*, **69**, 60–78.

British Nutrition Foundation Task Force (1990). *Complex Carbohydrates in Foods*. London: Chapman and Hall.

Burley, V. J. & Blundell, J. E. (1990). Action of dietary fiber on the satiety cascade. In *Dietary Fiber: Chemistry, Physiology and Health Effects*, Kritchevsky, D. Bonfield, C. & Anderson, J.W., eds, pp. 227–46, New York: Plenum.

Crapo, P. A., Reaven, G. & Olefsky, J. (1976). Plasma glucose and insulin responses to orally administered simple and complex carbohydrates. *Diabetes*, **25**, 741–7.

Cummings, J. H. (1981). Dietary fibre. *British Medical Bulletin*, **37**, 65–70.

Cummings, J. H. & Englyst, H. N. (1991a). What is dietary fibre? *Trends in Food Science Technology*, **2**, 99–103.

Cummings, J.H. & Englyst, H. N. (1991b). Measurement of starch fermentation in the human large intestine. *Canadian Journal of Physiology and Pharmacology*, **69**, 121–9.

Cummings, J. H. & Macfarlane, G. T. (1991). The control and consequences of bacterial fermentation in the human colon. A review. *Journal of Applied Bacteriology*, **70**, 443–59.

Department of Health (1991). *Dietary Reference Values for Food Energy and Nutrients for the United Kingdom*. Report of the Panel on Dietary Reference Values of the Committee on Medical Aspects of Food Policy. London: HMSO.

Englyst, H. N. & Cummings, J. H. (1985). Digestion of the polysaccharides of some cereal foods in the human small intestine. *American Journal of Clinical Nutrition*, **42**, 778–87.

Englyst, H. N. & Cummings, J. H. (1986). Digestion of the polysaccharides of banana (*Musa paradisiaca sapientum*) in man. *American Journal of Clinical Nutrition*, **44**, 42–50.

Englyst, H. N. & Cummings, J. H. (1987) Digestion of the polysaccharides of potato in the small intestine of man. *American Journal of Clinical Nutrition*, **45**, 423–31.

Englyst, H. N. & Cummings, J. H. (1988). Improved method for measurement of dietary fiber as non-starch polysaccharides in plant foods. *Journal of the Association of Official Analytical Chemists*, **71**, 808–14.

Englyst, H. N. & Cummings, J. H. (1990). Non-starch polysaccharides (dietary fibre) and resistant starch. In *New Developments in Dietary Fibre*, Furda, I. & Brine, C. J., eds, pp. 205–225. New York: Plenum.

Englyst, H. N. & Hudson, G. J. (1987). Colorimetric method for routine measurement of dietary fibre as non-starch polysaccharides. A comparison with gas–liquid chromatography. *Food Chemistry*, **24**, 63–76.

Englyst, H. N., Kingman, S. & Cummings, J. H. (1992). Classification and measurement of nutritionally important starch fractions. *European Journal of Clinical Nutrition*, in press.

Federal Register (1990). **5**, 29475–531.

Gibson, G. R., Cummings, J. H., Macfarlane, G. T., Allison, C. *et al.* (1990). Alternative pathways for hydrogen disposal during fermentation in the human colon. *Gut*, **31**, 679–83.

Hidaka, H., Eida, T., Takizawa, T., Tokunaga, T. & Tashiro, Y. (1986). Effects of fructo-oligosaccharides on intestinal flora and human health. *Bifidobacteria Microflora*, **5**, 37–50.

Jenkins, D. J. A., Wolever, T. M. S., Taylor, R. H., Barker, H. M. *et al.* (1981).
Glycemic index of foods: a physiological basis for carbohydrate exchange.
American Journal of Clinical Nutrition, **34**, 362–6.

Kritchevsky, D., Bonfield, C. & Anderson, J. W., eds. (1990). *Dietary Fiber:
Chemistry , Physiology and Health Effects.* New York: Plenum.

Marcus, S. N. & Heaton, K. W. (1986). Intestinal transit, deoxycholic acid and
the cholesterol saturation of bile – three inter-related factors. *Gut,* **27**,
550–8.

Morris, V. J. (1990). Starch gelation and retrogradation. *Trends in Food Science
& Technology,* **1**, 2–6.

Prosky, L., Asp, N-G., Schweizer, T. F., DeVries, J. W. & Furda, I. (1988).
Determination of insoluble, soluble and total dietary fiber in foods and
food products: interlaboratory study. *Journal of the Association of Official
Analytical Chemists,* **71**, 1017–23.

Roche, A. F, ed, (1991). *Short Chain Fatty Acids: Metabolism and Clinical
Importance.* Report of the Tenth Ross Research Conference on Medical
Issues. Columbus, Ohio: Ross Laboratories.

Selvendran, R. R. & Robertson, J. A. (1990). The chemistry of dietary fibre – an
holistic view of the cell wall matrix. In *Dietary Fibre: Chemical and
Biological Aspects.* Southgate, D. A. T., Waldron, K., Johnson, I. T. &
Fenwick, G. R., eds, pp. 27–43. Cambridge: Royal Society of Chemistry.

Southgate, D. A. T., Waldron, K., Johnson, I. T. & Fenwick, G. R., eds, (1990).
Dietary Fibre: Chemical and Biological Aspects. Cambridge: Royal Society
of Chemistry.

Stephen, A. M. (1991). Starch in human nutrition. Symposium Proceedings.
Canadian Journal of Physiology & Pharmacology, **69**, 53–136.

WHO (1990). *Diet, Nutrition and the Prevention of Chronic Diseases.* Tech. Rep.
Series 797. WHO, Geneva.

Wolever, T. M. S. & Jenkins, D. J. A. (1986). Effect of dietary fiber and foods
on carbohydrate metabolism. In *CRC Handbook of Dietary Fiber in Human
Nutrition,* Spiller, G. A., ed., pp. 87–119. Florida: CRC Press.

Wood, R., Englyst, H. N., Southgate, D. A. T. & Cummings, J. H. (1992).
Determination of dietary fibre in foods – collaborative trial. Part IV:
Comparison of Englyst GLC and colorimetric measurement with Prosky
procedure. *Journal of the Association of Official Analytical Chemists* (in
press).

Part three
Minerals and vitamins

13

Calcium metabolism

DAVID R. FRASER

A considerable body of knowledge about calcium in animal biology was already well established over 50 years ago. It was known that most (99 %) of the calcium in vertebrates was located in the mineralised hard tissues: bones and teeth. It was known that much of the calcium in the diet did not get absorbed from the alimentary tract (Leitch, 1937) but that, nevertheless, the efficiency of absorption increased as the need for calcium increased (Nicolaysen, 1943). Calcium was also known to be less available for absorption from plant foods (in comparison to milk), and particularly from cereals, because of being tightly bound by organic substances such as phytic acid (Harrison & Mellanby, 1939; McCance & Widdowson, 1942). But, perhaps the most important discovery which had been made over 50 years ago was the realisation that the fat-soluble vitamin D had some role in enabling dietary calcium to be absorbed and utilised (Nicolaysen, 1937).

Much of the research effort concerning calcium and nutrition over the past half a century has been attempting to answer questions related (a) to calcium in bone and (b) to the utilisation of calcium from food. Nutritionists have instigated numerous investigations to try to define, with reasonable certainty, the 'dietary requirement' for calcium at different ages and under various physiological circumstances.

Calcium and cell biology

Meanwhile, from general biological research over the last 50 years, calcium has been gaining in importance. Most, if not all, of the activities of cells have been found to be affected by changes in intracellular calcium concentration. Contraction of muscle (Ebashi *et al.*, 1980), the function of cytoplasmic microtubules in mitosis (Ratan & Shelanski, 1986), the activation of intracellular protease (Murachi *et al.*, 1981), the response of

141

cells to hormones (Blackmore *et al.*, 1982) and, conversely, the secretion of hormones in response to extracellular stimuli (Hellman & Gylfe, 1986) all have calcium as a pivotal component of their respective mechanisms. Calcium has become the doyen of the regulatory factors in cell biology. It is now recognised as the key intracellular signal or message which leads to the expression of many cell functions, necessary for the survival of the animal (Rasmussen & Barrett, 1984; Carafoli & Penniston, 1985).

The way in which all these messenger functions are executed by such a simple inorganic substance as the calcium ion is by large, controlled, fleeting swings in its concentration. The intracellular calcium ion concentration may undergo a transient, tenfold increase which can initiate a variety of sustained responses by the cell. This change in concentration is the essence of what is meant by the misnomer 'calcium metabolism'. Calcium does not take part in a series of enzyme-catalysed reactions with organic substrates: the classical definition of metabolism. It merely undergoes changes in concentration from about 0.1 μM to as high as 5 μM as a result of controlled transport across membranes. Because of the multiplicity of responses induced by this concentration change, the degree of change must be precisely controlled. Elevation of intracellular Ca^{2+} level to 10–50 μM causes cell damage and cell death (Campbell, 1987).

Calcium homeostasis

Thus, to function as an intracellular message, calcium concentration in all cells is regulated by highly efficient homeostatic mechanisms. This homeostasis, in turn, depends upon a constancy of extracellular Ca^{2+} concentration. One of the notable characteristics of vertebrates, both of aquatic and land species, is that the Ca^{2+} concentration in blood is maintained at close to 1.25 mM (Urist, 1963). Any tendency for this level to rise causes excretory processes to remove the excess. Conversely, when the extracellular Ca^{2+} concentration tends to decline below 1.25 mM, an adaptive capacity develops to enhance absorption of calcium from the diet or from the aquatic environment. Internal calcium stores in the calcified tissues may also be mobilised to assist in maintaining the constancy of extracellular Ca^{2+} concentration.

If there is a dietary deficiency of calcium during growth, there will be competition between the needs of the mineralising tissues and the needs of the extracellular fluid for the limited supply. Because of the importance of a constant extracellular Ca^{2+} level for the function of all cells, the maintenance of this level apparently takes precedence over the mineralisation of bone. Hence whole body calcium homeostasis has two components: (a) the regulation of the levels in intracellular compartments and (b) the maintenance of a constant extracellular concentration. The mechanisms of calcium homeostasis are those which regulate the transport of Ca^{2+} across cell membranes and which monitor its concentration both inside and outside cells. By this reasoning, and contrary to conventional nutritional ideas, the mechanisms for maintaining bone growth seem to be subordinate to these two processes which regulate the concentration of Ca^{2+} in body fluids.

The characteristics of calcium homeostasis have much in common with the homeostatic mechanisms for the two other extracellular constituents where constancy of concentration is important. These are the mechanisms for glucose and sodium homeostasis. Although the extracellular concentrations of sodium and glucose may fluctuate, particularly after meals, efficient controls soon return the levels to defined set points. For both sodium and glucose the mechanisms of homeostasis depend on the distinctly different functions of specific peptide and steroid hormones. The steroid hormones have a long-term influence and induce cells to synthesise the proteins required for homeostasis. In contrast, the peptide hormones provide short-term regulation. They are secreted in response to changes in concentration, monitored by the peptide-secreting cells, and their action produces a rapid correction to the normal level.

For glucose, the steroid hormone is an adrenal glucocorticoid which induces the formation of enzymes concerned with glucose metabolism. The peptide hormones, insulin and glucagon, activate these cellular mechanisms to enable respectively the uptake of glucose from, or its production and secretion into, the extracellular fluid. The dual control of extracellular sodium utilises in a very similar way the steroid hormone aldosterone and the renin/angiotensin peptide hormone system.

Calcium homeostasis has long been recognised to have parathyroid hormone as the agent which is secreted in response to a fall in the concentration of extracellular Ca^{2+} and which rapidly restores the concentration to the set-point level (Collip, 1925). In the 1960s another small peptide hormone, calcitonin, was discovered which has the opposite effect of lowering the extracellular Ca^{2+} concentration when it becomes elevated above the normal level (Copp *et al.*, 1962; Foster *et al.*, 1964). Although the significance of calcitonin in calcium homeostasis is still not clear, it nevertheless has a rapid effect on the transport of calcium by certain cells, notably osteoclasts. Now, other calcium regulating peptides: the calcitonin gene-related peptide (Girgis *et al.*, 1985) and parathyroid hormone-related protein (Martin *et al.*, 1989) have been discovered and these may also have specific, short-term regulatory functions in the transport of calcium by cells.

Regulation of calcium absorption

The identification of the endocrine role of vitamin D when metabolised to 1,25-dihydroxycholecalciferol [1,25(OH)$_2$D] has not so far prompted the question as to how it relates to the other calcium homeostatic hormones. When vitamin D-deficient animals are given 1,25(OH)$_2$D, there is enhanced absorption of calcium by the intestinal mucosa and calcium is also mobilised from bone. From these observations, 1,25(OH)$_2$D has been interpreted as a *stimulatory* hormone with comparable functions to parathyroid hormone in calcium homeostasis. Yet 1,25(OH)$_2$D has many of the properties of a steroid hormone. It has a secosteroid structure, it binds to a specific intranuclear receptor and it induces the synthesis of a number of proteins including a vitamin D-dependent calcium-binding protein (CaBP). The molecular function of CaBP is still open to question but it appears to play a role in the enhanced transport of calcium across the intestinal mucosal cell (Bronner, 1990).

This action of 1,25(OH)$_2$D in the small intestine and in bone raises the question of what is the real role of vitamin D in calcium homeostasis. Like parathyroid hormone, it appears to raise extracellular Ca^{2+} concentration. Yet why should there be duplication of this function of parathyroid hormone? All the evidence suggests that 1,25(OH)$_2$D is a steroid hormone, analogous to aldosterone and the glucocorticoids in sodium and glucose homeostasis. If this were so, then 1,25(OH)$_2$D would induce cells to produce the machinery of calcium transport – machinery which would then be controlled by other, short-term regulators. The endocrine factors regulating calcium homeostasis would then be entirely comparable to those maintaining glucose and sodium concentrations.

However, convincing evidence for such a steroid/peptide hormone homeostatic control mechanism is still missing. Nicolaysen (1960) postulated that there was some 'endogenous factor' which stimulated intestinal calcium absorption when there was an increased requirement. When 1,25(OH)$_2$D was discovered it was hailed as Nicolaysen's endogenous factor and human studies have shown that about 75 % of the calcium absorbed is transported by the 1,25(OH)$_2$D-dependent pathway (Sheikh *et al.*, 1988). Yet there is also much evidence that calcium absorption from the intestine is enhanced by the action of hormones other than 1,25(OH)$_2$D. These include parathyroid hormone (Hino *et al.*, 1986; Nemere & Norman, 1986), prolactin (Krishnamra, Thumchai & Limlomwongse, 1990; Balakir *et al.*, 1990), thyroid hormone (Cross, Polzleitner & Peterlik, 1986) and growth hormone (Chipman *et al.*, 1980). Intestinal calcium absorption capacity also declines rapidly when there is nutritionally induced cessation of growth (Adams *et al.*, 1974) and, in the laying hen, when egg shell secretion is complete (Nys, N'guyen & Garabedian, 1984). This change in absorption capacity cannot be explained simply by a change in the supply of 1,25(OH)$_2$D. These observations again suggest that some short-term regulatory factor is acting on the intestinal mucosal cells and is controlling the expression of the 1,25(OH)$_2$D-dependent calcium absorption pathway.

Recommended dietary allowances for calcium

Despite the better understanding in recent years of the role of vitamin D in calcium absorption, there is still much to learn about the way in which adaptive increases and decreases in absorptive capacity occur. In adults, a decrease in calcium supply can lead to an enhanced absorptive capacity, but this does not always occur, even in severe, negative calcium balance (Malm, 1958). This problem of predicting adaptation to variation in calcium supply has led to the pragmatic assumption when deciding calcium 'requirements' that only about 30% of dietary calcium is absorbed (Nordin *et al.*, 1979). Such an assumption is unlikely to apply to populations of many developing countries where calcium intake is very much lower than that recommended in the Western world. Furthermore, dietary calcium intake is often not only low, but it is also mainly from plant sources where the nutritional availability of calcium is presumed to be low.

Both these assumptions: a low absorption capacity and a low availability of calcium, need further investigation before realistic requirements can be defined. Comparative studies of populations on high and low calcium diets show little effect on the degree of bone mineralisation throughout the whole of adult life (Prentice *et al.*, 1991), although low calcium intake may be a cause of undermineralisation in early childhood (Prentice *et al.*, 1990). There is some evidence for an adaptive increase in the absorption of calcium from the large intestine under the influence of 1,25(OH)$_2$D (Grinstead, Pak & Krejs, 1984). Microbial action in the colon releases calcium from organic complexes so that absorption from this site could be a means by which adequate amounts of calcium are obtained, even when the dietary intake is low. Attempts to define calcium requirements have largely ignored the probability that calcium intakes during human evolution have been much lower than the levels now being considered for recommendation. More recognition should be given to the fact that calcium homeostasis is efficient and has evolved to cope with wide variation in calcium supply.

Calcium and osteoporosis

There are two reasons for trying to identify optimum calcium intakes. One reason is to ensure that the requirements for bone growth are met. The other reason is based on the belief that osteoporosis in the elderly, particularly in elderly women, is in some way able to be prevented or ameliorated by ensuring a high intake of calcium. The calcium content of bone at all stages of human growth is now well known so the minimum dietary requirements, assuming efficient absorption, can be accurately defined. Therefore, daily allowances of from 1000 to 1200 mg per day, which are recommended for adolescent children in many countries, have a reasonable physiological basis. However, there is fierce controversy over the rationale for the recommended allowances for calcium in adult life.

In the elderly, bone resorption occurs at a faster rate than bone formation so that there is an inevitable, gradual decline in bone mass. This imbalance is reflected by an increase in urinary calcium output, a decrease in the intestinal absorptive capacity for calcium and, indeed, a diminished responsiveness of the intestine for increased calcium absorption when $1,25(OH)_2D$ is administered (Need *et al.*, 1985). For some investigators (e.g. Nordin & Polley, 1987), the problem of bone loss is seen as one of negative calcium balance which, if corrected, would prevent the clinical effects of bone fragility in the elderly. Indeed, calcium supplementation has been shown to diminish the rate of bone loss (Need *et al.*, 1987). However, other studies have not supported the concept that it is an insufficiency of dietary calcium which leads to loss of bone in elderly women (Riis, Thomsen & Christiansen, 1987; Riggs *et al.*, 1987).

Any decrease in the rate of bone loss, as a result of dietary supplementation with calcium, is likely to have been brought about by a pharmacological effect of the excess calcium which may suppress parathyroid hormone secretion. If this effect of calcium supplementation were to occur during growth, then the diminution of parathyroid hormone secretion might lead to defective bone formation (Fraser, 1988). Hence, it may be unsound and unwise to believe the oft quoted justification: calcium supplements may do no harm, even if they do no good. The recommendation of high calcium intakes, which are unlikely to be achieved from conventional diets, should thus be assessed with caution.

The observations about the utilisation of calcium in osteoporosis of the elderly can be given an equally valid, alternative explanation to that of a defect in calcium homeostasis. If the primary abnormality were in the regulation of bone turnover, all the changes in calcium metabolism could be a consequence of this, and thus would be entirely normal. Because the rate of bone resorption is greater than that of formation then clearly the excess calcium passing into the extracellular fluid would have to be excreted by the kidney. Similarly, because of the decrease in the rate of bone formation, there would be a decrease in the amount of calcium moving out of the circulation to be incorporated into bone. Therefore, a compensatory decrease in calcium absorption from the alimentary tract would follow. The difficulty of deciding which of these two interpretations is correct, highlights again the need to identify whether there is some short-term regulatory factor which modulates the rate of calcium absorption by the vitamin D-dependent pathway.

Challenges for the future

Irrespective of any nutritional relevance, the cellular functions of calcium and the mechanisms of cellular calcium homeostasis will continue to be dominant fields in biological research. However, as with many other aspects of cell biology, the relationship of the calcium messenger system in cells to whole animal physiology has been rather overlooked. Although some components of whole-body calcium homeostasis have been identified, the way in which these endocrine controls are integrated is still poorly understood. The efficiency by which calcium homeostasis can adapt, either to changes in the requirement for calcium, to changes in calcium supply, or indeed to a persistent long-term, low level of intake is also uncertain.

The difficulties which many national advisory bodies have had in reaching agreement on 'calcium requirements' are mainly caused by a lack of knowledge about the efficiency of calcium homeostasis. To be heretical: it is possible, because of the ability to adapt to low levels of intake, that calcium is a nutrient for which dietary recommendations can never be accurately defined. Yet, there may still be reasons, other than the need to maintain calcium balance, as to why some recommendation is desirable. Epidemiological studies have shown beneficial effects of high calcium intakes on the prevalence of some diseases such as hypertension

(McCarron, 1985) and colon cancer (Sorenson, Slattery & Ford, 1988). The increase in knowledge about calcium in biology has made the significance of the level of dietary calcium even more puzzling and elusive than it was 50 years ago.

References

Adams, P. H., Hill, L. F., Wain, D. & Taylor, C. (1974). The effects of undernutrition and its relief on intestinal calcium transport in the rat. *Calcified Tissue Research*, **16**, 293–304.

Balakir, R. A., Cheng, L., Sacktor, B. & Liang, C. T. (1990). Age-dependent and sex-dependent stimulation of calcium uptake in duodenal cells by prolactin in vitamin D-deficient rats. *Life Sciences*, **47**, 77–83.

Blackmore, P. F., Hughes, B. P., Shuman, E. A. & Exton, J. H. (1982). α-Adrenergic activation of phosphorylase in liver cells involves mobilization of intracellular calcium without influx of extracellular calcium. *Journal of Biological Chemistry*, **257**, 190–7.

Bronner, F. (1990). Intestinal calcium transport – the cellular pathway. *Mineral and Electrolyte Metabolism*, **16**, 94–100.

Campbell, A. K. (1987). Intracellular calcium: friend or foe? *Clinical Science*, **72**, 1–10.

Carafoli, E. & Penniston, J. T. (1985). The calcium signal. *Scientific American*, **253**, 50–88.

Chipman, J. J., Zerwekh, J., Nicar, M., Marks, J. & Pak, C. Y. C. (1980). Effect of growth hormone administration: reciprocal changes in serum 1α,25-dihydroxyvitamin D and intestinal calcium absorption. *Journal of Clinical Endocrinology and Metabolism*, **51**, 321–4.

Collip, J. B. (1925). Extraction of a parathyroid hormone which will prevent or control parathyroid tetany and which regulates the level of blood calcium. *Journal of Biological Chemistry*, **63**, 395–438.

Copp, D. H., Cameron, E. C., Cheney, B. A., Davidson, A. G, F. & Henze, K. G. (1962). Evidence for calcitonin – a new hormone from the parathyroid that lowers blood calcium. *Endocrinology*, **70**, 638–49.

Cross, H. S., Polzleitner, D. & Peterlik, M. (1986). Intestinal phosphate and calcium absorption – joint regulation by thyroid hormones and 1,25-dihydroxyvitamin-D₃. *Acta Endocrinologica*, **113**, 96–103.

Ebashi, S., Nonomura, Y., Kohama, K., Kitazawa, T. & Mikawa, T. (1980). Regulation of muscle contraction by Ca ion. In *Chemical Recognition in Biology*, Chapville, F. & Haenni, H-L., eds, pp. 183–94, Berlin, Heidelberg, New York: Springer-Verlag.

Foster, G. W., Baghdiantz, A., Kumar, M. A., Slack, E., Soliman, H. A. & MacIntyre, I. (1964). Thyroid origin of calcitonin. *Nature*, **202**, 1303–5.

Fraser, D. R. (1988). Bone minerals and fat-soluble vitamins. In *Comparative Nutrition*, Blaxter, K. & Macdonald, I., eds, pp. 105–16, London: John Libbey.

Girgis, S., MacDonald, D. W. R., Stevenson, J. C., Bevis, P. J. R., Lynch, C., Wimalawansa, S. J., Self, C. H., Morris, H. R. & MacIntyre, I. (1985). Calcitonin gene-related peptide: potent vasodilator and major product of calcitonin gene. *Lancet*, **ii**, 14–15.

Grinstead, W. C., Pak, C. Y. C. & Krejs, G. J. (1984). Effect of 1,25-dihydroxyvitamin D₃ on calcium absorption in the colon of healthy humans. *American Journal of Physiology*, **247**, G189–92.

Harrison, D. C. & Mellanby, E. (1939). Phytic acid and the rickets-producing action of cereals. *Biochemical Journal*, **33**, 1660–81.

Hellman, B. & Gylfe, E. (1986). Calcium and the control of insulin secretion. In *Calcium and Cell Function*, Cheung, W. Y., ed., vol. 6, Chap. 8, New York: Academic Press.

Hino, M., Yamamoto, I., Shigeno, C., Aoki, J., Dokoh, S., Fukunaga, M., Morita, R. & Torizuka, K. (1986). Evidence that factors other than 1,25-dihydroxyvitamin D may play a role in augmenting intestinal calcium absorption in patients with primary hyperparathyroidism. *Calcified Tissue International*, **38**, 193–6.

Krishnamra, N., Thumchai, R. & Limlomwongse, L. (1990). Acute effect of prolactin on the intestinal calcium absorption in normal, pregnant and lactating rats. *Bone and Mineral*, **11**, 31–41.

Leitch, I. (1937). The determination of the calcium requirements of man. *Nutrition Abstracts and Reviews*, **6**, 553–78.

McCance, R. A., & Widdowson, E. M. (1942). Mineral metabolism of healthy adults on white and brown bread dietaries. *Journal of Physiology*, **101**, 44–85.

McCarron, D. A. (1985). Is calcium more important than sodium in the pathogenesis of essential hypertension? *Hypertension*, **7**, 607–27.

Malm, O. J. (1958). Calcium requirement and adaptation in adult men. *Scandinavian Journal of Clinical and Laboratory Investigation*, **10**, Suppl, 1–289.

Martin, T. Y., Allan, E. H., Caple, I. W., Care, A. D., Danks, J. A., Diefenbachjagger, H., Ebeling, P. R., Gillespie, M. T., Hammonds, G., Heath, J. A., Hudson, P. J., Kemp, B. E., Kubota, M., Kukreja, S. C., Moseley, J. M., Ng, K. W., Raisz, L. G., Rodda, C. P., Simmons, H. A., Suva, L. J., Wettenhall, R. E. H. & Wood, W. I. (1989). Parathyroid hormone-related protein – isolation, molecular cloning, and mechanism of action. *Recent Progress in Hormone Research*, **45**, 467–506.

Murachi, T., Tanaka, K., Hatanaka, M. & Murakami, T. (1981). Intracellular Ca^{2+}-dependent protease (calpain) and its high-molecular-weight endogenous inhibitor (calpastatin). *Advances in Enzyme Regulation*, **19**, 407–24.

Need, A. G., Horowitz, M., Philcox, J. C. & Nordin, B. E. C. (1985). 1,25-Dihydroxycalciferol and calcium therapy in osteoporosis with calcium malabsorption. *Mineral and Electrolyte Metabolism*, **11**, 35–40.

Need, A. G., Horowitz, M., Philcox, J. C. & Nordin, B. E. C. (1987). Biochemical effects of a calcium supplement in osteoporotic postmenopausal women with normal absorption and malabsorption of calcium. *Mineral and Electrolyte Metabolism*, **13**, 112–16.

Nemere, I. & Norman, A. W. (1986). Parathyroid hormone stimulates calcium transport in perfused duodena from normal chicks: comparison with the rapid (transcaltachic) effect of 1,25-dihydroxyvitamin D_3. *Endocrinology*, **119**, 1406–8.

Nicolaysen, R. (1937). Studies upon the mode of action of vitamin D. III. The influence of vitamin D on the absorption of calcium and phosphorus in the rat. *Biochemical Journal*, **31**, 122–9.

Nicolaysen, R. (1943). The absorption of calcium as a function of the body saturation with calcium. *Acta Physiologica Scandinavica*, **5**, 201–12.

Nicolaysen, R. (1960). The calcium requirement of man as related to diseases of the skeleton. *Clinical Orthopedics*, **17**, 226–34.

Nordin, B. E. C., Horsman, A., Marshall, D. H., Simpson, M. & Waterhouse, G. M. (1979). Calcium requirement and calcium therapy. *Clinical Orthopedics*, **140**, 216–46.

Nordin, B. E. C. & Polley, K. J. (1987). Metabolic consequences of the menopause. *Calcified Tissue International*, **41** (Suppl. 1), 1–59.

Nys, Y., N'guyen, T. M. & Garabedian, M. (1984). Involvement of 1,25-dihydroxycholecalciferol in the short- and long-term increase in intestinal calcium absorption in laying hens: stimulation by gonadal hormones is partly independent of 1,25-dihydroxycholecalciferol. *Comparative Biochemistry and Physiology, A*, **53A**, 54–9.

Prentice, A., Laskey, M. A., Shaw, J. M., Cole, T. J. & Fraser, D. R. (1990). Bone mineral content of Gambian and British children aged 0–36 months. *Bone and Mineral*, **10**, 211–24.

Prentice, A., Shaw, J. M., Laskey, M. A., Cole, T. J. & Fraser, D. R. (1991). Bone mineral content of British and rural Gambian women aged 18–80+ years. *Bone and Mineral*, **12**, 201–14.

Rasmussen, H. & Barrett, P. Q. (1984). Calcium messenger system: an integrated view. *Physiological Reviews*, **64**, 938–84.

Ratan, R. R. & Shelanski, M. L. (1986). Calcium and the regulation of mitotic events. *Trends in Biochemical Sciences*, **11**, 456–9.

Riggs, B. L., Wahner, H. W., Melton, L. J., Richelson, L. S., Judd, H. L. & O'Fallon, W. M. (1987). Dietary calcium intake and rates of bone loss in women. *Journal of Clinical Investigation*, **80**, 979–82.

Riis, B., Thomsen, K. & Christiansen, C. (1987). Does calcium supplementation prevent postmenopausal bone loss? *New England Journal of Medicine*, **316**, 173–7.

Sheikh, M. S., Ramirez, A., Emmett, M., Ana, C. S., Schiller, L. R. & Fordtran, J. S. (1988). Role of vitamin D-dependent and vitamin D-independent mechanisms in absorption of food calcium. *Journal of Clinical Investigation*, **81**, 126–32.

Sorenson, A. W., Slattery, M. L. & Ford, M. H. (1988). Calcium and colon cancer: a review. *Nutrition and Cancer*, **11**, 135–45.

Urist, M. R. (1963). The regulation of calcium and other ions in the serums of hagfish and lampreys. *Annals of the New York Academy of Science*, **109**, 294–311.

14

The metabolism of iron and its bioavailability in foods

SUSAN J. FAIRWEATHER-TAIT

Iron is an essential component of cellular respiration and oxygen transport, and plays a key role in erythropoiesis and haemoglobin metabolism. Iron deficiency anaemia is the most commonly recognised nutritional deficiency disease worldwide; there are also problems associated with iron overload. Investigators from a wide range of disciplines have studied iron metabolism, and some of our current knowledge originates from principles established more than 50 years ago. Since then major advances have been made, partly resulting from the development of isotopic methods, but a number of important aspects of iron metabolism and bioavailability are still not fully resolved. This chapter will briefly review major developments over the past 50 years, and outline problems dominating current research.

Iron absorption

Until the late 1930s it was generally accepted that body iron homeostasis was maintained primarily by excretion. McCance & Widdowson (1937) were amongst the first scientists to recognise that absorption controls iron balance. The role of the intestinal mucosa in the regulation of iron absorption was investigated further by Balfour et al. (1942) and Hahn et al. (1943) who showed that anaemia and pregnancy increased iron absorption whereas iron overload reduced absorption. These investigators were the first to use radioactive iron (Hahn et al., 1938), and the emerging use of isotopes at this time greatly facilitated more detailed investigations of iron metabolism. Granick's studies provided support for Hahn's work and led to the so-called 'mucosal block' theory of iron absorption (Granick, 1946), in which mucosal cell ferritin levels were purported to play a key role in the regulation of absorption.

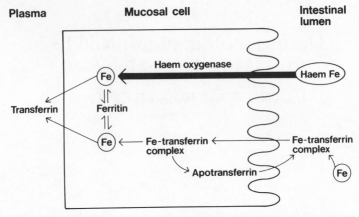

Fig. 14.1. Proposed model of iron absorption (from Huebers *et al.*, 1983).

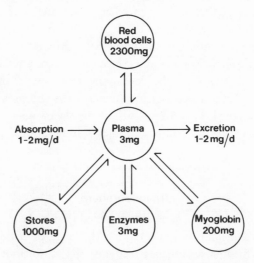

Fig. 14.2. The distribution of iron in the body.

The most active site of absorption is the duodenum and upper jejunum; absorption consists of two distinct steps, entry of iron into the mucosal cell from the lumen of the intestine, and transfer from the mucosal cell into the body. At least two pathways exist for the uptake of iron from the intestinal lumen (Fig. 14.1). Non-haem iron is chelated by an as yet unidentified transport protein, and the complex enters the mucosal cell via a transferrin-like receptor system (Huebers *et al.*, 1983*a*). Haem iron is absorbed into the mucosal cell as an intact porphyrin complex; specific receptors have been identified in laboratory animals (Grasbeck *et al.*, 1982) but not in humans. Once haem iron has entered the cell, it is rapidly degraded by haem oxygenase (Raffin *et al.*, 1974) and enters the common intracellular iron pool.

The body can adapt to a wide range of iron intakes and requirements by modifying the efficiency of gastrointestinal absorption. How the mucosal cells achieve adaptation is one of the most important unsolved questions in iron metabolism (Cook, 1990). Kinetic studies in dogs indicate that the rate-limiting step is mucosal uptake (Nathanson, Muir & McLaren, 1985), although Huebers (1986) contends that iron uptake in the mucosa is more rapid than its release, and favours serosal transfer as the rate-limiting step. When body demands for iron are high, a large fraction of the iron entering the mucosal cell is transported rapidly to the blood, but with increasing iron stores, more of the iron is sequestered in mucosal ferritin, and subsequently lost when the cell is exfoliated. The regulation of iron absorption may well lie in the partitioning of iron between these two pathways. However, although body iron status is the most important factor determining the efficiency of iron absorption, the regulatory signal has not been identified. Intestinal mucosal iron concentration, as affected by previous iron intake, has also been shown to play an important role in the day-to-day regulation of iron absorption (Hahn *et al.*, 1943; Crosby, 1966; Fairweather-Tait & Wright, 1984; Adams *et al.*, 1991). The molecular events that control absorption at the gene or receptor level remain to be determined.

Iron transport and distribution

The distribution of iron in the body of adult man is illustrated in Fig. 14.2. Much of it is found as iron porphyrin complexes, haemoglobin, myoglobin and a variety of enzymes. It is stored as ferritin and haemosiderin, mainly in the liver, but the amount is very variable depending on dietary and host-related factors.

Since the mid 1920s plasma has been known to contain a small amount of iron, and by 1937 adequate evidence had accumulated to establish that this fraction comprised a transport pool (Moore, Doan & Arrowsmith, 1937), namely transferrin. The purification of transferrin was performed independently in the mid-1940s by Holmberg & Laurell (1945) and Schade & Caroline (1946). Lactoferrin, another iron-binding protein, was isolated from human milk in 1960 (Montreuil, Tonnelat & Mullet, 1960), but its possible roles in iron absorption, and in resistance against bacterial infections in the newborn, have not been fully resolved. The transferrin molecule has two binding sites which were shown in 1977 to function differently (Aisen & Brown, 1977), and is found in the mono- and diferric forms. Iron is transported into cells by receptor mediated endocytosis (Iacopetta & Morgan, 1983). Once transferrin binds to its membrane receptor all the iron is delivered; therefore the contribution of the di- is twice as great as the monoferric molecule (Huebers *et al.*, 1983*b*). It is 40 years since the first characterisation of transferrin proteins and, in the last decade, a great deal has been found out about the structure and function of transferrins (Baker, Rumball & Anderson, 1987).

In 1937, a crystallisable iron protein, ferritin, the major storage form of iron in the body, was isolated from horse spleen (Laufberger, 1937), but it was nearly 50 years before its structure was resolved (Ford *et al.*, 1984). The presence of ferritin in blood was first reported by Reissmann & Dietrich (1956), but with the method used at that time it was only detected in patients with liver disorders. Sixteen years later Addison *et al.* (1972) developed a sensitive immunoradiometric assay and they were able to measure ferritin in serum from normal subjects. It soon became clear that serum ferritin could be used to measure body iron stores (Jacobs *et al.*, 1972). However, at lower levels of storage, before the haemoglobin concentration falls, serum ferritin cannot be used to assess the degree of iron deficiency. With this in mind, a new technique is being developed and validated for measuring serum transferrin receptors as an indicator of tissue iron (Skikne, Flowers & Cook, 1990).

Iron excretion

Some 50 years ago it was generally considered that any absorbed iron not immediately needed by the body was excreted in the large intestine, but this was challenged by McCance & Widdowson (1937), and subsequent work led to the firm conclusion that iron was not actively excreted by any organ of the body (McCance & Widdowson, 1943). Dubach, Moore & Callender (1949) injected human subjects intravenously with radio-iron and followed the excretion of radio-iron for 140 days. Normal individuals excreted 0.03–0.7% of the dose per day 4–24 post-injection, falling to 0.01% of the dose once the isotope had reached a constant level in the blood. Hypochromic anaemia reduced, and sickle cell anaemia increased, isotope excretion. Assuming complete mixing of isotope and haemoglobin iron, the authors calculated the total faecal excretion to be 0.2–0.9 mg/d for normal subjects. Ten years later, again with the aid of radio-iron, Finch studied body iron turnover in men and women and calculated daily losses of iron to be 0.38–0.52 mg (Finch & Loden, 1959).

A study on body iron excretion in the mid-1960s by Green *et al.* (1968) provided data on iron excretion which is still in use for calculating iron requirements. The authors concluded from their experiments that excessive sweating does not represent a major route for iron excretion. Urinary iron loss was about 0.1 mg/d, and faecal loss about 0.76 mg/d (comprising 0.1 mg from desquamated mucosal cells, 0.4 mg from blood and 0.26 mg from bile). Menstrual losses were studied comprehensively in Swedish women by Hallberg *et al.* (1966), but further data are required to establish the distribution of losses amongst women using current methods of birth control.

Disorders of iron metabolism

The pathological and clinical implications of iron-deficiency anaemia are not fully understood or agreed. Overt symptoms of iron deficiency are generally inconspicuous; compensatory mechanisms make up for the deficit in oxygen transport when anaemia is moderate, but they do reduce the capacity of the individual to meet other kinds of stress. Functional abnormalities of both lymphocytes and neutrophils have been shown in anaemic children (Srikantia *et al.*, 1976), although the exact effect of iron deficiency upon the immune system is not clear. A marked decrease in haemoglobin concentration reduces physical work capacity (Viteri & Torun, 1974), thermoregulation is impaired (Martinez-Torres *et al.*, 1984) and blood and urinary catecholamines are raised (Voorhess *et al.*, 1975).

There is now substantial evidence that iron deficiency has an adverse effect on brain function. Oski & Honig (1978) found that iron therapy improved mental development and behaviour of iron-deficient children aged 9–26 months. Similar results were obtained by Walter, Kovalskys & Steel (1983) in Chile, where the most striking behavioural characteristic of the 15 month-old anaemic children was that they were noticeably less happy than their non-anaemic counterparts. Improvements in mental performance in school children have been demonstrated with iron treatment (Pollitt *et al.*, 1985). The effect of degree of iron depletion and its long-term effects on brain function are currently under investigation.

At the other end of the spectrum there is the clinical condition of iron overload. Idiopathic haemochromatosis was the only variety recognised when Sheldon (1935) concluded that haemochromatosis was due to an inborn error of metabolism. Since then it has become apparent that iron overload may also arise from the intake of excess oral iron, a prime example being that of the South African blacks who used to consume home-brewed alcoholic beverages that contained large amounts of iron (Bothwell et al., 1964), or from repeated blood transfusions. During the past two decades it has become apparent that haemochromatosis in some racial groups is not as rare as previously thought (Olsson et al., 1983), which has implications for food iron fortification policies, since the disease will manifest itself earlier in life when dietary iron intakes are high.

Bioavailability

One of the first human iron bioavailability experiments originated from a study of rationing carried out during the first six months of war (Widdowson & McCance, 1942). At that time, for economic reasons, the extraction rate of flour was raised, and investigations into the nutritional effects of this showed that the iron from bread made with 92 % extraction (brown) flour was very poorly absorbed compared with iron from white flour. This was attributed, quite correctly, to the higher levels of phytate in brown than white flour. Since then many factors, both dietary and host-related, have been shown to affect iron bioavailability (Table 14.1).

Various techniques have been used to assess iron bioavailability, such as rat haemoglobin repletion (Fritz et al., 1974), in vitro solubility (Jacobs & Greenman, 1969), in vitro dialysability (Miller et al., 1981), and calculated 'available' iron using a predictive model (Monsen et al., 1978). However, undoubtedly the most appropriate and informative methods are based on the use of isotopes. Amongst the major advances that have been made in the study of iron bioavailability are the measurement of haemoglobin incorporation of iron using a dual isotope technique (Brise & Hallberg, 1962), and the use of extrinsic labelling techniques (Cook et al., 1972, Hallberg & Björn-Rasmussen, 1972). Added inorganic radio-iron tracers were found to label rapidly and uniformly the various non-haem but not haem iron compounds in a meal, by isotopic exchange. Thus the concept of two separate pools of iron in the gastrointestinal tract was introduced. Since the non-haem pool is fully exchangeable, it follows that the bioavailability of iron in any one food is dependent upon the composition of any dietary constituents consumed with it, as well as the physico-chemical form of the iron and the nature of the foodstuff itself. More recently, ethical approval for the administration of radio-isotopes is becoming very restricted due to the increasing awareness of the hazards of ionising radiation, and iron absorption in particularly vulnerable groups,

Table 14.1. *Factors affecting iron bioavailability*

+	−
Dietary	
Ascorbic acid	Phytate
Citric acid	Polyphenols
Animal protein	Calcium
Haem iron	Eggs
Alcohol	Other trace elements
Some amino acids	(Cu, Zn, Mn, Co)
Fructose	
Host-related	
Iron deficiency	Iron overload
Gastric acid	Achlorhydria
Previous low-iron diet	Previous high-iron diet
Anabolic condition	Malabsorption syndromes
(e.g. pregnancy)	

such as infants, children and pregnant women, can only be studied with the aid of stable isotopes, as pioneered by Dyer & Brill (1972) and further developed by other groups, such as Janghorbani, Ting & Young (1980) and Fairweather-Tait & Minski (1986).

One major problem with estimating iron bioavailability from different foods and diets is the wide inter-subject variation. Much of this is attributable to differences in iron status and hence efficiency of iron absorption, although there are significant, and as yet unexplained, day-to-day variations in iron absorption in the same individual. A method commonly employed to obtain comparable data from different foods/ meals is to give subjects a standard dose, generally 3 mg iron, in the form of ferrous ascorbate or sulphate, and to compare absorption of iron from the unknown with absorption from the reference dose.

Estimates of iron bioavailability are needed to assess the adequacy of dietary iron intakes and to set Recommended Dietary Allowances. The figure used has a dramatic effect on the calculated dietary iron requirement; FAO/WHO (1988) have published iron requirements for diets of low (5 %), intermediate (10 %) and high (15 %) bioavailability. Unfortunately, despite a great deal of experimental work measuring iron absorption from different meals, there are not enough data to ascribe accurate figures for iron bioavailability for different diets. An alternative approach to studying nutrient bioavailability is to relate body status to dietary intake. However, for iron it may take weeks or months to attain equilibrium when introducing a dietary change, and intake measurements must be carried out over a very long time period for results to be meaningful.

The complex question of iron bioavailability, particularly the relationship between diet and host-related variables, needs detailed consideration. Public health programmes to improve the iron status of vulnerable groups depend upon reliable information on factors affecting iron bioavailability and bioavailable nutrient density (Hallberg, 1981). As we move forward into the 21st century, one important objective is to instigate appropriate eating patterns, to promote good health and prevent disease. A better understanding of iron metabolism and bioavailability will undoubtedly help us achieve this goal.

References

Adams, P. C., Zhong, R., Haist, J., Flanagan, P. R. & Grant, D. R. (1991). Mucosal iron in the control of iron absorption in a rat intestinal transplant model. *Gastroenterology*, **100**, 370–4.

Addison, G. M., Beamish, M. R., Hales, C. N., Hodgkins, M., Jacobs, A. & Llewellin, P. (1972). An immunoradiometric assay for ferritin in the serum of normal subjects and patients with iron deficiency and iron overload. *Journal of Clinical Pathology*, **25**, 326–9.

Aisen, P. & Brown, E. B. (1977). The iron-binding function of transferrin in iron metabolism. *Seminars in Haematology*, **14**, 31–53.

Baker, E. N., Rumball, S. V. & Anderson, B. F. (1987). Transferrins: insights into structure and function from studies on lactoferrin. *Trends in Biochemical Science*, **12**, 350–3.

Balfour, W. M., Hahn, P. F., Bale, W. F., Pommerenke, W. T. & Whipple, G. H. (1942). Radioactive iron absorption in clinical conditions: normal, pregnancy, anemia, and hemochromatosis. *Journal of Experimental Medicine*, **76**, 15–30.

Bothwell, T. H., Sefte, H., Jacobs, P., Torrance, J. D. & Baumslag, N. (1964). Iron overload in Bantu subjects. Studies on the availability of iron in Bantu beer. *American Journal of Clinical Nutrition*, **14**, 47–51.

Brise, H. & Hallberg, L. (1962). A method for comparative studies on iron absorption in man using two radio-iron isotopes. *Acta Medica Scandinavica Supplement* **376, 59**, 7–21.

Cook, J. D. (1990). Adaptation in iron metabolism. *American Journal of Clinical Nutrition*, **51**, 301–8.

Cook, J. D., Layrisse, M., Martinez-Torres, C., Walker, R., Monsen, E. & Finch, C. A. (1972). Food iron absorption measured by an extrinsic tag. *Journal of Clinical Investigation*, **51**, 805–15.

Crosby, W. H. (1966). Mucosal block: an evaluation of concepts relating to the control of iron absorption. *Seminars in Haematology*, **3**, 299–313.

Dubach, R., Moore, C. V. & Callender, S. (1949). Iron excretion in human subjects as measured by the isotope technique. *Federation Proceedings*, **8**, 353.

Dyer, N. C. & Brill, A. B. (1972). Use of the stable tracers [58]Fe and [50]Cr for the study of iron utilization in pregnant women. In *Nuclear Activation Techniques in the Life Sciences*, pp. 469–477, International Atomic Energy Agency: Vienna.

Fairweather-Tait, S. J. & Minski, M. J. (1986). Studies on iron availability in man, using stable isotope techniques. *British Journal of Nutrition*, **55**, 279–85.

Fairweather-Tait, S. J. & Wright, A. J. A. (1984). The influence of previous iron intake on the estimation of bioavailability of Fe from a test meal given to rats. *British Journal of Nutrition*, **51**, 185–91.

FAO/WHO. (1988). Requirements of vitamin A, iron, folate and vitamin B12. *FAO Food and Nutrition Series No. 23*, Food and Agricultural Organisation of the United Nations: Rome.

Finch, C. A. & Loden, B. (1959). Body iron exchange in man. *Journal of Clinical Investigation*, **38**, 392–6.

Ford, G. C., Harrison, P. M., Rice, D. W., Smith, J. M. A., Treffry, A., White, J. L. & Yariv, J. (1984). Ferritin: design and formation of an iron-storage molecule. *Philosophical Transactions of the Royal Society, London B*, **304**, 551–65.

Fritz, J. C., Pla, G. W., Harrison, B. N. & Clark, G. A. (1974). Collaborative study of the rat haemoglobin repletion test for bioavailability of iron. *Journal of the Association of Official Analytical Chemists*, **57**, 513–17.

Granick, S. (1946). Ferritin. *Journal of Biological Chemistry*, **164**, 737–46.

Grasbeck, R., Majuri, R., Kouvonen, I. & Tenhunen, R. (1982). Spectral and other studies on the intestinal haem receptor of the pig. *Biochimica et Biophysica Acta*, **700**, 137–42.

Green, R., Charlton, R., Seftel, H., Bothwell, T., Mayet, F., Adams, B., Finch, C. and Layrisse, M. (1968). Body iron excretion in man. *American Journal of Medicine*, **45**, 336–53.

Hahn, P. F., Bale, W. F., Lawrence, E. O. & Whipple, G. H. (1938). Radioactive iron and its metabolism in anaemia. *Journal of the American Medical Association*, **111**, 2285–6.

Hahn, P. F., Bale, W. F., Ross, J. F., Balfour, W. M. & Whipple, G. H. (1943). Radioactive iron absorption by the gastrointestinal tract: influence of anemia, anoxia and antecedent feeding distribution. *Journal of Experimental Medicine*, **78**, 169–88.

Hallberg, L. (1981). Bioavailable nutrient density: a new concept applied in the interpretation of food iron absorption data. *American Journal of Clinical Nutrition*, **34**, 2242–7.

Hallberg, L. & Björn-Rasmussen, E. (1972). Determination of iron absorption from whole diet. A new two-pool model using two radioiron isotopes given as haem and non-haem iron. *Scandinavian Journal of Haematology*, **9**, 193–7.

Hallberg, L., Högdahl, A-M., Nilsson, L. & Rybo, G. (1966). Menstrual blood loss – a population study. *Acta Obstetricia et Gynecologia Scandinavica*, **45**, 320–51.

Holmberg, C. G. & Laurell, C. B. (1945). Studies on the capacity of serum to bind iron. A contribution to our knowledge of the regulation mechanism of serum iron. *Acta Physiologica Scandinavica*, **10**, 307–19.

Huebers, H. A. (1986). Iron absorption: molecular aspects and its regulation. *Acta Haematologica Japonica*, **49**, 1528–35.

Huebers, H., Csiba, E., Huebers, E. & Finch, C. A. (1983*b*). Competitive advantage of diferric transferrin in delivering iron to reticulocytes. *Proceedings of the National Academy of Sciences USA*, **80**, 300–4.

Huebers, H., Huebers, E., Csiba, E., Rummel, W. & Finch, C. A. (1983*a*). The significance of transferrin for intestinal iron absorption. *Blood*, **61**, 283–90.

Iacopetta, B. J. & Morgan, E. H. (1983). The kinetics of transferrin endocytosis and iron uptake from transferrin in rabbit reticulocytes. *Journal of Biological Chemistry*, **25B**, 9108–55.

Jacobs, A. & Greenman, D. A. (1969). Availability of food iron. *British Medical Journal*, **1**, 673–6.

Jacobs, A., Miller, F., Worwood, M., Beamish, M. R. & Wardrop, C. A. (1972). Ferritin in the serum of normal subjects and patients with iron deficiency and iron overload. *British Medical Journal*, **4**, 206–8.

Janghorbani, M., Ting, B. T. G. & Young, V. R. (1980). Accurate analysis of stable isotopes ^{68}Zn, ^{70}Zn, and ^{58}Fe in human feces with neutron activation analysis. *Clinica Chimica Acta*, **108**, 9–24.

Laufberger, M. V. (1937). Sur la cristallisation de la ferritine. *Bulletin de la Societé de Chimie Biologique*, **19**, 1575–82.

McCance, R. A. & Widdowson, E. M. (1937). Absorption and excretion of iron. *Lancet*, **ii**, 680–4.

McCance, R. A. & Widdowson, E. M. (1943). Iron excretion and metabolism in man. *Nature*, **152**, 326–7.

Martinez-Torres, C., Cubeddu, L., Dillmann, E., Brengelmann, G. L., Leets, I., Layrisse, M., Johnson, D. G. & Finch, C. (1984). Effect of exposure to low temperature on normal and iron-deficient subjects. *American Journal of Physiology*, **246**, R380–3.

Miller, D. D., Schricker, B. R., Rasmussen, R. R. & Van Campen, D. (1981). An *in vitro* method for estimation of iron availability from meals. *American Journal of Clinical Nutrition*, **34**, 2248–56.

Monsen, E. R., Hallberg, L., Layrisse, M., Hegsted, D. M., Cook, J. D., Mertz, W. & Finch, C. A. (1978). Estimation of available dietary iron. *American Journal of Clinical Nutrition*, **31**, 134–41.

Montreuil, J., Tonnelat, J. & Mullet, S. (1960). Préparation et propriétés de la lactosidérophiline (lactotransferrine) du lait de femme. *Biochimica et Biophysica Acta* **45**, 413–21.

Moore, C. V., Doan, C. A. & Arrowsmith, W. R. (1937). Studies on iron transportation and metabolism. II. The mechanism of iron transportation: its significance in iron utilization in anemic states of varied etiology. *Journal of Clinical Investigation*, **16**, 627–48.

Nathanson, M. H., Muir, A. & McLaren, G. D. (1985). Iron absorption in normal and iron-deficient beagle dogs: mucosal iron kinetics. *American Journal of Physiology*, **249**, G439–48.

Olsson, K. S., Ritter, B., Rosen, U., Heedman, P. A. & Staugard, F. (1983). Prevalence of iron overload in central Sweden. *Acta Medica Scandinavica*, **213**, 145–50.

Oski, F. A. & Honig, A. S. (1978). The effects of therapy on the developmental scores of iron deficient infants. *Journal of Pediatrics*, **92**, 21–5.

Pollit, E., Soemantri, A. G., Yunis, F. & Scrimshaw, N. S. (1985). Cognitive effects of iron deficiency anaemia. *Lancet*, **i**, 158.

Raffin, S. B., Woo, C. H., Roost, K. T., Price, D. C. & Schmid, R. (1974). Intestinal absorption of haemoglobin iron – heme cleavage by mucosal heme oxygenase. *Journal of Clinical Investigation*, **54**, 1344–52.

Reissmann, K. R. & Dietrich, M. R. (1956). On the presence of ferritin in the peripheral blood of patients with hepatocellular disease. *Journal of Clinical Investigation*, **35**, 588–95.

Schade, A. L. & Caroline, L. (1946). An iron-binding component in human blood plasma. *Science*, **104**, 340–1.

Sheldon, J. H. (1935). *Haemochromatosis*. London: Oxford University Press.
Srikantia, S. G., Prasad, J. S., Bhaskram, C. & Krishnamachari, K. A. V. R. (1976). Anaemia and the immune response. *Lancet*, i, 1307–9.
Skikne, B. S., Flowers, C. H. & Cook, J. D. (1990). Serum transferrin receptor: a quantitative measure of tissue iron deficiency. *Blood*, 75, 1870–6.
Viteri, F. E. & Torun, B. (1974). Anaemia and physical work capacity. *Clinics in Haematology*, 3, 609–26.
Voorhess, M. L., Stuart, M. J., Stockman, J. A. & Oski, F. A. (1975). Iron deficiency anaemia and increased urinary norepinephrine excretion. *Journal of Paediatrics*, 86, 542–7.
Walter, T., Kovalskys, J. & Steel, A. (1983). Effect of mild iron deficiency on infant mental development scores. *Journal of Paediatrics*, 102, 519–22.
Widdowson, E. M. & McCance, R. A. (1942). Iron exchanges of adults on white and brown bread diets. *Lancet*, i, 588–90.

15

Trace element investigations in man and animals

COLIN F. MILLS

The last 50 years have seen a remarkable growth in the range of trace elements regarded as nutritionally essential. This brief chapter can only consider some important milestones of this progress. Many other aspects are considered in the review volumes edited by Mertz (1987*a*). At the start of the half century, iron and iodine were very firmly established as essential elements with convincing demonstrations of their importance for health in animals and human subjects. Evidence obtained previously from studies with laboratory animals that demonstrated the essentiality of zinc and of copper was just beginning to be exploited in the detection and correction of deficiencies of these elements in commercial livestock production. The essentiality of cobalt for ruminants had just been revealed by a series of systematic investigations that led in the late 1940s to discovery of its role as a component of vitamin B_{12}. Manganese was known to be essential but its importance in the nutrition of commercial livestock had yet to be appreciated.

The elements selenium, chromium, molybdenum, nickel and silicon must now be added to the lists of known essential trace elements. Boron is emerging as a likely candidate for essentiality and recent reappraisals of data which led to claims of the essentiality of fluorine appear likely to support this case. Controversy continues to surround recent claims of the nutritional essentiality of lead, a concept that is supported by a limited range of studies with rats and pigs but at a time when environmental agencies are debating the suggestion that there is no intake of lead that is not toxic. The elements arsenic, tin and cadmium have each had their brief periods of fame conferred by putative essentiality but much more convincing evidence is needed before this trio of elements is accepted into the family of essential nutrients.

Spectacular improvements in analytical techniques in the past 50 years have made much of this progress possible. The development of atomic absorption and fluorimetric analytical procedures have increased, by almost two orders of magnitude, the daily output of trace element analyses that can be achieved by reasonably equipped laboratories. This potential has been exploited both in the development of procedures for effective control of adventitious contaminants of experimental diets and for monitoring the progress of such studies by frequent analyses of the trace element composition of animal tissues. The output and quality of studies of trace element bioavailability and metabolism is certain to increase following the wider application of stable isotope techniques made possible by recent developments in plasma emission mass spectrometric techniques.

Experimental studies of trace element essentiality

The intrinsic scientific importance of defining the full range of nutritionally essential trace elements justifies the application of extreme measures for the control of dietary and environmental contamination in the experimental work serving this objective. Improvements in the purification of consti-tuents and in the formulation of synthetic and semi-synthetic diets have drastically reduced the basal trace element levels that can be achieved. They have also reduced the opportunities of confusion that in the past have arisen from the inadvertent induction of multiple deficiencies in ex-perimental subjects. Typical of such developments during the last fifty years has been the progress in studies of copper deficiency. Initially these were based on the use of iron-fortified milk diets, sometimes treated with sulphide, but more recently employing fully supplemented synthetic diets based on purified casein or synthetic amino acids as nitrogen sources. Such changes have halved the time taken to produce copper deficiency in the young rat, have reduced the chances of concurrent development of other deficiencies such as those of manganese or of vitamin E and have eliminated the problems created by prolonged exposure to milk 'diets' high in their content of water and lactose. Such refinements in experimental techniques have been adopted enthusiastically, and, especially when searching for the 'newer' trace elements, have sometimes been applied to successive generations of experimental animal. While they serve these purposes admirably it must be emphasised that the adoption of extreme experimental procedures strongly influences the relevance of such studies to the less rigorous conditions normally encountered in the nutrition of man and animals.

The adoption of more efficient techniques for excluding trace element contaminants from experimental diets or environments has had some disadvantages. Investigators have sometimes tended to disregard the fact that our greatest need in the context of the detection and control of trace element-related problems in man and animals is to improve our ability to detect early pathological changes and metabolic responses to relatively mild degrees of deficiency. Although the clinical data derived from such studies are frequently less dramatic than those from investigations involving more severe challenges, and thus less likely to excite the continued interest of financial sponsors, the biochemical and pathological results of studies of the early phases of deficiency or excess have particular value in the circumstances in which pathological manifestations of deficiency or excess are so rarely accompanied by unequivocally diagnostic clinical signs.

For many trace elements, the greatest sensitivity to deficiency is exhibited during early post-natal growth, at puberty and during pregnancy. With absolutely no possibility that such interrelationships can be defined by direct experimentation with human subjects, progress in such a topic will depend on careful interpretation of the data derived from work with appropriate animal models. The effectiveness of such model studies will be governed by the physiological timing and severity of the deficiency induced, by the duration of exposure to the deficient diet and by due consideration of any metabolic differences which may vitiate extrapolation of data between species. Examples abound in which failure to consider such aspects has led to confusion. Thus detection of copper deficiency in the human infant (for review, see Danks, 1988) was delayed 20 years by failure to appreciate that the development of anaemia in the severely copper depleted rat model was a late, but certainly not definitive, feature of the copper deficiency syndromes in other species, especially where they were not depleted as severely. Similar considerations influence the interpretation of model studies of the influence of zinc deficiency on reproductive performance. In addition to possible species differences in response, the severity and timing of depletion determines whether the response to zinc depletion is total failure of conception, a high incidence of fetal malformations, delayed parturition with a high perinatal death or merely a reduced birth weight (Hurley, 1981; Keen & Hurley, 1989). The severity of depletion of the rat needed to inhibit conception or give rise to a marked increase in the incidence of teratogenic defects is extreme and, as reasonably suggested by studies with laboratory primates, is unlikely to be an outcome of zinc deficiency in human subjects. Evidence that the pathological outcome of selenium deficiency in terms of its effects either upon growth, when it is the sole limiting nutrient, or upon oxidative damage promoting liver necrosis or dystrophy of muscle tissue when vitamin E supply is concurrently restricted, provides additional illustration of the importance of precisely defining the conditions under which trace element investigations are conducted with animal models. Equally, it points to the importance of covering both aspects of responses to low tissue selenium when endeavouring to define the effects of selenium deficiency in man.

Developments in studies of trace element bioavailability

Coincidentally, 50 years have elapsed since it was first suspected that dietary constituents acting as antagonists or synergists of trace element utilisation could have a profound influence upon susceptibility to trace element related-disorders (for review, see Mills, 1985). The first antagonistic interaction to be discovered, the antagonistic influence of molybdenum upon copper utilisation by ruminants, undoubtedly has the greatest worldwide significance for animal health and productivity and has proved particularly difficult to understand. The almost complete species specificity of this interaction reflects interactions between dietary sources of soluble molybdenum with sulphide generated microbiologically within the rumen. The thiomolybdates thus formed interact with copper either within the digestive tract to restrict its absorption or are themselves absorbed to render unavailable the copper already present in many tissues. Studies of this sulphur/molybdenum interaction with a variety of animal models have revealed the outstanding potency of the thiomolybdates as copper antagonists. However, inadequate understanding of the factors governing intraruminal levels of the free sulphide involved in their biosynthesis has so far precluded satisfactory quantitative prediction of the effects of dietary intakes of molybdenum and sulphur sources on the requirements of ruminants. High intakes of iron have a similar inhibitory effect on copper utilisation by ruminants but, in this instance, by mechanisms as yet unresolved. Although quantitative understanding of these relationships restricting copper utilisation is incomplete, recognition of dietary or environmental circumstances likely to promote excessive exposure to molybdenum or to iron is usually considered sufficient to justify prophylactic or therapeutic administration of copper to ruminants.

The antagonistic potency of the thiomolybdates has been exploited by their use as very effective therapeutic agents for control of the dramatic consequences of copper poisoning in ruminants. Also used prophylactically for control of excessive copper accumulation in cases of the genetically related Wilson's disease in man, they provide effective alternatives to the longer established practices of chelate therapy or the use of high doses of zinc as a competitive inhibitor of copper absorption and metabolism in this otherwise fatal disorder.

Appreciation of the significance of some organic dietary constituents as trace element antagonists has grown significantly since discovery of the inhibitory effect of goitrogens on iodine utilisation in 1928. Principal developments during the period under review have centred around the limiting effects of dietary phytates on the bioavailability of zinc and iron and more recently of lead. Surprisingly in view of their likely significance, little has been done to *quantify* relationships between the dietary content of these inhibitors and their effects on essential element requirements. *Ad hoc* experimentation provided the data upon which were defined the increments of zinc needed to protect pigs and poultry against the development of zinc deficiency when corn/soya rations were fed. These studies also provided the first indication that phytate-based interactions were potentiated by increases in dietary calcium. From data on dietary calcium and phytate (in its hexa- and penta-phosphoinositol forms) it has proved feasible to predict whether dietary zinc is adequate to meet the requirements of rats.

Such relationships have not yet been investigated adequately in human subjects so that it is still uncertain as to the significance of dietary phytate in the zinc nutrition of man. Interest in the topic is high because of the increase in phytate intake when high fibre diets are consumed. It is heightened by evidence from studies with rats indicating that the phytate content of soya protein-based 'meat expanders', when used as the sole protein source, can increase requirements for zinc more than fivefold. Little doubt surrounds evidence that high phytate foods are involved in the aetiology of some instances of zinc deficiency in the Middle East and that the phytate of soya-based milk formulas reduces the efficiency of zinc absorption by infants. However, in the absence of direct experimentation, it remains arguable whether the calcium content of most human diets has sufficient potentiating influence on the inhibitory effect of phytate to increase, significantly, the risks of zinc deficiency. Whether this applies to phytate-rich vegan diets fortified with calcium is less questionable.

Studies during the last 10 years indicate that the adverse effects of phytate are likely to be reduced by food processing techniques that partially degrade the active hexa- and penta-phospho forms of this inositol derivative to its less phosphorylated analogues; it has also been shown that its effects as a zinc and calcium binder decline if dietary protein or amino acids competitively remove zinc from its insoluble products (for review, see Sandström and Lönnerdal, 1989). Its effect as an inhibitor of iron absorption is reduced by dietary ascorbate.

The mutually antagonistic effects of iron, copper and zinc have been demonstrated in a variety of animal species and in human subjects. They are strongly evident when these mutually competitive elements are administered in aqueous solution. Their relevance to solid diets is mostly confined to situations in which extensive environmental pollution has occurred. The tolerance of excessive environmental exposure to cadmium and to lead may well be directly proportional to the iron status of exposed subjects.

With the exception of the above examples and metabolic interactions involving the essential and toxic trace metals and the protein metallo-thionein (Bremner & Beattie, 1990), the multitude of other interactions that can be demonstrated should perhaps be regarded as interesting biological phenomena, but nevertheless of questionable relevance to normal conditions of nutrition or environmental exposure.

The assessment of trace element requirements and tolerance

Provocatively perhaps, it is suggested that virtually all estimates of trace element requirement that have been found to stand the test of time have been based on pragmatic consideration of the doses of trace element observed to protect against the development of clinical or covert metabolic evidence of deficiency. Almost without exception, estimates based on data derived from balance trials or derived by 'factorial' techniques are being revised downwards, sometimes by more than 50%. Usually this is not promoted by the appearance of new balance or factorial data but by evidence that very significant numbers of healthy, ostensibly normal populations have intakes well below the recommended minima. However, the superiority of the dose/response trial over input/output balance trials or factorial methods of estimating requirements is confined to situations in which the physiological response has been monitored under specific dietary conditions. Extrapolation to other circumstances may be invalid if changes occur in dietary composition or in those physiological parameters controlling bioavailability.

The relatively slow progress in defining trace element requirements is attributable, first, to the difficulty in developing reliable techniques for monitoring the early covert pathological effects of deficiency and secondly, to the frequent failure to define adaptive increases in absorptive efficiency or decreased endogenous loss as trace element status declines. Unless adaptive responses to changes in status can be monitored, the data from most 'balance' or bioavailability trials may be of value for comparative studies (e.g. between foods as trace element sources) but are virtually uninterpretable for the purpose of quantifying requirements (for review see Mertz, 1987*b*).

The latter criticism can be levelled at most earlier studies of the utilisation of zinc, copper, molybdenum and chromium, with the consequence that human requirements for these elements are poorly defined. The more reliable estimates of the requirements of farm animals have been derived either from studies of pathological responses to changes in intake or from epidemiological data.

Fortunately it is now becoming feasible to use stable isotope kinetic techniques to calibrate both the initial element status of experimental subjects and their adaptive responses to changes in element intake (Jackson, 1989; King, 1986). Their use in metabolic balance of bioavailability studies may well yield data that can be used with greater confidence for the estimation of trace element requirements.

Demands for closer definition of 'basal' requirements – the supply needed solely to maintain essential biological functions – are also increasing. Their improved definition requires closer agreement on the question 'requirement for what?', and the development of relatively non-invasive procedures for detecting functional defects in the target tissues of interest. Aspects of these problems are considered in the next section.

Significance of trace element deficiencies

Copper deficiency

Few instances of copper deficiency occur in non-ruminant farm animals. Requirements are well defined; instances of deficiency arising from low dietary copper availability are confined to occasions when accidental oversupplementation with zinc competitively inhibits copper absorption. In contrast, copper deficiency in ruminants is much more frequent, reflecting their much less efficient utilisation of dietary copper and the frequency with which metabolic events in the rumen involving molybdenum, sulphur, iron and other, poorly identified, antagonists further restrict copper bioavailability. For unknown reasons, deficiency is rare in animals receiving high concentrate diets or dried forages. The ataxia of neonatal deficiency in lambs and goats is characteristic, but absence of this feature does not imply that copper status is normal; deficiency restricts growth rate and induces structural defects of wool at later stages of development. Skeletal and cardiovascular and connective tissue lesions in bovine copper deficiency reflect its involvement in collagen and elastin crosslinking. Reasons for the extreme sensitivity of Type IV basement membrane collagen synthesis of pancreas, kidney and muscle tissue, including that of the heart, to copper deficiency are unknown as is the pathological significance of this very early lesion (Farquharson & Robins, 1991; Fell, 1987). Neutrophil microbicidal activity also declines at early stages of deficiency (Babu & Failla, 1990).

The metabolic defect responsible for growth failure in young animals and human infants due to copper deficiency is unknown as is the pathological importance of defects in catecholamine metabolism and neuropeptide synthesis (for review see Prohaska, 1990). The latter, and decreases in the activities of the enzymes superoxide dismutase and caeruloplasmin involved in tissue protection against reactive oxygen free radical-induced peroxidation, appear to be the most characteristic and consistent features preceding tissue damage early in copper deficiency. On the basis of this conclusion it appears likely that the pathological expression of a low copper status may be partly contingent upon the extent to which other variables promote free radical generation. Although not all results of studies with human subjects consistently agree, it appears probable from dietary surveys in UK and US that mean intakes of copper are declining to the point that significant proportions of these populations are at risk of developing the above functional defects.

Evidence of such responses, reversible by copper supplementation, is much more convincing in situations where a low copper status has developed in infants as a consequence of generalised malnutrition (Macdonald & Warren, 1961; Danks, 1988). Sometimes this arises from the inadvertent selection of low-copper foods during rehabilitation or when ignorance of their nutritional limitations has led to excessively prolonged infant feeding with low copper dairy products and refined cereals.

The significance of copper deficiency in ruminant animals is beyond doubt; its importance in human nutrition is being investigated with increasing interest in the light of recent downward trends in dietary copper intakes and increased awareness of the covert consequences of deficiency.

Zinc deficiency

Although not exclusively and specifically indicative of zinc deficiency, the skin lesions of parakeratosis and hyperkeratosis that develop if deficiency is severe appear in most species, including man. Nevertheless studies conducted during the last 10 years indicate, increasingly, the wide range of defects of function, growth and development that arise if dietary zinc, while suboptimal, is not sufficiently low to induce overt clinical symptoms (for review see Prasad, 1991).

Sensitivity to deficiency is highest in all species at stages when the potential for growth and development is high. At such stages the response to deficiency is virtually immediate unless other nutrient deficiencies limit growth. If so, clinical signs of zinc deficiency may only appear when correction of the primary nutrient deficit permits a brief resumption of tissue growth with, in consequence, an increase in zinc demands.

Adequate understanding of the types of diet likely to limit zinc utilisation, provoke deficiency, and thus require fortification, has led to the virtual disappearance of zinc-related deficiency disorders in the livestock industry. Disregard of such relationships when formulating phytate-rich, calcium fortified diets has recently provoked clinical signs of zinc deficiency in dogs. Zinc deficiency has been identified in grazing ruminants when arid conditions restrict forage growth and thus limit dietary zinc supply.

Apart from clinical manifestations of zinc deficiency that have developed as a consequence of surprisingly frequent errors in the formulation of parenteral infusates, most manifestations of human zinc deficiency have arisen in rural communities subsisting on monotonous, phytate-rich cereal diets. It has been identified in infants from socially disadvantaged urban communities arbitrarily selecting diets low in their content of available zinc. Manifestations of deficiency include defective immunocompetence and retarded growth and development, particularly in males. Recent data suggest that a suboptimal zinc status during pregnancy results in delayed and prolonged parturition with a higher perinatal mortality. Other studies, initially questioned but now more widely accepted, suggest that the rate of healing of superficial skin wounds is significantly retarded by a low zinc status, particularly of old people.

Despite discoveries of an extensive range of zinc-containing enzymes, it has proved difficult to relate changes in their activity during depletion to the pathological changes that ensue (Chester & Arthur, 1988). This failure to detect a specifically selective index of an optimal zinc status has proved to be particularly unfortunate since interpretation of plasma zinc data is hindered by the fact that tissue catabolism during general malnutrition or brief deprivation of food, can markedly increase plasma zinc concentration. Conversely, many infections or rehabilitation from a previous deficiency are accompanied, typically, by a fall in plasma zinc. Until the search for more suitable indices of zinc status proves successful the most effective means of detecting a suboptimal status remains the monitoring of responses to supplementation (Golden & Golden, 1985).

Other trace elements

The significance of recent achievements in studies of the essentiality of the trace elements iron, fluorine, iodine and selenium is considered in accompanying contributions to this volume; see pp. 151, 174.

Studies of chromium and manganese deficiencies, temporarily hindered by severe analytical difficulties, have, despite this, confirmed the essentiality of both during the last 30 years. Manganese deficiency, a problem principally in the intensive nutrition of pigs and poultry, is manifested by impaired skeletal maturation, inhibition of chondroitin sulphate synthesis and by infertility. In contrast, interest in chromium centres around its suspected role in the potentiation of insulin activity and thus in the decrease of glucose tolerance in human subjects observed after depletion of tissue chromium reserves. Human requirements for both elements have yet to be defined quantitatively.

Indications of the essentiality of nickel for ruminants and of silicon and, it is claimed, of boron, lead and arsenic, merit additional verification and definition of their likely roles before it can be claimed with confidence that human or animal health is likely to be prejudiced by deficiencies of these elements.

Future prospects

Much has been achieved in studies of the trace elements during the last 50 years. However, those facing problems of achieving a satisfactory diagnosis of trace element-related problems or having to improve estimates of requirement are left in no doubt that the greatest priority for future work should be the systematic description of early preclinical indices of metabolic dysfunctions attributable to deficiency. Many such defects have been described. Although their precise functional relevance may not yet be clear, the frequency with which covert pathological lesions are detected during many such experimental deficiency studies convincingly indicates the need for investigation of their influence upon health. Such studies will eventually yield more appropriate indices of trace element status than, for example, the trace element content of plasma or liver tissue, neither of which is usually indicative of the functional adequacy of supply (Mills, 1981). Furthermore, they will bring to human clinical studies a much needed re-emphasis of the fact that, although frequently lacking in specificity, the covert lesions of trace element deficiency can rarely be ignored – an attitude long accepted and acted upon by veterinarians and animal nutritionists because of the economic importance of maintaining animal health and productivity even in the absence of gross clinical symptoms. Such pathologically relevant indicators of imminent deficiency are needed urgently to provide more satisfactory bases for the estimation of trace element requirements.

Previously, human requirements for zinc, copper and some other trace elements may well have been overestimated. Estimates for zinc and copper have been 'pruned' rigorously in the UK (Committee on Medical Aspects of Food Policy, 1991) and elsewhere (National Research Council, 1989). Meanwhile, comparisons between non-ruminant species of trace element intakes per unit body weight or dietary energy suggest from UK survey data (Gregory et al., 1990) that the copper and zinc intakes of at least 1% of the UK population are low and likely to be prejudicial to health. Further investigation is warrantable.

In the fields of trace elements and animal production, the priorities are now largely educational and advisory, coupled with more effective exploitation of evidence illustrating how factors modifying trace element flux through soils and cropping systems can modify the risks of deficiency.

Both sets of priorities are best served by the interdisciplinary meetings that have been encouraged by this Society.

References

Babu, V. & Failla, M. L. (1990). Copper status and function of neutrophils are reversibly depressed in marginally and severely copper deficient rats. *Journal of Nutrition*, **120**, 1700–9.

Bremner, I. & Beattie, J. H. (1990). Metallothionein and the trace metals. *Annual Reviews of Nutrition*, **10**, 63–83.

Chesters, J. K. & Arthur, J. R. (1988). Early biochemical defects caused by dietary trace element deficiencies. *Nutrition Research Reviews*, **1**, 39–56.

Committee on Medical Aspects of Food Policy (1991). *Dietary Reference Values for Food Energy and Nutrients for the United Kingdom*. Report on Health and Social Subjects, **41**, London: HMSO.

Danks, D. M. (1988). Copper deficiency in humans. *Annual Reviews of Nutrition*, **8**, 235–57.

Farquharson, C. & Robins, S. P. (1991). Immunolocalisation of collagen types

I, III and IV, elastin and fibronectin within the hearts of normal and copper deficient rats. *Journal of Comparative Pathology*, **104**, 245–55.

Fell, B. F. (1987). The pathology of copper deficiency in animals. In *Copper in Animals and Man*, Howell, J. M. & Gawthorne, J. M., eds, vol. 2, pp. 1–28, Boca Raton: CRC Press.

Golden, M. H. N. & Golden, B. (1985). Problems with the recognition of human zinc-responsive conditions. In *Trace Elements in Man and Animals* (*TEMA*) 5. Momcilovic, B., ed., pp. 933–938, University of Zagreb, Zagreb: Institute of Medical Research and Occupational Health.

Gregory, J., Foster, K., Tyler, H. & Wiseman, M. (1990). *The Dietary and Nutritional Survey of British Adults*. London: HMSO.

Hurley, L. S. (1981). Teratogenic aspects of manganese, zinc and copper nutrition. *Physiology Reviews*, **61**, 249–95.

Jackson, M. J. (1989). Physiology of zinc: general aspects. In *Zinc in Human Biology*, Mills, C. F., ed., pp. 1–14, London: Springer.

Keen, C. L. & Hurley, L. S. (1989). Zinc and reproduction: effects of deficiency on foetal and postnatal development. In *Zinc in Human Biology*, Mills, C. F., ed., pp. 183–220, London: Springer.

King, J. C. (1986). Assessment of techniques for determining human zinc requirement. *Journal of the American Dietetic Association*, **86**, 1523–8.

Macdonald, I. & Warren, P. J. (1961). The copper content of the liver and hair of African children with kwashiorkor. *British Journal of Nutrition*, **15**, 593–6.

Mertz, W. (1987*a*). *Trace Elements in Human and Animal Nutrition*. 5th edn, Mertz, W., ed., vols 1 and 2. Academic Press: New York.

Mertz, W. (1987*b*). Use and misuse of balance studies. *Journal of Nutrition*, **117**, 1811–13.

Mills, C. F. (1981). Some outstanding problems in the detection of trace element deficiency diseases. *Philosophical Transactions of the Royal Society*, **B294**, 199–213.

Mills, C. F. (1985). Dietary interactions involving the trace elements. *Annual Reviews in Nutrition*, **5**, 173–93.

National Research Council (1989). *Recommended Dietary Allowances*. 10th ed. Washington: National Academy Press.

Prasad, A. S. (1991). Discovery of human zinc deficiency and studies in an experimental animal model. *American Journal of Clinical Nutrition*, **53**, 403–412.

Prohaska, J. R. (1990). Biochemical changes in copper deficiency. *Journal of Nutritional Biochemistry*, **1**, 452–61.

Sandström, B. & Lönnerdal, B. (1989). Promoters and antagonists of zinc absorption. In *Zinc in Human Biology*, Mills, C. F., ed., pp. 57–78, London: Springer-Verlag.

16

Recent investigations on trace elements, particularly selenium

MARION F. ROBINSON

Nothing could have been further from the minds of my forbears when they set out almost 150 years ago from UK for New Zealand than the exciting trace element environment which their progeny were to inherit. They came to the South Island of NZ and maybe some of them developed simple goitres as some of us did as adolescents. Goitre or tenga was known to occur amongst the Maoris too. Early this century other trace elements harassed some of my farming ancestors, such as the cobalt responsive Moreton Mains Disease, named from the small township south of Dunedin. Introduction of liberal liming and fertilisation of the land brought forth a host of agricultural problems.

During the past 50 years the international trace element field has become exceedingly complex with the interplay of many dietary, host and environmental factors. For the cationic trace elements (iron, zinc, copper, manganese) dietary and host factors influence greatly their absorption, bioavailability and status, whereas the geochemical environment is of minor importance. Their nutritional problems in NZ are essentially similar to those in other western countries.

New Zealand, with its unusually low iodine, fluorine and selenium environment, has provided a natural laboratory for studying these anionic trace elements. They are readily absorbed, with little homeostatic regulation, perhaps only at excretion, and the body's status as regards them reflects the geochemical environment.

Hence there are risks of deficiency and overexposure, and the margins between too much and too little may be quite narrow. This chapter is restricted to iodine, fluorine and selenium, and their relevance to human nutrition, concentrating on the NZ scene.

Fluorine

Fluorine provided my first personal contact with the Nutrition Society, through the Journal. Soon after arriving in UK as a research student in 1948 to work with Professor R. A. McCance I submitted two papers on fluorine to the British Journal of Nutrition. My NZ supervisor Muriel Bell had suspected that NZ's alarmingly high prevalence of dental caries might be caused by too little fluorine. Our fluorine results were so extraordinarily low for teeth, for urinary excretion and for fluorine status that the editor suspected poor analytical techniques and kindly suggested that I spend a Saturday morning with Professor Margaret Murray at Bedford College to discuss my methodology and findings. I am deeply indebted to her for that rich experience (Harrison, 1949).

All our natural water supplies were low, mainly less than 0.3 ppm fluoride. Fluoridation began in 1954 and was accompanied by a remarkable decline in caries prevalence. Half of NZ 5 year olds have caries-free teeth compared to 14% in 1950. For 12–13 year olds, 28% are caries free compared to 2% in 1973, and DMF (decayed, missing, filled teeth) has decreased from 10.8 to 2.5. Today, over half of NZ's population receives fluoridated water; several communities have recently discontinued it, whereas others have reinstated it. The fluoridation controversy fails to languish in NZ.

The very marked difference in caries prevalence between fluoridated and non-fluoridated areas has narrowed since the widespread introduction of fluoride toothpaste, and children in non-fluoridated areas have their teeth routinely painted with fluoride solutions. Some New Zealanders have claimed that much of the decline in dental decay in non-fluoridated areas is independent of fluorine. Nevertheless, evidence strongly endorses the major role fluorine plays in preventing dental decay throughout life. Thus the real issue has become, not whether fluorine should be part of a preventative programme, but in what form it is to be used. Fluoridation has the great advantage of being both cost effective and available to all members of the community, particularly to those with poor dental health, who otherwise might not seek the benefits of fluorine.

Ingestion of too much fluorine while teeth are developing may result in mottling of the tooth enamel (dental fluorosis). Children living in both non-fluoridated and fluoridated areas can have these white patchy markings on their teeth and some are likely to be related to fluorine. Most toothpastes contain fluorine and children are at risk from overexposure if they regularly swallow large amounts of toothpaste.

It is widely agreed that fluoridation to a level of 1.0 ppm fluoride is not associated with any known adverse health effects: no association with cancer mortality has been found in NZ or other countries at these levels. Large fluorine doses are sometimes used in the treatment of osteoporosis, but the bone quality tends to be poor and fractures may increase.

After re-examining the data, the NZ Nutrition Taskforce (1991) recommended that fluoride concentration of water supplies be kept within the range of 0.7 to 1.0 ppm fluoride.

Iodine

Goitre, which had been endemic in many areas, rapidly disappeared with the successful implementation of iodine supplementation in 1939 with iodised salt (40 ppm iodine; 1:25000 parts of salt). Only domestic salt was iodised contributing about 1.6 μmol/d (200 μg/d) based on a daily use of 4–6 g/d salt in the home, whereas non-iodised salt was used for commercially processed foods such as bread, butter, cheese and canned foods, and more recently in takeaways and for other pre-prepared foods.

However, an additional and unpredictable iodine supplement appeared in 1962 from contamination of dairy products with iodophors used as equipment sanitisers. This raised the iodine intake of regular milk and dairy produce users, sometimes to undesirable levels, close to 8 μmol/d compared to the recommended dietary intake (RDI) of 1.2 μmol/d (150 μg/d), and approaching the potentially harmful level of 16 μmol/d if kelp tablets or other iodine-containing medication were taken regularly. About 15 years ago, a non-iodine containing sanitiser (quaternary ammonium compound) was introduced; but iodophors are still used by some.

Two recent surveys of urinary iodide (indicator of iodine intake) have suggested that people are not receiving too much or too little iodine. For healthy Auckland women, the mean daily iodide excretion was 2.4 μmol/d (95% range: 0.9–5.8 μmol), equivalent to twice RDI, with no subject less than 0.4 μmol/d (potentially a deficient intake) or greater than 8 μmol/d. Further, the incidence of thyrotoxicosis in Auckland remained stable between 1966 and 1981 (Cooper, Croxson & Ibbertson, 1984).

New Zealanders are encouraged to restrict their salt intakes, thereby also reducing this form of iodine supplement. In a 1-year salt restriction study, subjects living in a previously goitrous Otago area (with iodide excretions 0.2–0.5 μmol/d before iodised salt was introduced) had reduced their salt intake by using almost no salt in the home (Simpson *et al.*, 1984). Their 24 h sodium excretions were almost all below 100 mmol/d, sodium coming mainly from non-iodised salt in bread, butter and other processed foods. Their iodide excretions, though reduced to 1.3 μmol/d and 1.1 μmol/d for the men and women, compared to 1.8 and 1.7 μmol/d respectively for the controls, were close to RDI for adults. Much iodine was apparently coming from dairy products; the local milk contained about 1.3 μmol/l, equivalent to 0.8 μmol per pint. Thus the adequacy of their iodine intakes did not depend upon the consumption of iodised salt.

However, the iodine intake and status could be inadequate for people whose consumption of dairy products or fish is negligible, particularly if they use very little salt or only non-iodised salt. Few people recall why salt is iodised. Clearly, the NZ situation needs continual surveillance because nothing has happened to alter the extraordinarily low iodine environment.

New Zealand's problems with iodine appear minor compared with those of third world countries like Zaire, India, Indonesia, China and Papua New Guinea, with millions of people affected by iodine deficiency disorders (IDD): goitre, cretinism, impaired brain function and hypothyroidism in children and adults. The severe deficiency is often aggravated by goitrogens in staple foods such as cassava, and by other antithyroid agents. Largely through the initiative of Hetzel, iodine deficiency is recognised as a major international public health problem, and United Nations Agencies have adopted a 10-year global programme for prevention and control of IDD (Hetzel & Dunn, 1989).

Selenium

Selenium was described by Krehl as 'perverse, contradictory and yet all the while vastly intriguing'. It was recognised 60 years ago that selenium was the toxic agent in cereals causing alkali disease in livestock. Basic studies on the role of selenium in nutrition developed quickly.

After 1957, when Schwarz established selenium as an essential trace element, preventing dietary liver necrosis in vitamin E deficient rats, selenium responsive diseases were identified quickly in sheep, cattle, horses, swine and poultry in low soil selenium areas. Extensive selenium supplementation rapidly began in NZ and some farmers convinced themselves that self-dosing relieved their own muscular aches and pains. This prompted Christine Thomson and myself in the late 1960s to begin studies of the fate of such mega doses of selenium (Thomson & Robinson, 1980). In 1979, selenium became an essential trace element for humans with the discovery in China of selenium-responsive cardiomyopathy, Keshan disease (Yang *et al.*, 1984), and selenium deficiency in a NZ patient from Otago on total parenteral nutrition.

The questions we are now trying to answer are whether New Zealanders are at a disadvantage healthwise from their low selenium status, and whether selenium supplementation should be considered as for iodine and fluorine (Robinson, 1988)? This becomes more remote with the many current developments:

(a) fascinating revelations of more seleno-functions and of how selenium is handled within the body, with the potential for more sensitive measures of selenium status and bioavailability of the different forms of dietary selenium;

(b) recommended dietary selenium intakes from other countries approaching New Zealand's average intake;

(c) trends in epidemiological studies towards weaker associations, if any, between selenium status and western-type diseases.

Functions of selenium

Identification in 1973 of glutathione peroxidase (GSHPx) as a seleno-enzyme provided a basis for the antioxidant effect of selenium and its relationship with vitamin E; with glutathione it removed hydrogen peroxide and other free hydroperoxides, thereby preventing the initiation of peroxidation of membranes and oxidative damage. Recent re-examination of GSHPx has identified two enzymatically, structurally, and antigenically different forms in cells (including erythrocytes) and in plasma, and these two forms may have different functions (Avissar *et al.*, 1989).

Although a major part of body selenium is in the form of GSHPx, and its enzyme activity falls when dietary selenium is restricted, Burk (1990) considers there is no evidence that it is an oxidant defence; glutathione peroxidase may serve as a storage form of selenium, to be released for use in other selenoproteins when selenium is in short supply. The year before, Burk (1989) had pointed out that some functions of selenium such as its strong protection against diquat injury may be exerted through an oxidant defence role of selenium other than through GSHPx.

Another selenoprotein, phospholipid hydroperoxide glutathione per-oxidase from rat liver cytosol, is quite different from the classic GSHPx because it can metabolise fatty acid hydroperoxides esterified in cell membranes. It can inhibit microsomal lipid peroxidation and may provide some of the antioxidant roles of selenium (Ursini, Maiorino & Gregolin, 1985; Sunde, 1990).

A rat plasma selenoprotein P with no GSHPx activity has been purified and characterised. It is a glycoprotein containing selenocysteine; its concentration falls to less than 10 % of control in selenium deficient rats. It may have an antioxidant role or be a transport protein (Burk, 1989).

The deiodinases are the most recent selenoenzymes identified, also with selenocysteine at the active site: Type I deiodinase (liver and kidney) and probably also Type II deiodinase (brain, brown adipose tissue). Arthur, Nicol & Beckett (1990) showed that these enzymes are necessary to convert the prohormone thyroxine (T4) to 3':35 triiodothyronine (T3). Selenium deficiency in the rat has a similar inhibitory effect on both deiodinases, resulting in decreased plasma T3 and increased plasma T4. These workers made the interesting observation that both thyroid hormone deiodinase and GSHPx activities were decreased at a similar stage of selenium deficiency. Full implications are being sought.

Protein chemists are fascinated that the mRNA for Type 1 deiodinase contains a UGA codon for selenocysteine, as also for GSHPx; in other contexts this codon serves to terminate protein synthesis (Berry, Banu & Larsen, 1991).

This iodine/selenium relationship must be relevant to iodine deficiency diseases. Combined selenium and iodine deficiencies have been associated in Zaire with elevated frequency of endemic myxoedematous cretinism (Vanderpas *et al.*, 1990). Selenium supplementation raised serum selenium and erythrocyte GSHPx activity of school children and cretins, but its effect upon thyroid hormone function is not known, or whether any changes were irreversible.

The coincidence of the low selenium and iodine areas of the South Island of NZ has always intrigued us. Was the incidence of goitre in NZ aggravated by the low selenium status? This needs investigating especially with any downward trend in iodine status, particularly in infants, adolescents, and women during pregnancy.

Little is known about the functions of the many other selenoproteins (Behne *et al.*, 1988). In addition, selenium has an extraordinarily long list of interacting nutrients and other factors, and may protect against the toxic effects of mercury and cadmium.

Metabolism of selenium

New Zealand's environment was exploited to provide base line information about how selenium in its various forms is handled. All studies confirmed the low selenium status of NZ subjects, beginning with metabolic studies of young NZ women consuming their usual self-selected diets with mean selenium intake of 24 μg/d (Thomson & Robinson, 1980). Zero balances indicated these were habitual intakes, equal to one-third intakes of US women, but they were still double the intake for Chinese men from low selenium Keshan areas. However, the NZ intake approached these low levels when selenium rich foods were excluded, such as fish, liver and kidney and also eggs and poultry reflecting selenium supplementation of NZ poultry feeds. The Chinese were consuming almost entirely locally grown cereals and plant foods, very different from the Western style diets of US and NZ subjects, and were metabolising quite a different mixture of chemical forms of selenium.

Selenoamino acids are the main dietary forms of selenium, seleno-methionine from plants accounting for 50% or more in cereals, and selenocysteine the major component of animal foods. Selenate occurs in some green vegetables and like selenite is often used for selenium supplements. It is doubtful whether selenite is a natural food component or a human metabolite and yet it is commonly used as reference standard in measuring bioavailability of food selenium. Although the Chinese selenium intake was predominantly from cereals and plant foods, 92% compared with 18% from NZ intake, their actual intakes of selenomethionine were probably similar, whereas the NZ diet would have contained much more selenocysteine from animal foods and also more methionine, sparing the selenomethionine.

Over 15 years, the responses to selenium provided in the prime forms, selenite, selenate, selenomethionine, food selenium (bread, fish) were followed and the findings were summarised recently (Robinson, 1988). Early studies with tracers had shown considerable differences between rats and humans in metabolism of selenium, so that studies of human selenium metabolism were made on human subjects, mainly young women volun-teers in the NZ studies.

Briefly, selenium was readily absorbed, about 80% from food selenium, with selenomethionine and selenate better than selenite. Absorption was unaffected by selenium status and, as with fluorine and iodine, there appeared to be no homeostatic regulation of absorption or faecal output. Food selenium and selenomethionine were more effective in raising blood selenium than selenite and selenate. Urinary output was much greater from selenate than from selenomethionine.

Metabolism of selenium within the body was outlined recently by Levander and Burk (1990) (Fig. 16.1). Most selenium in tissues is associated with protein, and the tissue selenium levels are influenced by the dietary selenium intake. Selenomethionine, derived only from the diet, is in-corporated in place of methionine in proteins and is not regulated by selenium status of the animal. This selenium containing protein has no physiological function and is not available for synthesis of the functional forms of selenium until the protein is catabolised; whereas selenocysteine, selenite and selenate are directly available.

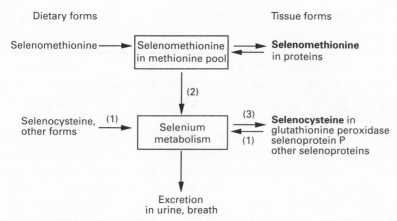

Fig. 16.1. Outline of selenium metabolism. (1) indicates selenocysteine-*β*-lysase which catabolises selenocysteine, and (2) indicates processes that catabolise selenomethionine. Both processes make selenium available to the organism. (3) indicates incorporation of selenium into serine during translation with formation of selenocysteine in selenoproteins. Modified from Levander, O. A. & Burk, R. F. (1990). Selenium. In *Present Knowledge of Nutrition*, Brown, M. L., ed., 6th ed., pp. 268–273. Washington, DC: International Life Sciences Institute-Nutrition Foundation.

Selenocysteine, the active form in selenoproteins, is believed to be tightly regulated. Selenide selenium from reduction of selenate or selenite or from catabolism of selenocysteine or selenomethionine is incorporated by replacement of oxygen into serine to form selenocysteine, while serine is attached to a unique tRNA. Selenocysteine is then incorporated into a selenoprotein.

Homeostasis of body selenium is achieved by regulation of urinary excretion of selenium; its daily excretion is closely associated with plasma selenium and dietary selenium. Renal plasma clearances of selenium show that kidneys of NZ residents excrete selenium more sparingly than those of US residents; Chinese from low selenium areas are even more thrifty, indicating possible adaptation of NZ and Chinese residents to their low selenium status.

Tri-methylselenonium (TMSe), the only urinary metabolite identified as yet, is only a minor metabolite, barely detectable in control NZ urines, but, when intake is supplemented, it rises to about 1 % TMSe/selenium excreted as in US urines.

Selenium status continues to be assessed by a variety of parameters: dietary intake, 24 h urine, blood, plasma (short-term changes), erythrocyte (long-term changes), hair, toenails and biopsy tissues; each has limitations and their relationship to body pools is not clear.

For functional indices, GSHPx activity goes with selenium levels only up to a plateau of 1.3 μmol/l blood or 1.8 μmol/l erythocytes, well below the US blood levels; this makes GSHPx measurements useful for subjects only from low selenium environments. However platelet GSHPx seems not so limited and also it is related to liver GSHPx and selenium content. More sensitive indices of selenium status may be derivable from newer functions which are being discovered.

Many diseases have been linked with low selenium status, but epidemiological studies within NZ are hampered because we are so uniformly low and have no truly high selenium areas for comparison. NZ blood selenium values are less than half values found in USA and many European countries excluding the Nordic countries. If a low selenium status was a risk factor for coronary heart disease, hypertension or cancer, the prevalence of these diseases in NZ should be greater than almost anywhere else. In fact, NZ disease patterns are not very different. Furthermore, no relationship was found between blood selenium and risk factors for cardiovascular disease in the New Zealand Milton survey; although in a recent Auckland study the effects of low selenium level on the risk of myocardial infarction were confined to cigarette smokers (Beaglehole et al., 1990). It is still uncertain whether selenium protects against cancer, and Willett and Stampfer (1988) have recommended against the use of dietary supplements.

Hence it seems selenophiles can report substantial progress, but mainly towards uncovering the tip of a large iceberg of ignorance requiring further work towards understanding:

(a) the real role of GSHPx, and other selenoproteins;
(b) functional indices of selenium status;
(c) in what ways if any a low selenium status as in NZ leads to any impairment in health;
(d) whether it is deemed desirable for countries like NZ to raise the selenium intake, preferably by dietary means such as by consuming more fish, and beans, cereals and other plant foods grown elsewhere on higher selenium soils or by selenium fertilisation of NZ soils as in Finland.

Discovering what may be the requirement of selenium for NZ residents of all ages remains an intriguing challenge.

References

Arthur, J. R., Nicol, F. & Beckett, G. J. (1990). Hepatic iodothyronine 5'deiodinase. *Biochemical Journal*, **272**, 537–40.

Avissar, N., Whitin, J. C., Allen, P. Z., Wagner, D. D., Liegey, P. & Cohen, H. J. (1989). Plasma selenium-dependent glutathione peroxidase. *Journal of Biological Chemistry*, **264**, 15850–5.

Beaglehole, R., Jackson, R., Watkinson, J., Scragg, R. & Yee, R. Y. (1990). Decreased blood selenium and risk of myocardial infarction. *International Journal of Epidemiology*, **19**, 918–22.

Behne, B., Hilmert, H., Scheid, S., Gessner, H. & Elger, W. (1988). Evidence for specific selenium target tissues and new biologically important selenoproteins. *Biochimica et Biophysica Acta*, **966**, 12–21.

Berry, M. J., Banu, L. & Larsen, P. R. (1991). Type I iodothyronine deiodinase is a selenocysteine-containing enzyme. *Nature*, **349**, 438–40.

Burk, R. F. (1989). Recent developments in trace element metabolism and function: newer roles of selenium in nutrition. *Journal of Nutrition*, **119**, 1051–4.

Burk, R. F. (1990). Protection against free radical injury by selenoenzymes. *Pharmacological Therapeutics*, **45**, 383–5.

Cooper, G. J. S., Croxson, M. S. & Ibbertson, H. K. (1984). Iodine intake in an urban environment. *New Zealand Medical Journal*, **97**, 142–5.

Harrison, M. F. (1949). Urinary excretion of fluorine in some New Zealand subjects. *British Journal of Nutrition*, **3**, 166–70.

Hetzel, B. S. & Dunn, J. T. (1989). The iodine deficiency disorders. *Annual Reviews of Nutrition*, **9**, 21–38.

Levander, O. A. & Burk, R. F. (1990). Selenium. In *Present Knowledge of Nutrition*, 6th edn, Brown, M. L. ed., pp. 268–273. Washington DC: International Life Sciences Institute-Nutrition Foundation.

NZ Nutrition Taskforce Report (1991). *Food for Health*. Wellington NZ: Department of Health.

Robinson M. F. (1988). The New Zealand selenium experience. *American Journal of Clinical Nutrition*, **48**, 521–34.

Simpson, F. O., Thaler, B. I., Paulin, J. M., Phelan, E. L. & Cooper, G. J. S. (1984). Iodide excretion in a salt-restriction trial. *New Zealand Medical Journal*, **97**, 890–3.

Sunde, R. A. (1990). Molecular biology of selenoproteins. *Annual Reviews of Nutrition*, **10**, 451–74.

Thomson, C. D. & Robinson, M. F. (1980). Selenium in human health and disease with emphasis on those aspects peculiar to New Zealand. *American Journal of Clinical Nutrition*, **33**, 303–23.

Ursini, F., Maiorino, M. & Gregolin, C. (1985). The selenoenzyme phospholipid hydroperoxide glutathione peroxidase. *Biochimica et Biophysica Acta*, **839**, 62–70.

Vanderpas, J. B., Contempré, B., Duale, N. L., Goossens, W., Bebe, N., Thorpe, R., Ntambue, K., Dumont, J., Thilly, C. H. & Diplock, A. T. (1990). Iodine and selenium deficiency associated with cretinism in northern Zaire. *American Journal of Clinical Nutrition*, **52**, 1087–93.

Willett, W. C. & Stampfer, M. J. (1988). Selenium and cancer. *British Medical Journal*, **297**, 573–4.

Yang, G., Chen, J., Wen, Z., Ge, K., Zhu, L., Chen, X. & Chen, X. (1984). The role of selenium in Keshan disease. *Advances in Nutritional Research*, **6**, 203–31.

17

Fat soluble vitamins

DAVID R. FRASER

It is surprising that at the end of the twentieth century nutritionists persist in grouping together as the 'fat-soluble vitamins' the four substances known as vitamins A, D, E and K. Apart from their hydrophobic physical property, their basic isoprenoid chemical structure and the historical links in their discovery, they appear to have little in common. One of them, vitamin D, is not even a nutrient in natural circumstances, but is produced by the photochemical action of ultraviolet sunlight on the vitamin D precursor, 7-dehydrocholesterol, in skin. Vitamin A also, for most vertebrate species, is a metabolic derivative and the true 'vitamin' nutrient is β-carotene or other similar carotenoid.

However, these fat-soluble vitamins do have another link through the enormous human effort which has been expended in seeking to discover their respective functions and mechanisms of action. In comparison with the enzyme cofactor vitamins, the identification of the function of each of these fat-soluble substances has proved to be a most difficult task. More than 50 years after their chemical characterisation, knowledge of what they do in biology and how they do it is, at best, rudimentary and incomplete. Lines of investigation have tended to be opportunistic and based on studies of nutritional deficiency rather than being biochemically imaginative. Yet for each of these problem substances there have been major triumphs of research in nutritional biochemistry.

The search for the function of vitamin A has made the most progress because a specific molecular biological event has been defined (Wald, 1968). The vitamin A metabolite, 11-*cis*-retinaldehyde, is isomerised to all-*trans*-retinaldehyde by the action of light. When this occurs with the 11-*cis* isomer bound to opsin as the visual pigment rhodopsin in the retina of the eye, the consequent conformational change in opsin structure leads to a neurological signal being transmitted to the visual centres in the brain. This discovery has given rise to the global hypothesis that the fat-soluble vitamins may act in association with specific proteins and may, through allosteric effects on the structure of those binding proteins, perform their biological function. Despite the success of defining a role for vitamin A in this way in the visual cycle, there has been much less progress made in identifying the systemic functions of vitamin A.

In the case of vitamin E, the vitamin/specific-protein hypothesis does not seem to be easily supported. Vitamin E has the distinct chemical property of being a chain-breaking antioxidant and is converted by peroxyl radicals *in vitro* to the free radical, α-tocopherol quinone (Green, 1972). Its biological role may therefore be to prevent the peroxidation of polyunsaturated fatty acids in cell membranes: a concept reinforced by the observation that there is increased lipid peroxidation *in vivo* in vitamin E deficiency (Hafeman & Hoekstra, 1977). The relatively large quantities of vitamin E supplied in the diet and the apparently high nutritional requirement for adults of about 10 mg per day, are compatible with the idea that vitamin E could be a component of all cells in the body perhaps having a structural and antioxidant function in cell membranes (Lucy, 1972).

The discovery of vitamin K clearly linked it with a role in the blood clotting mechanism. Deficiency of this nutrient gives rise to a haemorrhagic disease because there is defective functioning of prothrombin and three other blood clotting factors: factors VII, IX and X. The function of vitamin K has now been identified as that of a co-factor in the post-translational gamma carboxylation of glutamic acid residues during the formation of these blood clotting proteins (Nelsestuen & Suttie, 1973; Stenflo *et al.*, 1974). Hence, vitamin K has a quite specific enzyme-linked role in which it may mediate the incorporation of CO_2 at the gamma carbon of the glutamyl residue. This again is a quite different function from those suggested for vitamins A or E. A generalised mechanism of action for the hydrophobic vitamins by allosteric protein interaction now seems rather unlikely, and what is known of their respective functions yet again emphasises the dissimilarity between them.

Perhaps the fat-soluble vitamin function which many consider to be best elucidated is that of vitamin D. Certainly the fact that more than 10000 papers have been published in the last 20 years on aspects of its function would attest to this concept of great progress. Yet, in terms of understanding what it does and how it does it, this impression of progress is illusory.

The daily requirements for vitamin D are minute – a few micrograms per day. Therefore, when this 'nutritional' requirement became known, it was apparent that only with the use of radioactively-labelled vitamin D could this small quantity be located in the body, and its function investigated. The pioneer in this type of study was Egon Kodicek in Cambridge who first prepared ^{14}C-labelled ergocalciferol from biologically labelled ergosterol produced in yeast (Kodicek, 1959). Subsequently, with R. K. Callow, a tritiated form, [1 α-^{3}H]cholecalciferol, was chemically synthesised and this had a higher specific activity (141 mCi mmol^{-1}) than was possible with a ^{14}C-label (Callow, Kodicek & Thompson, 1966). In Madison, USA, Hector DeLuca also synthesised tritiated [1,2-^{3}H]cholecalciferol with a specific activity of 180 mCi mmol^{-1} (Neville & DeLuca, 1966).

Using the classical experiments of vitamin research, these labelled forms of vitamin D were administered to vitamin D-deficient rats and chickens. However, the working hypotheses in the experiments of the Cambridge and Madison groups were different. Kodicek had previously shown that vitamin D, when added to cultures of *Lactobacillus helveticus* and other Gram-positive bacteria, antagonised a growth inhibition caused by unsaturated fatty acids (Kodicek, 1956). He had also shown that when large doses of ^{14}C-ergocalciferol were given to rachitic rats, most of the dose was metabolically inactivated within 24 hours (Kodicek, 1960). It was therefore postulated that vitamin D itself was the functional form and acted as a 'catalytic surfactant' in membranes to modify the calcium transporting activities of cells.

In contrast, DeLuca postulated that because there was a long lag of several hours between the administration of vitamin D to deficient animals and the observation of any biological response in calcium transport, the fat-soluble substance may require to be metabolised to an active form. From this basis he then discovered a metabolite in plasma which had higher biological activity than the parent vitamin D. This was identified as 25-hydroxyvitamin D (25(OH)D$_3$) (Blunt, DeLuca & Schnoes, 1968). It was found to have been synthesised in the liver and it seemed to become concentrated in the nuclei of intestinal mucosal cells (Stohs & DeLuca, 1967; Haussler, Myrtle & Norman, 1968).

Accepting that their functional vitamin D hypothesis had been disproven, Lawson and his colleagues in Cambridge nevertheless consistently failed to find any tritium in the nuclei of intestinal cells of animals dosed with [1 α-^{3}H]cholecalciferol (Lawson, Wilson & Kodicek, 1969a). The discrepancy between Cambridge and Madison was finally resolved when doubly labelled [4-^{14}C, 1 α-^{3}H]cholecalciferol was given to vitamin D-deficient chickens. The mucosal cell nuclei were then found to contain a 'tritium-deficient' ^{14}C-labelled metabolite which was more polar than 25(OH)D$_3$, was a metabolite of 25(OH)D$_3$, had greater biological activity than 25(OH)D$_3$ and had lost the tritium from carbon-1. Therefore, from these observations, it was suggested that the new metabolite was a vitamin D molecule with oxygen atoms inserted both at carbon-25 and at carbon-1 and that it was probably the functional form of vitamin D (Lawson, Wilson & Kodicek, 1969b).

The site of formation of this second metabolite was not readily apparent. Although the highest concentrations were in the nuclei of the intestinal mucosal cells, traces of this substance were present in most other tissues and a very small amount was also found in blood plasma. After an extensive search by means of tissue incubation experiments and surgical extirpation of organs, the Cambridge group eventually stumbled on the fact that the metabolite was produced solely by the kidney (Fraser & Kodicek, 1970). The identity of this active metabolite as 1,25-dihydroxy-cholecalciferol (1,25(OH)$_2$D$_3$) was then confirmed from kidney enzyme preparations (Lawson *et al.*, 1971) and from extracts of large numbers of chicken intestines (Holick *et al.*, 1971).

Meanwhile, Wasserman and his colleagues at Cornell University had discovered that administration of vitamin D to vitamin D-deficient chickens induced the formation *de novo* of a specific calcium-binding protein in the mucosa of the small intestine (for review see Wasserman, Fullmer & Taylor, 1978). This finding, along with the metabolic activation of vitamin D, suggested that 1,25(OH)$_2$D$_3$ was a steroid hormone that acted in the intestinal mucosa to provide an enhanced capacity for calcium absorption as part of whole body calcium homeostasis. The metabolic addition of the two hydroxyl groups to the parent vitamin D molecule gave this secosteroid structure the essential polar groups required for steroid hormone function and also, in the specifically controlled 1-hydroxylation reaction, provided a means of regulating the supply of this steroid hormone according to the requirements of calcium homeostasis.

This function as a steroid hormone was further reinforced by the discovery of a specific 'receptor' protein which binds 1,25(OH)$_2$D$_3$ with high affinity and specificity and which then associated with DNA in the chromatin of cells (for review see Franceschi, Simpson & DeLuca, 1981). Thus, 1,25(OH)$_2$D$_3$ has all the functional attributes of the classical steroid hormones such as aldosterone, corticosterone and oestradiol. Its synthesis is increased whenever the extracellular Ca^{2+} concentration tends to fall, such as during rapid bone growth, during lactation, and when there is a dietary deficiency of calcium. By its action in target tissue cells, most notably those of the mucosa of the small intestine, the bone and the renal tubules, there is a resultant increased transport of Ca^{2+} into the extracellular fluid to maintain the constant concentration.

Despite this apparent leap forward in understanding of the mechanism of action of vitamin D, there are two enormous problems which remain. One of these is that the cellular function(s) which vitamin D modifies in its calcium homeostatic role are still largely unknown. This homeostatic action undoubtedly involves the participation of the vitamin D-dependent calcium-binding protein. However, the function of this protein itself is not yet understood and, besides, knowledge of this function would be unlikely to reveal the entire molecular mechanism through which the cellular action of vitamin D is expressed.

The other major problem in the function of vitamin D is that the receptor protein for $1,25(OH)_2D_3$ is present in most cells, many of which are not concerned at all with whole body calcium homeostasis. Also, studies with cells *in vitro* have demonstrated that $1,25(OH)_2D_3$ induces a wide range of changes in function. These include changes in the differentiated properties of cells, the induction of hormone secretion, the fusion of cell membranes and the depression of mitotic rate. Little attention has been paid to the problem of how these 'new' functions of $1,25(OH)_2D_3$ can co-exist with the traditional one of being a major regulatory factor in whole body calcium homeostatis.

This lack of understanding of what vitamin D is really doing has been compounded by a lack of awareness of the nature of recent research on the biology of vitamin D. Although this research has generated many thousands of publications, the field has been characterised by an unfortunate absence of predictive ideas. Practically every discovery has been serendipitous and could eventually have been made by any one of the many investigators who have been performing standard experiments in the hope of stumbling on to the mechanism of action of vitamin D.

The challenge in the future for studies on all the fat-soluble vitamins is for investigators to develop imaginative hypotheses, soundly based on existing information, and which attempt to define the real functions and molecular mechanisms of action. For vitamin K, this goal of understanding may soon be reached. However, for the systemic function of vitamin A, the membrane action of vitamin E and for the general cell function of vitamin D the answers to the questions: (1) what are these molecules doing and (2) how are they doing it, are still far away. From the enormous pool of data which has accumulated from past research, it should be possible to devise predictive and testable hypotheses to determine the real functions for all that disparate group of fat-soluble vitamins.

References

Blunt, J. W., DeLuca, H. F. & Schnoes, H. J. K. (1968). 25-Hydroxycholecalciferol. A biologically active metabolite of vitamin D_3. *Biochemistry*, **7**, 3317–22.

Callow, R. K., Kodicek, E. & Thompson, G. A. (1966). Metabolism of tritiated vitamin D. *Proceedings of the Royal Society of London B*, **164**, 1–20.

Franceschi, R. T., Simpson, R. U. & DeLuca, H. F. (1981). Binding proteins for vitamin D metabolites; serum carriers and intracellular receptors. *Archives of Biochemistry and Biophysics*, **210**, 1–13.

Fraser, D. R. & Kodicek, E. (1970). Unique biosynthesis by kidney of a biologically active vitamin D metabolite. *Nature*, **228**, 764–6.

Green, J. (1972). Vitamin E and the biological antioxidant theory. *Annals of the New York Academy of Science*, **203**, 29–44.

Hafeman, D. G. & Hoekstra, W. G. (1977). Lipid peroxidation *in vivo* during vitamin E and selenium deficiency in the rat as monitored by ethane evolution. *Journal of Nutrition*, **107**, 666–72.

Haussler, M. R., Myrtle, J. F. & Norman, A. W. (1968). The association of a metabolite of vitamin D_3 with intestinal mucosal chromatin *in vivo*. *Journal of Biological Chemistry*, **243**, 4055–64.

Holick, M. F., Schnoes, H. K., DeLuca, H. F., Suda, T. & Cousins, R. J. (1971). Isolation and identification of 1,25-dihydroxycholecalciferol, a form of vitamin D_3 metabolically active in the intestine. *Proceedings of the National Academy of Science of USA*, **68**, 803–4.

Kodicek, E. (1956). The effect of unsaturated fatty acids, of vitamin D and other sterols on Gram-positive bacteria. In *Biochemical Problems of Lipids*, Popják, G. & Le Breton, E., eds, pp. 401–6, London: Butterworths Scientific Publications.

Kodicek, E. (1959). Biosynthesis of yeast sterols and the preparation of ^{14}C-labelled vitamin D_2. In *Biosynthesis of Terpenes and Sterols (A Ciba Foundation Symposium)*, Wolstenholme, G. E. W. & O'Connor, C. M., eds, pp. 173–83, London: J. & A. Churchill.

Kodicek, E. (1960). The metabolism of vitamin D. In *Fourth International Congress of Biochemistry, Vienna, 1958*, vol. 9 *Vitamin Metabolism* Umbreit, W. & Molitor, H., eds, pp. 198–208, London: Pergamon Press.

Lawson, D. E. M., Wilson, P. W. & Kodicek, E. (1969a). New vitamin D metabolite localized in intestinal cell nuclei. *Nature*, **222**, 171–2.

Lawson, D. E. M., Wilson, P. W. & Kodicek, E. (1969b). Metabolism of vitamin D. A new cholecalciferol metabolite, involving loss of hydrogen at C-1, in chick intestinal nuclei. *Biochemical Journal*, **115**, 269–77.

Lawson, D. E. M., Fraser, D. R., Kodicek, E., Morris, H. R. & Williams, D. H. (1971). Identification of 1,25-dihydroxycholecalciferol, a new kidney hormone controlling calcium metabolism. *Nature*, **230**, 228–30.

Lucy, J. A. (1972). Functional and structural aspects of biological membranes: a suggested structural role for vitamin E in the control of membrane permeability and stability. *Annals of the New York Academy of Science*, **203**, 4–11.

Nelsestuen, G. L. & Suttie, J. W. (1973). The mode of action of vitamin K. Isolation of a peptide containing the vitamin K-dependent portion of prothrombin. *Proceedings of the National Academy of Science of USA*, **70**, 3366–70.

Neville, P. F. & DeLuca, H. F. (1966). The synthesis of [1,2-^{3}H]-vitamin D_3 and the tissue localization of a 0.25 μg (10 i.u.) dose per rat. *Biochemistry*, **5**, 2201–7.

Stenflo, J., Fernlund, P., Egan, W. & Roepstorff, P. (1974). Vitamin K dependent modifications of glutamic acid residues in prothrombin. *Proceedings of the National Academy of Science of USA*, **71**, 2730–3.

Stohs, S. J. & DeLuca, H. F. (1967). Subcellular location of vitamin D and its metabolites in intestinal mucosa after a 10 i.u. dose. *Biochemistry*, **6**, 3338–49.

Wald, G. (1968). The molecular basis of visual excitation, *Nature*, **219**, 800–7.

Wasserman, R. H., Fullmer, C. S. & Taylor, A. N. (1978). The vitamin D-dependent calcium-binding proteins. In *Vitamin D*, Lawson, D. E. M., ed., pp. 133–66, London: Academic Press.

18

Water-soluble vitamins

C. J. BATES

'Vitamin' means one has to eat it

Albert Szent-Gyorgyi, who achieved the first unequivocal isolation of vitamin C from a biological material, exclaimed: 'Vitamin means that one has to eat it. What one has to eat is the first concern of the chef, not the scientist!' Why have solid scientific advances been so infuriatingly elusive in nutrition? The subject stands at a crossroads, impinging on many areas of human endeavour, many of which have proved difficult to investigate or to quantitate.

Ascorbic acid: the chameleon of the vitamins

Sir Richard Hawkins wrote in his 'Voyage into the South Sea' of 1593: 'Betwixt three or foure degrees of the equinoctiall line, my company within a fewe dayes began to fall sicke of a disease which sea-men are wont to call the scurvy' (Hawkins, 1847). 'Sower oranges and lemmons' were one of his favoured antidotes, but a further three centuries had to pass before this idea was given a sound experimental basis.

Medical practitioners for many centuries shied away from the idea that there might be a *dietary* cause and cure for scurvy. Starvation or diseases caused by putrid food were easy to comprehend, but the delayed deterioration produced by a subtle micronutrient deficiency was not. The difficulty was compounded by the rapid destruction of the curative factor, by air or metal surfaces.

Dame Harriette Chick and Solomon Zilva at the Lister Institute found that the antiscorbutic substance obtained from plant tissues was unstable to heat, to metals and to high pH. They measured the antiscorbutic potency of many foods, but failed to isolate the vitamin. Holst and

Frölich's (1907) observation that guinea-pigs share with humans an absolute requirement for a dietary antiscorbutic was a vital advance, leading to the isolation and an animal model for scurvy and hence to characterisation of vitamin C in 1928–33. Szent-Györgyi was not actually seeking the antiscorbutic substance in the 1920s, but he believed that the powerful reducing properties of adrenal glands might be central to energy release, or might represent a new hormone, so he proceeded to purify the reducing substance. Without even realising it, he thus succeeded in isolating the antiscorbutic, and in measuring its elemental composition and molecular weight (Szent-Györgyi, 1928). The final piece of the jigsaw fell into place in several places almost simultaneously, and Szent-Györgyi's reducing 'hexuronic acid' could be renamed as 'vitamin C', or 'ascorbic acid'.

Stepwise degradation revealing the structure of vitamin C, and its chemical synthesis from common sugars, were then achieved remarkably quickly: by Norman Haworth in Birmingham (Haworth & Hirst, 1933), and by Tadeus Reichstein in Switzerland. Excellent summaries of the history of scurvy and discovery of vitamin C can be found in The Lind Bicentenary Symposium of the Nutrition Society (Proceedings of the Nutrition Society, 1958) and the account by Carpenter (1986).

Food rationing during World War II demanded precise definition of human nutrient requirements. A classic and heroic study was performed in Sheffield (Krebs, 1953), in which nine men and one woman put up with diets containing less than 1 mg vitamin C/d for up to 39 weeks (Table 18.1)! Less than 10 mg of vitamin C per day was sufficient to prevent and cure any signs of incipient scurvy. Later studies (Table 18.1) using isotope-labelled vitamin C were able to define the rate of turnover of the vitamin in 'normal' adults, and the intake needed to maintain a defined body pool or to saturate the degradation pathway. However, they have not yet answered the more difficult questions: how much is needed for tissue protection in situations of metabolic stress or increased free radical production, and what critical indices need to be measured to define this amount?

There is good evidence for vitamin C involvement in connective tissue synthesis and repair (Padh, 1990). Failure of wound healing, breakage of old wounds, bleeding gums and capillary haemorrhages: all are characteristic of scurvy. These lesions are preventable by daily intakes of a few mg of vitamin C in adult man. The principal biochemical lesion is a failure of collagen synthesis. This requires two 'oxygenase' enzymes: prolyl and lysyl hydroxylases, which are both 'dioxygenases', in which the two halves of an oxygen molecule are inserted into two different substrates. Ascorbate

Table 18.1. *Studies of adult human vitamin C requirements*

	Bartley, Krebs & O'Brien (1953)	Baker et al. (1971)	Kallner, Hartmann & Hörnig (1979)	Leggott et al. (1986)
Subjects	9 men, 1 woman	6 men	14 men	11 men
Type of study	Controlled depletion and repletion	Depletion/repletion + labelled ascorbate	Kinetic study; labelled ascorbate; constant intakes	Controlled depletion/repletion
Outcome measures	Scorbutic lesions Wound healing. Plasma and white cell vit. C	Scorbutic lesions. Psychological Body pool from sp. activity	Turnover rate, body pool, rates of catabolism, excretion	Gingival lesions; blood vit. C
Basis of estimate	Prevention/cure of lesions	Body pool $\geqslant$ 300 mg	Max. turnover rate	Not addressed
Min. daily requirement:	5–10 mg	6.5–10 mg	Not addressed	Results suggest 5 mg is inadequate for full gingival health
Acceptable intake (suggested)	30 mg	45 mg (for 1500 mg body pool)	100 mg to achieve max. turnover and 20 mg/kg body wt	Not addressed

Table 18.2. *Protective functions of vitamin C* in vivo

1. Removal of oxidising free radicals (e.g. ·OH, ·OOH) and hence chain
   termination:

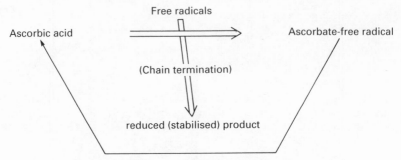

Pyridine nucleotide-linked reductase, or comproportionation
to ascorbic + dehydroascorbic acids

2. Recycling of oxidised vitamin E, hence reduced lipid peroxidation (Niki,
   1987).
3. Protection of tetrahydrofolate and tetrahydrobiopterin derivatives.
4. Chelation and removal of potentially toxic metal ions, (e.g. Cd^{2+}).

is essential, but is not consumed in the reaction. Other ascorbate-dependent
enzymes are 'mono-oxygenases'; here ascorbate is consumed, but is then
recycled, either by a pyridine nucleotide-linked semidehydroascorbate
reductase, or by 'comproportionation' to yield ascorbate plus dehydro-
ascorbate (Table 18.2).

This leads to a paradox. Vitamin C clearly acts as a reducing agent, and
hence as an *anti*oxidant in most *in vivo* situations (Table 18.2). Indeed, Frei,
Stocker & Ames (1988) have shown that ascorbate is the first line of
defence against pro-oxidants, at least in human plasma *in vitro*, and that its
oxidation precedes that of other natural antioxidants. Yet this chameleon
of vitamins can act also as a *pro*-oxidant, by participating in oxygenase
reactions, or in ferrous iron-driven Fenton chemistry, whereby potent
oxidising free radicals are formed (Halliwell, 1990).

In vivo, ascorbate maintains the reduced forms of iron or copper at the
active centre of essential ascorbate-dependent mono- or di-oxygenases.
Without these scurvy is contracted and people die. Ferrous iron, like the
spark in an internal combustion engine, is an essential catalyst, but it can
also be a harbinger of destruction for DNA and other macromolecules, if
the reaction gets out of control. If vitamin C levels are too high in

situations of iron-overload, or in other disease processes which release free, unchelated transition metal ions into the tissues *in vivo*, enhanced tissue damage may ensue.

Vitamin C may protect against cataractogenesis (Taylor, 1989), or carcinogenesis (Block, 1991; Tannenbaum, Wishnok & Leaf, 1991), possibly by its capacity to scavenge free radicals. Like the sailors of the seventeenth and eighteenth centuries in their quest for a scurvy cure, researchers are, still searching for the right instruments and experimental approaches to show where real benefits can occur.

The vitamin B group: snows of yesteryear?

Beriberi, pellagra, megaloblastic and pernicious anaemia all yielded up their principal biochemical secrets during the first half of this century. There are eight currently recognised B-vitamins in human nutrition, all of which are enzyme cofactors or cofactor precursors (Table 18.3). The metabolic processes which they control span a spectrum from lipids, through carbohydrates and proteins, to nucleic acids. They are essential for all tissues: muscle, bone, blood vessels, internal organs, brain and nerves. Nutritionally it is necessary to know not only what are their precise biochemical functions, but also which sites are especially sensitive to dietary depletion, because of intense competition for available supplies. Minute amounts can be absorbed from the diet, and are efficiently retained against massive concentration gradients. The fetus and suckling infant concentrate them at the expense of the maternal tissues. Darwinian demands of survival have placed a high premium upon frugality and efficiency.

What still needs to be unravelled? Clinical signs of B-vitamin deficiencies are not well explained by their known biochemical functions. Skin lesions typical of pellagra, riboflavin deficiency, etc, and loss of lingual papillae in nearly all B-vitamin deficiencies, are unexplained.

Certain B-vitamins exhibit the same paradox as vitamin C. Riboflavin is an antioxidant in most cells, by its role as cofactor of glutathione reductase (Bates, 1987). In neonatal hyperbilirubinaemia (jaundice), however, riboflavin as prooxidant can enhance light-catalysed removal of bilirubin, but may also cause DNA strand breakage (Speck & Rosenkranz, 1979). Thus it may be unsafe to combine phototherapy with riboflavin supplements.

Like vitamin C, riboflavin interacts with iron. Recent studies (Powers, Wright & Fairweather-Tait, 1988) show that riboflavin can benefit iron economy by assisting transport of iron across several barriers. In

Table 18.3. *Functions of coenzymes derived from B-vitamins*

Vitamin (Year of isolation)	Area of involvement	Type of reaction
Thiamine (B_1) (1932)	Intermediary metabolism	Decarboxylations and group transfers
Riboflavin (B_2) (1933)	Carbohydrates, lipids and other small molecules	Reduction, electron transport
Pyridoxine (B_6) (1938)	Protein turnover; many other metabolic processes	Group transfers involving $-NH_2$, $-COOH$, $-SH$, etc
Niacin (1935)[a]	Electron transport	Precursor of pyridine nucleotide coenzymes
Biotin (1935)	Lipid biosynthesis	Carboxylation of lipid intermediates
Panthothenic acid (1940)	Fatty acid metabolism	Precursor of coenzyme A
Folic acid (1941)	Nucleic acid synthesis, methionine synthesis, etc	C_1-group transfers
Vitamin B_{12} (1947)	Methionine synthesis, valine degradation	Synergistic with folate

[a] Chemical synthesis was achieved in 1894, but vitamin status was not recognised until 1935.

developing countries both nutrients are in short supply, and a combination is more effective than either alone in correcting iron-deficiency (Powers & Bates, 1987). Such micronutrient interactions need further study.

Vitamin supplies during pregnancy are critical for normal development of the fetus, and the recently identified importance of folate in reducing the prevalence of neural tube defects (spina bifida and anencephaly) in high-risk human subjects is a good example of this (Wald, 1991). Some people can benefit dramatically from high-level vitamin supplementation, because they suffer from a metabolic error which impairs the use of specific vitamins from a normal diet, and they need to be identified and treated.

Folate antagonists such as methotrexate are powerful anticancer drugs, starving cancerous cells of DNA precursors. Yet paradoxically, a localised folate deficiency in the *pre*malignant state in bronchial metaplasia of smokers apparently increased neoplastic transformation (Heimburger *et al.*, 1987). Folate is needed for DNA repair, critical for reversal of

Table 18.4. *Accessory food factors which are not vitamins for man*

	Function
Carnitine	Mitochondrial fatty acid activation
Choline, inositol	Components of phospholipids
Taurine	Bile acid conjugation, anti-oxidant in retina
Biopterin	Aromatic amino acid metabolism
Bioflavinoids	Anti-oxidants
Pyrroloquinoline quinone (PQQ)	?Cofactor for amine oxidases (Smidt, Steinberg & Rucker, 1991).

precancerous lesions. Such anticancer protective roles of nutrients in non-neoplastic tissues may, not infrequently, be replaced by tumour-promoting properties in the cancerous state, with obvious therapeutic implications.

A close relationship between folate and vitamin B_{12} is well established, but the explanation is uncertain. Deficiency of either nutrient results in megaloblastic anaemia because lack of thymidine formation impairs DNA synthesis. Adenosyl cobalamin is required for reaction of methyltetrahydrofolate with homocysteine, to give methionine and tetrahydrofolate. This proceeds to methylene tetrahydrofolate, and hence to the thymidine methyl. Without B_{12} folates may become 'trapped' as methyltetrahydrofolate. However, in animals treated with nitrous oxide, and thus B_{12}-depleted, tetrahydrofolate was unable to stimulate DNA synthesis, whereas formyltetrahydrofolate was strikingly effective (Chanarin, 1990). C_1 unit economy is of central importance in several key vitamin-dependent pathways, but the precise mechanisms remain controversial.

Several vitamins affect neurological function and disease, especially in the elderly. Certain kinds of neurological dysfunction or degeneration may be linked either with disturbances in vitamin-dependent reactions, or with free radical-mediated tissue damage, and this requires new investigations. Likewise, vitamins and other micronutrients interact with immune function, in ways that remain poorly understood (Beisel, 1982).

Other accessory food factors (Table 18.4) may confer benefits, either because they are essential cofactors which are synthesised too slowly in some population groups, or because they have long-term, subtle protective effects, e.g. against oxidative stress, or toxins.

Thus the B-vitamins continue to challenge us, and pose important practical problems, 50 years after their discovery.

C. J. Bates

Future challenges

A major challenge exists, to correct the shortfall of many vitamins in the developing world. In western society, a better recognition of the benefits of fresh fruit and vegetables may help to protect against degenerative disease. Looking further ahead, it may be possible to tailor nutrient intakes according to individual genetic maps. Different people clearly have individual requirements, and different set-points for 'optimum nutrition'. Possibly vitamin requirements will one day be met by implanted genes obtained from other species, permitting *de novo* synthesis within the body, thus dispensing with the need for exogenous dietary sources.

This chapter has inevitably become idiosyncratic: a flower picked here and there from a huge carpet! There have been incredible advances during this century: from deficiency disease to animal model, to metabolic pathway, and thence to nutrient isolation and nutrient synthesis. The jigsaw has been taken apart, and its elements analysed in some detail. Now it has to be put back together, in order to comprehend the subtleties of interaction, and to apprehend long-term protective possibilities. Accessory food factors will then truly have come of age.

References

Baker, E. M., Hodges, R. E., Hood, J., Sauberlich, H. E., March, S. C. & Canham, J. E. (1971). Metabolism of ^{14}C- and ^{3}H-labelled L-ascorbic acid in human scurvy. *American Journal of Clinical Nutrition*, **24**, 444–54.

Bartley, W., Krebs, H. A. & O'Brien, J. R. P. (1953). Vitamin C requirements of human adults. *MRC Special Report Series 280*. London: HMSO.

Bates, C. J. (1987). Human riboflavin requirements, and metabolic consequences of deficiency in man and animals. *World Review of Nutrition and Dietetics*, **50**, 215–65.

Beisel, W. R. (1982). Single nutrients and immunity. *American Journal of Clinical Nutrition*, **35** (Suppl.), 416–68.

Block, G. (1991). Vitamin C and cancer prevention: the epidemiological evidence. *American Journal of Clinical Nutrition*, **53** (Suppl.), 270S–82S.

Carpenter, K. J. (1986). *The History of Scurvy and Vitamin C*. Cambridge: Cambridge University Press.

Chanarin, I. (1990). *The Megaloblastic Anaemias*. 3rd edn. Chap. 8, pp. 68–76, Oxford: Blackwell Scientific Publications.

Frei, B., Stocker, R. & Ames, B. N. (1988). Antioxidant defenses and lipid peroxidation in human blood plasma. *Proceedings of the National Academy of Sciences, USA*, **85**, 9748–52.

Halliwell, B. (1990). How to characterize a biological anti-oxidant. *Free Radical Research Communications*, **9**, 1–32.

Haworth, W. N. & Hirst, E. L. (1933). Synthesis of ascorbic acid. *Chemistry and Industry (London)*, **52**, 645–6.

Hawkins, R. (1847). *Voyage into the South Sea, in the Year 1593*. London: Haklyt Society. Original edition. London, Jaggard, 1622.

Heimburger, D. C., Krumdieck, C. L., Alexander, B., Birch, R., Dill, S. R. & Bailey, W. C. (1987). Localized folic acid deficiency and bronchial metaplasia in smokers: hypothesis and preliminary report. *Nutrition International*, **3**, 54–60.

Holst, A. & Frölich, T. (1907). Experimental studies relating to ship-beri-beri and scurvy. II. On the etiology of scurvy. *Journal of Hygiene (Cambridge)*, **7**, 634–71.

Kallner, A., Hartmann, D. & Hörnig, D. (1979). Steady-state turnover and body pool of ascorbic acid in man. *American Journal of Clinical Nutrition*, **32**, 530–9.

Krebs, H. A. (1953). The Sheffield experiment on the vitamin C requirement of human adults. *Proceedings of the Nutrition Society*, **12**, 237–55.

Leggott, P. J., Robertson, P. B., Rothman, D. L., Murray, P. A. & Jacob, R. A. (1986). The effect of controlled ascorbic acid depletion and supplementation on periodontal health. *Journal of Periodontology*, **57**, 480–5.

Lind Bicentenary Symposium. (1953). *Proceedings of the Nutrition Society*, **12**, 201–344.

Niki, E. (1987). Interaction of ascorbate and tocopherol. *Annals of the New York Academy of Sciences*, **498**, 186–99.

Padh, H. (1990). Cellular functions of ascorbic acid. *Biochemical and Cellular Biology*, **68**, 1166–73.

Powers, H. J. & Bates, C. J. (1987). Micronutrient deficiencies in the aetiology of anaemia in a rural area in The Gambia. *Transactions of the Royal Society of Tropical Medicine and Hygiene*, **81**, 421–5.

Powers, H. J., Wright, A. J. A. & Fairweather-Tait, S. J. (1988). The effect of riboflavin deficiency in rats on the absorption and distribution of iron. *British Journal of Nutrition*, **59**, 381–7.

Smidt, C. R., Steinberg, F. M. & Rucker, R. B. (1991). Physiologic importance of pyrroloquinoline quinone. *Proceedings of the Society of Experimental Biology and Medicine*, **197**, 19–25.

Speck, W. T. & Rosenkranz, H. S. (1979). Phototherapy for neonatal hyperbilirubinemia – a potential environmental health hazard to newborn infants: a review. *Environmental Mutagenesis*, **1**, 321–36.

Szent-Györgyi, A. (1928). Observations on the function of the peroxidase systems and the chemistry of the adrenal cortex. Description of a new carbohydrate derivative. *Biochemical Journal*, **22**, 1387–409.

Tannenbaum, S. R., Wishnok, J. S. & Leaf, C. D. (1991). Inhibition of nitrosamine formation by ascorbic acid. *American Journal of Clinical Nutrition*, **53** (Suppl.), 247S–50S.

Taylor, A. (1989). Associations between nutrition and cataract. *Nutrition Reviews*, **47**, 225–34.

Wald, N. (1991). Prevention of neural tube defects. Results of the Medical Research Council Vitamin Study. *Lancet*, **i**, 131–6.

Part four

Pregnancy, lactation and growth

19

Nutrition and pregnancy in animals

J. J. ROBINSON

At the first meeting of the Nutrition Society Sir John Hammond (Hammond, 1944a) drew attention to the importance of nutrition during pregnancy in a way that prompted much of the research that was to follow by pointing out that after undernutrition during the last 2 months of pregnancy the birthweight of twin lambs was 30 % less than that of lambs of ewes adequately fed. From this observation came the classical Cambridge studies of Wallace (1948) on the effects of nutrition on the growth and development of the sheep fetus. At the same time the ability of the fetus to draw on its mother's tissues to supply its needs was recognised (Hammond, 1944b); so too was the importance to normal fetal growth of specific dietary nutrients (Bourne, 1944).

The earliest meetings of the Society also illustrate the curiosity of researchers about the role of the placenta. In his paper 'Nutritional Functions of the Placenta', Sir Joseph Barcroft reflects on whether the placenta might simply be an ultra-filter or whether it possesses any functions in the active sense (Barcroft, 1944). Thanks to the early pioneering research of Barcroft at Cambridge and the stimulus that it generated, the high metabolic activity of the placenta is now well recognised, its ultrastructure well defined and the details of transplacental nutrient transfer documented (see Faber & Thornburg, 1983; Bassett, 1991).

Current knowledge on nutrition during pregnancy is built on data from a wide range of mammalian species in which the size and appearance of the newly fertilised ovum are the most uniform interspecies features. Thereafter, the diversity between species in the rate of cell multiplication and thus the rate of prenatal growth is enormous. It is not surprising, therefore, that the quantitative expression of pregnancy across the mammalian species reveals little uniformity when scaled for body size by allometry

(Martin & MacLarnon, 1985). It can be argued, why should it? After all, the methods by which different species meet the nutrient demands for pregnancy are also diverse. For example, there are many species (red deer, feral sheep and arctic reindeer) in which the demand for nutrients at certain stages of pregnancy is well in excess of that available to the mother, and maternal tissue has to play a major role in nutrient supply. The Polar bear, albeit not burdened with a particularly demanding pregnancy, is an even more extreme example; late pregnancy coincides with an extended period of natural starvation and around a 30 % reduction in metabolic rate while the mother confines herself to her maternity den (Watts and Hansen, 1987). At the other extreme, where there is an ample supply of food, there is the tendency, particularly in the rat, mouse and pig, to deposit fat in the maternal body during pregnancy and lose it during lactation.

The embryo

Despite the tiny size of the newly fertilised mammalian egg (100 to 150 μ in diameter) and its minute requirement for nutrients, many of the early studies concentrated on the influence of undernutrition on embryo survival. Most of the observations were equivocal and failed to distinguish between fertilisation failure and embryo loss. Indeed, despite the availability since the mid-1950s of embryo transfer techniques which enable this distinction to be made, it is only recently that they have been employed in this role. What is now emerging is contrary to the long-accepted recommendation, albeit based more on notional than scientific evidence, that high-plane feeding should be adopted in the postmating period to ensure maximal embryo survival. In species as diverse as the sheep and pig, high-plane feeding can reduce embryo survival; the mechanisms appear to involve increases in hepatic blood flow and the metabolic clearance rate of progesterone which reduce circulating pro-gesterone to concentrations that impede embryo growth and survival (for review see Robinson, 1990). This nutritionally-induced fall in progesterone may influence embryo growth via a modification in the production of the endometrial secretory proteins (Ashworth & Bazer, 1989). In the pig one of these proteins, uteroferrin, is involved in transporting iron to the conceptus and two others, which have sequence homology with a retinol-binding protein of human plasma, may be involved in the uptake of vitamin A by the conceptus (Roberts & Bazer, 1988; Simmen & Simmen, 1990).

The embryo also plays an active role. The trophoblast is rich in growth factor receptors (de Pablo, Scott & Roth, 1990). At the same time its secretions, which exhibit some degree of species specificity (Bazer, 1989) and which may well be influenced by the nutrition of the mother, provide the signal for the maternal recognition of pregnancy.

The placenta

Over the last 50 years data have accumulated to show that across the species there is a remarkably close association between fetal and placental weights (Bassett, 1991). Within a species the association has been noted so early in pregnancy (day 60 in the case of the highly prolific ewe) that it has prompted the idea that in the ewe, within-litter variation in the size of the placenta and lamb birthweight (Dingwall *et al.*, 1987) may be governed by the variation between embryos in the ability of their rapidly expanding trophoblasts to compete for the caruncular attachment points on the uterine epithelium. In this context, the intriguing question that remains unanswered, is 'does maternal nutrition in early pregnancy influence this within-litter variability in prenatal growth?'.

In all species severe undernutrition causes a reduction in placental growth, and there is evidence in laboratory (guinea pig; Young & Widdowson, 1975) and farmed species (sheep; Robinson & McDonald, 1989) that the placenta may be more vulnerable to a protein than an energy deficiency. In the last decade there have been a number of reports for the ewe showing that a mild degree of undernutrition in mid-pregnancy can enhance placental size (see McCrabb, Egan & Hosking, 1991 for the latest of these). The mechanisms of this response are not yet understood, but the effect appears to be linked to the body condition of the ewe; mature ewes in good condition exhibit the response while immature ones and those in poor condition do not; indeed the latter often show the opposite effect. Such observations provide a sharp reminder of how little we still know about the nutritional factors controlling the growth of the conceptus during the time when placental size is increasing rapidly and the fetus, albeit still only 5% of its birthweight, is undergoing rapid changes in the ontogeny of its metabolic and endocrine systems. The importance of the role played by the uteroplacental tissues of the ewe at this stage is reflected in the fact that they account for > 80% of the total oxygen consumption of the pregnant uterus. Similarly, the high metabolic activity of the fetus at this time is seen in fetal oxygen consumption which, per unit weight, is about 40% higher than in late gestation (Bell *et al.*, 1986).

For many years nutritional influences on placental growth were dominated by the concept that they were unidirectional, i.e. from the maternal circulation to the placenta. In 1986 Bassett proposed that the fetal endocrine system may play an important role in integrating the responses of the fetal and placental tissues to alterations in maternal nutrition. His hypothesis was based on the close association between the circulating insulin concentrations in the fetal plasma and fetal and placental weights and on the observation that infusions of insulin into fetal monkeys and rabbits increased placental weight. In this context the observations of Charlton and Johengen (1987) are intriguing. Following embolism of the uterine artery, these authors found that an intravenous infusion of glucose and amino acids directly into the fetal lamb not only maintained normal fetal growth but enhanced the growth of the placenta. Recently, Hay *et al.* (1990) have shown that uteroplacental glucose metabolism, of which the placenta is by far the major contributor, is a function of fetal rather than maternal glucose concentrations. Thus a direct effect of fetal nutrition on placental growth and function is now established.

The fetus
Growth

Following the early observations of the adverse effects of low feed intakes on size at birth, considerable effort went into defining normal values for the rates of accretion of nutrients in the fetus as these are an integral part of the factorial method of estimating dietary needs. Often the studies were limited to the period of rapid fetal growth and the equations used to describe nutrient accretion were invariably empirical. Thus their accuracy in providing estimates of accretion rates by differentiation with respect to time were often suspect. In terms of its accuracy in describing prenatal growth, the logarithmic form of the Gompertz equation is now regarded as superior to all other equations. Its general form is: $\ln(w) = A - Be^{-Ct}$ where t is time from conception, $\ln(w)$ is the natural logarithm of the weight of the fetal tissue or nutrient in question and A, B and C are constants. The inherent feature of the Gompertz equation which distinguishes it from all other growth equations is that it accommodates an important attribute of fetal growth, namely that specific growth rate decreases exponentially with time.

As a result of the precision which now exists in the data for the rates of accretion of nutrients in the gravid uterus, the nutrient requirements for pregnancy in many species are well defined (Agricultural Research Council, 1980, 1981). In practice, however, the exact nutrient needs at each point in pregnancy are seldom met from the diet. It is therefore essential to consider some of the more important influences of dietary inadequacies or nutrient imbalances on fetal growth and development. The ewe again provides a useful example in that her natural environment invariably results in abrupt changes in food intake. Here the development of a novel technique by Mellor and Matheson (1979) for the continuous monitoring of the changes in the crown–rump length of the fetus marked a major advance in detecting the effects of short-term changes of nutrition on fetal growth. Mellor and his coworkers showed that abruptly imposed severe under-nutrition around day 120 of gestation reduced fetal growth to 50% of normal within 3 days. They also demonstrated that a nutritionally imposed cessation in growth for a period of one week was followed by a return to normal growth rates when feed intake was increased, but for longer periods this was not the case. For example, after 16 days of undernutrition, characterised by prefeeding concentrations of glucose in maternal plasma that were only 50% of well-fed controls, fetuses lacked the ability to revert to normal growth rates when food intake was increased.

One aspect of fetal metabolism in the ovine that has remained controversial for almost half a century relates to the view expressed by Barcroft (1946) that during reductions in maternal glucose production caused by undernutrition, the demands of the fetus take priority over those of the mother. Such a concept was understandable not only in terms of thinking at that time on the high priority of the fetus for nutrients (Hammond, 1944*b*) but also from the recognition that hypoglycaemic-induced pregnancy toxaemia was common in undernourished pregnant ewes. Now a consensus view on the subject appears to be emerging. In starved or severely undernourished ewes there appears to be no evidence to support the idea that the conceptus exercises a priority for glucose over that of the maternal tissues. In contrast, for ewes subjected to a less severe degree of undernutrition a glucose-sparing action in favour of the conceptus appears to operate, possibly via a homeorhetic modulation of insulin sensitivity in maternal tissues (Leury *et al.*, 1990). Additional observations in this experiment and in other recent studies show that during undernutrition fetal gluconeogenesis from amino acids plays a significant role in fetal energy metabolism.

Of the many observations on the effects of specific dietary nutrients on fetal growth one of the most intriguing relates to the inherent dangers of gross imbalances of dietary nutrients. Here the zinc content of the diet provides a good example. When pregnant rats were fed restricted amounts of a zinc-deficient diet the release of zinc from maternal tissues prevented the fetal abnormalities normally seen in zinc deficiency (Masters *et al.*, 1983). In contrast, high intakes of the zinc-deficient diet prevented tissue catabolism and resulted in a high incidence of zinc-deficiency terato-genicity. Such a finding implies that anorexia, arising from dietary nutrient imbalances, may act as an inherent safety mechanism to protect the fetus.

Development

For over 40 years the question of prenatal nutritional influences on contemporary and long-term development has aroused considerable debate. Obviously the long-term effects contain a between-animal genetic component that only recently could be overcome by the ability to 'split' embryos for the production of identical genotypes. At the same time many of the early results are confounded by carry-over effects of pregnancy nutrition on lactation performance, and for these reasons are difficult to interpret. Where newborn lambs have been reared artificially, there is little evidence that undernutrition in prenatal life has a permanent effect on organ size or chemical composition. For sheep breeds such as the Merino, with a propensity for high wool production, a reduction in the number of secondary wool follicles arising from prenatal growth retardation has been variously reported to reduce subsequent wool production by as much as 8% or to have no effect. In the pig, Widdowson (1976) reported that if well nourished, the 'runt' in the litter does not grow to quite the same size as its larger littermates and retains, at maturity, its birth characteristics of less DNA and fewer cells in its organs.

With regard to nutritional influences on contemporary development, the interpretation of the observations should be relatively easy, but this has not been the case. Many researchers still use comparisons between the ratios of organ and tissue weights to total bodyweight in control and undernourished fetuses to identify differential effects of nutrition on development. This approach ignores the fact that, because of the allometric relationships that exist between the total weight of the fetus and the weights of its tissues and organs, these ratios inevitably change as the fetus grows. Therefore a true assessment of nutritional influences on fetal development must combine both the temporal and allometric relationships (Robinson & McDonald, 1979). Combining the relationships shows that in growth-retarded fetuses some body components, e.g. the skeleton, which is essential for the attainment of functional competence, are more developed than the overall allometric relationships would imply while others, in particular the energy reserves that are so essential to survival between birth and first feed, are less developed.

The maternal body

When, in her paper to the Society in 1968, Dr Widdowson pointed out that in late pregnancy fetal guinea-pigs and rats deposit in their bodies every hour amounts of calcium and phosphorus equivalent to the total quantities of these elements circulating in their mother's serum, she vividly captured the enormously dynamic role played by the maternal body in meeting the nutrient needs of the fetus. When this information is viewed alongside the recent concept that a novel parathyroid hormone-related protein of the fetal parathyroid sustains fetal hypercalcaemia (Loveridge *et al.*, 1988), it is not surprising that maternal hypocalcaemia still remains an important practical problem in high producing animals.

In recent years a number of the early theories regarding changes in the maternal body during pregnancy have been revised. Pregnancy anabolism is no longer regarded as a permanent beneficial effect of pregnancy on the maternal body, but merely the storage of extra nutrients in early pregnancy to be used later in pregnancy or lost soon after parturition (for review see Robinson, 1986). Early suggestions of an improved energetic efficiency in pregnancy have not been substantiated in pair-feeding studies, although in those species that exhibit hyperphagia in pregnancy the extra intake appears to be deposited with high efficiency (Trayhurn, 1989). At the same time attempts to improve prolificacy in some farm species, notably the sheep, have created a demand for nutrients that is well beyond the capacity of the digestive tract to provide, thus placing even greater demands on the maternal body. The formulation of diets and feeding strategies in such a way that they complement the role of the maternal body in meeting the continuous and inescapable needs of the fetus in a diverse range of environments and production systems is a problem that we have only begun to address.

The future

Changes in reproduction potential and in the nature and availability of feed resources, together with welfare considerations, will inevitably place more stringent demands on those researching nutrition during pregnancy in farm animals. The ability to make a quantum leap in litter size in sheep through the incorporation of the Booroola gene for prolificacy is already with us and is raising many questions regarding optimal feeding strategies during pregnancy for animals that have the gene. At the same time neonatal mortality, which is a welfare issue, remains unacceptably high. Already there are encouraging new lines of investigation which suggest that the selenium status of the mother during pregnancy may be important in triggering thermogenesis from brown adipose tissue in the neonate (Arthur *et al.*, 1991). Similarly there is evidence that in ewes subclinical cobalt deficiency, even if it is restricted to the first half of gestation, results in less vigorous lambs at birth and a depression in passively-acquired immunity to disease (Fisher & MacPherson, 1991). These observations imply that there may be subtle influences of the micronutrients on the success of pregnancy that have yet to be identified. At the other extremity, unacceptably high embryo mortality exists. It is to be hoped that the current upsurge of research activity on the cellular and molecular mechanisms involved in the bidirectional signalling between the embryo and the mother will provide a much clearer picture of the role of specific nutrients in the growth and survival of the embryo.

References

Agricultural Research Council (1980). *The Nutrient Requirements of Ruminant Livestock*. Slough: Commonwealth Agricultural Bureaux.

Agricultural Research Council (1981). *The Nutrient Requirements of Pigs*. Slough: Commonwealth Agricultural Bureaux.

Arthur, J. R., Nicol, F., Beckett, G. J. & Trayhurn, P. (1991). Impairment of iodothyronine 5'-deiodinase activity in brown adipose tissue and its acute stimulation by cold in selenium deficiency. *Canadian Journal of Physiology and Pharmacology*, **69**, 782–5.

Ashworth, C. J. & Bazer, F. W. (1989). Changes in ovine conceptus and endometrial function following asynchronous embryo transfer or administration of progesterone. *Biology of Reproduction*, **40**, 425–33.

Barcroft, Sir Joseph (1944). Nutritional functions of the placenta. *Proceedings of the Nutrition Society*, **2**, 14–18.

Barcroft, J. (1946). *Researches in Prenatal Life*, Oxford: Blackwell.

Bassett, J. M. (1986). Nutrition of the conceptus: aspects of its regulation. *Proceedings of the Nutrition Society*, **45**, 1–10.

Bassett, J. M. (1991). Current perspectives on placental development and its integration with fetal growth. *Proceedings of the Nutrition Society*, **50**, 311–19.

Bazer, F. W. (1989). Establishment of pregnancy in sheep and pigs. *Reproduction, Fertility and Development*, **1**, 237–42.

Bell, A. W., Kennaugh, J. M., Battaglia, F. C., Makowski, E. L. & Meschia, G. (1986). Metabolic and circulatory studies of fetal lamb at mid-gestation. *American Journal of Physiology*, **250**, E538–44.

Bourne, A. W. (1944). Foetal development. *Proceedings of the Nutrition Society*, **2**, 1–6.

Charlton, V. & Johengen, M. (1987). Fetal intravenous nutritional supplementation ameliorates the development of embolization-induced growth retardation in sheep. *Pediatric Research*, **22**, 55–61.

de Pablo, F., Scott, L. A. & Roth, J. (1990). Insulin and insulin-like growth factor I in early development: peptides, receptors and biological events. *Endocrine Reviews*, **11**, 558–77.

Dingwall, W. S., Robinson, J. J., Aitken, R. P. & Fraser, C. (1987). Studies on reproduction in prolific ewes. 9. Embryo survival, early foetal growth and within-litter variation in foetal size. *Journal of Agricultural Science, Cambridge*, **108**, 311–19.

Faber, J. J. & Thornburg, K. L. (1983). *Placental Physiology*, New York: Raven Press.

Fisher, C. E. J. & MacPherson, A. (1991). Effect of cobalt deficiency in the pregnant ewe on reproductive performance and lamb viability. *Research in Veterinary Science*, **50**, 319–27.

Hammond, J. (1944*a*). Nutrition of farm animals. *Proceedings of the Nutrition Society*, **1**, 15–16.

Hammond, J. (1944*b*). Physiological factors affecting birth weight. *Proceedings of the Nutrition Society*, **2**, 8–12.

Hay, W. W. (Jr.), Molina, R. A., DiGiacomo, J. E. & Meschia, G. (1990). Model of placental glucose consumption and glucose transfer. *American Journal of Physiology*, **258**, R569–77.

Leury, B. J., Bird, A. R., Chandler, K. D. & Bell, A. W. (1990). Glucose partitioning in the pregnant ewe: effects of undernutrition and exercise. *British Journal of Nutrition*, **64**, 449–62.

Loveridge, N., Caple, I. W., Rodda, C., Martin, T. J. & Care, A. D. (1988). Further evidence for a parathyroid hormone-related protein in fetal parathyroid glands of sheep. *Quarterly Journal of Experimental Physiology*, **73**, 781–4.

McCrabb, G. J., Egan, A. R. & Hosking, B. J. (1991). Maternal undernutrition during mid pregnancy in sheep. Placental size and its relationship to calcium transfer during late pregnancy. *British Journal of Nutrition*, **65**, 157–68.

Martin, R. D. & MacLarnon, A. M. (1985). Gestation period, neonatal size and maternal investment in placental mammals. *Nature*, **313**, 220–3.

Masters, D. G., Keen, C. L., Lönnerdal, B. & Hurley, L. S. (1983). Zinc deficiency teratogenicity: the protective role of maternal tissue catabolism. *Journal of Nutrition*, **113**, 905–12.

Mellor, D. J. & Matheson, I. C. (1979). Daily changes in the curved crown-rump length of individual sheep foetuses during the last 60 days of pregnancy and effects of different levels of maternal nutrition. *Quarterly Journal of Experimental Physiology*, **64**, 119–31.

Roberts, R. M. & Bazer, F. W. (1988). The functions of uterine secretions. *Journal of Reproduction and Fertility*, **82**, 875–92.

Robinson, J. J. (1986). Changes in body composition during pregnancy and lactation. *Proceedings of the Nutrition Society*, **45**, 71–80.

Robinson, J. J. (1990). Nutrition in the reproduction of farm animals. *Nutrition Research Reviews*, **3**, 253–76.

Robinson, J. J. & McDonald, I. (1979). Ovine prenatal growth, its mathematical description and the effects of maternal nutrition. *Annales de Biologie Animale, Biochimie, Biophysique*, **19(1B)**, 225–34.

Robinson, J. J. & McDonald, I. (1989). Ewe nutrition, foetal growth and development. In *Reproduction, Growth and Nutrition in Sheep*, Dýrmundsson, Ó. R. & Thorgeirsson, S., eds, pp. 57–77, Reykjavik: Agricultural Research Institute and Agricultural Society of Iceland.

Simmen, R. C. M. & Simmen, F. A. (1990). Regulation of uterine and conceptus secretory activity in the pig. *Journal of Reproduction and Fertility*, **40** (Suppl.), 279–92.

Trayhurn, P. (1989). Thermogenesis and the energetics of pregnancy and lactation. *Canadian Journal of Physiology and Pharmacology*, **67**, 370–5.

Wallace, L. R. (1948). The growth of lambs before and after birth in relation to level of nutrition. *Journal of Agricultural Science, Cambridge*, **38**, 243–302.

Watts, P. D. & Hansen, S. E. (1987). Cyclic starvation as a reproductive strategy in the polar bear. In *Reproductive Energetics in Mammals. Symposia of the Zoological Society of London, Publication* no. 57, Loudon, A. S. I. & Racey, P. A., eds, pp. 305–318, Oxford: Clarendon Press.

Widdowson, E. M. (1968). Nutrition of the foetus and the newly born. *Proceedings of the Nutrition Society*, **28**, 17–24.

Widdowson, E. M. (1976). Environmental control of growth: the maternal environment. In *Meat Animals, Growth and Productivity*, Lister, D., Rhodes, D. N., Fowler, V. R. & Fuller, M. F., eds, pp. 273–84. London: Plenum Press.
Young, M. & Widdowson, E. M. (1975). The influence of diets deficient in energy, or in protein, on conceptus weight, and the placental transfer of a non-metabolisable amino acid in the guinea pig. *Biology of the Neonate*, **27**, 184–91.

20

The endocrine control of lactation

IAN C. HART

Introduction

In contrast with most other foods, milk supplies a wide range of nutrients. Five hundred millilitres of milk each day will supply a moderately active man with one-quarter of his recommended intake of protein, all his calcium and at least one tenth of his energy requirements. The earliest record of the use of cattle for dairy purposes dates from 3100 BC (Parau, 1975); by 1660 a high-yielding English cow was said, by Markham, to give approximately 9 litres of milk per day, and selective breeding caused this to rise to 23 litres per day by 1838 (Youatt, 1838). However, it is only in the present century that the consumption of liquid milk has become widespread, stimulating even more intensive selection such that in 1987/89 the average British Friesian and American Holstein cows yielded 5800 and 6461 litres of milk throughout lactation respectively. (Figures obtained from United States Department of Agriculture, Agricultural Statistics, 1990, United States Government Printing Office, Washington, DC and Dairy Facts and Figures 1990, Federation of UK Milk Marketing Boards.)

The involvement of the endocrine system in controlling mammary growth, development and lactation was suspected by Marshall in 1910, but it was not until the 1930s, and the availability of ovarian steroids, that research started unravelling the exquisitely integrated hormonal mechanisms controlling mammary function in all its phases. As with the elucidation of most endocrine mechanisms, progress has been largely dependent upon technological and analytical advances which have led to new and valuable discoveries. This chapter endeavours to review the important milestones which, over the last 50–60 years, have contributed to our understanding of the hormonal control of lactation and to cite two examples which illustrate how nutrition and diet composition can influence those hormones intimately involved in the process both at the mammary gland and in the partitioning of nutrients. Although some data will be drawn from the human and rat literature, the importance of the dairy industry is such that an enormous amount of research has concentrated on the economics of feeding dairy cows. This has meant that hormonal studies could be carried out against a well-defined nutritional background, and it is for this reason that the majority of information relating nutrition to mammary development and lactation will be derived from farm animal experiments.

When considering progress in this area it is convenient to subdivide mammary events into mammary gland development (mammogenesis), the initiation of milk secretion at parturition (lactogenesis) and the maintenance of lactation (galactopoiesis).

Mammogenesis

While fetal mammary development continues during gestation, the majority of growth occurs during the last trimester of pregnancy resulting, at birth, in a sparsely differentiated lobuloalveolar structure. Growth resumes at puberty and is accompanied by considerable branching and differentiation of the duct system and, in humans, some lobuloalveolar development. However, the greatest morphological changes in the gland occur during pregnancy when the mammary stromal tissue is progressively displaced by the lobuloalveolar system, which matures into the functional secretory tissue of the gland. Extension and branching of the duct system occurs during the first trimester of pregnancy in humans; mature alveoli are present early in the second trimester and milk secretory material is evident in the alveoli a few weeks later.

Early studies

It is now known that mammary gland growth and differentiation are influenced by a variety of hormones including prolactin (PRL), growth hormone (GH), thyroxine (T_4), adrenal glucocorticoids, insulin, oestrogen and progesterone. In fact, the number of hormones makes it difficult to define their relative importance. The initial availability of pure preparations of ovarian steroids made it possible to confirm results formerly obtained with only crude ovarian extracts, and it was rapidly established that oestrogen alone stimulated growth of the duct system while lobuloalveolar formation appeared to require the presence of both oestrogen and progesterone (for review see Folley, 1952). The studies of Stricker and

Grueter (1928, 1929) then focused attention on the involvement of the anterior pituitary gland in mammary growth, and it became evident that an intact anterior pituitary was essential for the ovarian steroids to exert their mammogenic function. However, major elucidation of the roles of ovarian and pituitary hormones in mammogenesis awaited the efforts of Lyons and colleagues (for reviews see Lyons, 1958; Lyons & Dixon, 1966) who worked on the hypothesis that hormones from both sources synergised to induce both ductal and lobuloalveolar development. Using hormone replacement therapy in double (hypophysectomy, ovariectomy) and triple (hypophysectomy, ovariectomy, adrenalectomy) operated rats they conducted a classical series of studies which showed that the minimal hormonal requirements for duct growth were oestrogen, adrenal steroids and bovine GH (bGH), whereas lobuloalveolar development required the addition of progesterone and ovine PRL. Subsequent extensive studies in mice by Nandi (1959) suggested that species may differ in their endocrine requirements for the different phases of mammary development; this was later confirmed by Cowie *et al.* (1966) who demonstrated that the hormone combinations which were effective in rats did not stimulate satisfactory lobuloalveolar or duct growth in goats.

Placental lactogen

It had been known for some years that a functional fetal placental unit was essential for the normal development of the mammary gland during pregnancy (for references see Forsyth, 1974; & Cowie, Forsyth & Hart, 1980). Subsequent work showed that, starting at 8–10 weeks of gestation, the placenta becomes the primary source of oestrogen and progesterone in women (Simpson & MacDonald, 1981) and that the placenta of humans, and several other mammals, produces a protein hormone, placental lactogen (PL) with structural and biological similarities to GH and PRL (Talamantes, 1975; Talamantes *et al.*, 1980). There is no doubt that the placentae of several mammalian species contain one or more mammogenic substances. This is supported by a number of studies demonstrating that pregnant women, goats and rats can maintain normal mammary development after hypophysectomy, and also by the fact that the secretory activity of mouse mammary tissue is stimulated by coculture with bovine placental tissue (for references see Forsyth, 1974; del Pozo & Fluckiger 1973). However, despite this evidence, unequivocal proof that placental lactogen plays an important role during normal pregnancy remains to be established. Byatt and Bremel (1986) failed to demonstrate an effect of different bovine PL preparations on the synthesis of milk fat, casein and α-lactalbumin in mammary tissue taken from mid-pregnant heifers, whereas the same preparations were effective in mammary tissue taken from pregnant rabbits. It is clear that much remains to be learned of the role of PL in mammary development, particularly in relation to species specificity.

Growth factors

Looking to the future, Dembinski and Shiu (1987) contend, in their review, that the greatest progress in the future will be in understanding the manner in which mammary development may be influenced by both paracrine and apocrine growth factors. Drawing upon diverse sources of evidence they postulate roles for epidermal growth factor, a specific mammary growth factor and pituitary-derived mammary mitogens (estromedins) which may mediate or potentiate the growth-promoting action of oestrogen on the mammary epithelium.

Lactogenesis

Lactogenesis is defined as the initiation of milk secretion, but this definition has led to some confusion because the timing of the event depends upon the species studied and the criteria used to establish its occurrence. Fleet *et al.* (1975) divided lactogenesis more conveniently into Stage I, the formation of pre-colostrum by enhanced activity of the pre-secretory differentiated alveolar cells prior to parturition, and Stage II, the onset of copious milk secretion from the fully differentiated terminal alveolar cells which normally occurs at parturition. At this time there is not only an increase in the proteins secreted into milk (e.g. casein and α-lactalbumin) but also an increase in cellular proteins such as biosynthetic enzymes and the secretory membrane proteins involved in the production and release of milk components. Association of specific hormones with these two stages of lactogenesis has been difficult, but it has now been established that the minimal endocrine requirement for lactogenesis is increased secretion of PRL, adrenocorticotrophin (ACTH; to stimulate secretion of gluco-corticoids), oestrogen and the relative absence of progesterone.

Early studies

As with mammogenesis, Stricker and Grueter (1928) were again the first to implicate the anterior pituitary in lactogenesis by noting the onset of copious milk secretion in pseudopregnant rabbits injected with anterior pituitary extract. Lyons and colleagues later stimulated mammogenesis in triply operated rats (see above) with oestrogen, progesterone, bGH, adrenal steroids and ovine PRL (oPRL) and showed that lactogenesis occurred when treatment with the former three was stopped and injections of the latter two continued (see Lyons, Li & Johnson, 1953). There is also species specificity in the endocrine requirements for lactogenesis. In some strains of mice, GH can be substituted by, or have an additive effect to that of PRL (Nandi, 1959). However, one of the most convincing pieces of evidence supporting a role for PRL in lactogenesis originates from work carried out in the 1960s at the National Institute for Research in Dairying, UK where Cowie and colleagues showed that hypophysectomy of the lactating goat caused an almost complete cessation of lactation. Some degree of milk production was restored by treatment with triiodothyronine, dexamethasone (adrenal steroid) and bGH. However, it was not until oPRL was added to this combination that milk yield was completely restored (Fig. 20.1; for references see Cowie, 1969).

Initiation of lactogenesis

The period around parturition is characterised by falling blood concentrations of progesterone and PL and by increases in PRL, oestrogen, prostaglandin-$F_2\alpha$, oxytocin and adrenal corticoids. As a result of this and much supporting evidence, two basic hormonal mechanisms have been invoked to account for the initiation of lactogenesis. The first suggested that progesterone has an inhibitory influence on the lactogenic capacity of the mammary gland and that this is removed by the decline in circulating concentrations of the hormone at parturition. The second ascribed a role to increasing blood levels of lactogenic hormones, particularly PRL and possibly also adrenal corticoids. A combination of these mechanisms is likely (see Cowie, 1969; Kuhn, 1977; Kleinberg et al., 1982 for references). Progesterone withdrawal is undoubtedly the best candidate for a lactogenic trigger in eutherian mammals and this view is supported by studies in women (Kulski, Smith & Hartmann, 1977), pigs (Martin, Hartmann & Gooneratne, 1978) and goats (Davis et al., 1979). Furthermore, such a role is compatible with the ability of progesterone to inhibit the normal induction of mammary lactose, α-lactalbumin and casein synthesis during pregnancy and to block the action of PRL on increased synthesis of these and other milk constituents. It has been suggested that this effect of progesterone may be exerted via its ability to compete with glucocorticoids for binding to mammary receptors or by inhibiting the ability of PRL to induce its own receptors (Hayden, Bonney & Forsyth, 1979).

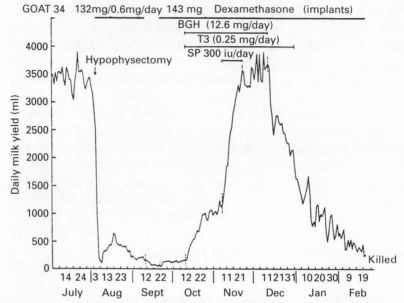

Fig. 20.1. Daily milk yields of a goat before and after complete hypophysectomy and during replacement therapy. BGH: bovine growth hormone, T3: tri-iodothyronine, SP: sheep prolactin. Horizontal lines indicate periods over which the hormones were administered. (From Cowie, A. T., 1969.)

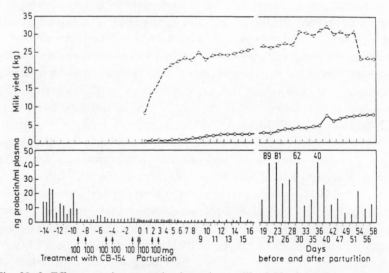

Fig. 20. 2. Effects on plasma prolactin and on milk yield of treating a cow with bromocryptine (CB 154) before and after parturition. Solid line, milk yield after treatment; broken line, milk yield of previous year (Schams, Reinhardt & Karg, 1972).

However, it has become evident that falling progesterone alone does not initiate successful lactogenesis in the absence of adequate quantities of lactogenic hormones, particularly PRL. Suppression of PRL to basal circulation levels with bromocryptine before and after parturition almost completely abolished milk secretion in cows (Schams, Reinhardt & Karg, 1972; Fig. 20.2) and women (Venturini *et al.*, 1981). The mechanism by which PRL exerts its lactogenic activity is, as yet, unknown. The hormone binds to high affinity receptors on mammary epithelial cells (Shiu & Friesen, 1980), and receptor binding appears to be essential to initiate milk protein production, possibly by its action on RNA synthesis (Rillema, 1980; Shiu & Friesen, 1980).

Galactopoiesis

The term galactopoiesis was originally applied to the enhancement of an established lactation. However, more recently it has been used synonymously with the maintenance of lactation (see Cowie & Tindal, 1971) and it is in that context it is used here. Galactopoiesis requires the maintenance of alveolar cell numbers, the synthetic capacity of each mammary cell and the efficacy of the milk ejection reflex. Depending on the species studied, a hormonal complex consisting of PRL, GH, ACTH (or glucocorticoids), TSH (or thyroid hormones), insulin, parathyroid hormone and oxytocin have all been implicated in these processes. However, unless milk is frequently removed from the gland, milk synthesis will not persist despite the presence of an adequate hormonal supply. Numbers of studies have examined, in several species, the galactopoietic role of these hormones in both intact and endocrinectomised animals (for references see Cowie & Tindal, 1971) and it is clear that most attention has focused on PRL, GH and oxytocin. It is aspects of this work that represent the major milestones defining the hormonal control of galactopoiesis.

Prolactin

Although a number of factors concentrated attention on the role of PRL in established lactation it was clear from an early stage that the situation differed with species, particularly between monogastric and ruminant mammals.

Early radioimmunoassay measurement of the hormone circulating in blood rapidly confirmed indirect studies which had suggested that PRL was released from the pituitary by the stimulus of suckling in rats and

I. C. Hart

women (Kwa & Verhofstad, 1968; Ostrom, 1990). Furthermore, the treatment of rats and women with a variety of ergot alkaloids, such that circulating PRL declined to basal concentrations at various stages of lactation, was almost invariably accompanied by a complete cessation of milk secretion (Nagasawa & Meites, 1970; Taylor and Peaker, 1975; DeGezelle *et al.*, 1979; Venturini *et al.*, 1981). Conversely, when PRL release was stimulated in lactating women by treatment with dopaminergic antagonists (e.g. metoclopramide) or thyrotropin-releasing hormone (TRH) milk secretion was enhanced (Tyson, Friesen & Anderson, 1973; McNeilly *et al.*, 1983), even after 18 months of lactation (Tyson *et al.*, 1975). Evidence from *in vitro* studies have shown that PRL binds to specific receptors on mammary epithelial cells and is internalised to induce casein mRNA at the nuclear level. Biosynthesis of mammary α-lactalbumin, lactose and lipids are also induced by the action of PRL.

Despite the foregoing evidence, and the fact that early rat experiments established a relationship between the PRL response to suckling and milk production (Krulich *et al.*, 1970), recent studies have failed to establish convincingly a correlation between basal blood PRL concentrations and milk yield in women (Aono *et al.*, 1977; Howie *et al.*, 1980). Whilst Aono *et al.* (1977) observed a positive correlation between milk volume and the quantity of PRL released at suckling, others have failed to establish such a relationship (Howie & McNeilly, 1980; Bohnet & Kato, 1985). However, it should be noted that Aono *et al.*, 1977) estimated milk more accurately from pre- and postnursing infant weight plus residual milk removed by a breast pump. The work of Grosvenor and colleagues, on rats, has made it clear that the relationship between blood PRL concentrations and milk yield may not be a simple correlation. They found that the stimulatory effect of the hormone on milk secretion does not fully express itself until 8–12 hours after PRL release at suckling (Grosvenor & Mena, 1973). Furthermore, it was determined that the PRL released during the first 5 minutes of suckling was sufficient to stimulate the refilling of the previously emptied mammary glands (Grosvenor, Whitworth & Mena, 1975). This might explain why it is difficult to establish a direct correlation between circulating PRL and production and suggests that after lactogenesis PRL may play a more permissive role. This conclusion is supported by the fact that abundant milk production continues in women, while basal levels of prolactin decrease to near normal levels after 3–4 months (Tyson, Friesen & Anderson, 1972).

The situation in cows and goats contrasts markedly with that in non-ruminants in that PRL plays virtually no role in the maintenance of

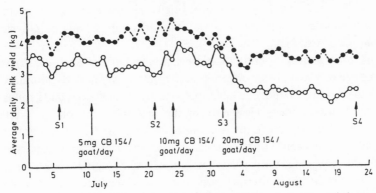

Fig. 20.3. Mean milk yields of three control goats (closed circle), and three goats treated with bromocryptine (CB 154) (open circle). S, date of blood sampling (Hart, 1973).

lactation. Once milk secretion is established both basal circulating PRL and the release of the hormone at milking can be reduced to very low levels with bromocryptine without affecting the yield to any great extent (Fig. 20.3; Karg, Schams & Reinhardt, 1972; Hart, 1973). These results were not entirely unexpected as it had been shown some years previously that once lactation had been restored in hypophysectomized goats using a hormonal combination including PRL, milk secretion could be maintained for several weeks in the absence of the hormone, using bGH, triiodothyronine and dexamethasone (Fig. 20.1; Cowie, 1969). Radioimmunoassay of PRL in blood failed to establish any correlation between basal PRL and stage of lactation (Koprowski & Tucker, 1973; Hart *et al.*, 1978). Furthermore no significant difference was found between circulating PRL in high-and low-yielding cows (Hart *et al.*, 1978), and supplementary PRL, whether given exogenously (Folley & Young, 1940) or by stimulating the endogenous hormone (Karg and Schams, 1974) failed to stimulate milk production in cows. Although initial efforts established a positive correlation between milk yield and the quantity of PRL released at milking in cows and goats (Johke, 1970; Hart, 1975) it rapidly became clear that secretion of the hormone is markedly influenced by day length in ruminants such that this confounded the relationship with stage of lactation (Cowie, Forsyth & Hart, 1980).

Oxytocin

The importance of the milk-ejection reflex for the efficient removal of milk from the mammary gland has been recognised for over 5000 years, and research into its physiological mechanisms spans much of the present century. It is sufficient here to describe briefly the role played by oxytocin in the process of expelling milk from the mammary alveoli and ducts towards the nipple or teat.

The first significant observation was made by Ott and Scott (1910) who showed that, when posterior pituitary extracts were injected, milk flowed from the cannulated teat of a lactating goat. By 1915, Gaines had proposed that milk was actively ejected from the mammary alveoli by a reflex contraction in response to the stimulus of milking, but he did not make the connection between tactile stimulation of the teat and the posterior pituitary. It was not until 1930 that Turner and Slaughter took that step and postulated that pituitary secretions may mediate the contractile changes in the mammary gland. Ely and Petersen (1941) finally obtained clear evidence of the neuro-endocrine nature of the milk-ejection reflex by demonstrating milk expulsion in cows in which one half of the udder had been denervated. Further confirmation of the hormonal component of the milk ejection reflex was obtained by perfusing the isolated cow udder with blood taken from a cow at milking and demonstrating expulsion of milk from the teats (Peeters, Massart & Coussens, 1947). The subsequent determination of the structure and synthesis of oxytocin (see du Vigneaud, 1956) confirmed that this was the milk-ejection hormone.

The neuro-endocrine nature of the milk-ejection reflex has been exhaustively researched over the last 30 years (for reviews see Cowie & Tindal, 1971; Cowie, Forsyth & Hart, 1980). It is clear that milking/suckling activates pressure receptors in the skin of the teat/nipple. Those impulses, destined to release oxytocin, enter the spinal cord bilaterally, via the dorsal roots. The nerve fibres ascend the spinal cord in the dorsal funiculus to the mid-brain, where the bilateral pathway projects into the dorsal and ventral paths and into the posterior hypothalamus. Here it is likely that the afferent neural pathway innervates the paraventricular nucleus and/or the pituitary stalk. Oxytocin is synthesised in both the paraventricular and supraoptic nuclei and secretory granules move down axons to the posterior pituitary where they are stored in Herring bodies. At the time of milking/suckling, oxytocin is released by exocytosis into the blood stream and is carried to the mammary gland where it causes the contraction of the myo-epithelial cells.

The final demonstration of elevated blood concentrations of oxytocin in response to suckling/milking was an important piece of evidence firmly supporting the validity of the neuro-endocrine nature of the milk-ejection reflex. This vital link took some time to demonstrate owing to the lack of suitable sensitive and specific assay techniques. Satisfactory measurement of oxytocin originally stemmed from bioassay procedures based on pressure changes in the mammary gland of lactating guinea-pigs (Tindal & Yokoyama, 1960), and was later followed by radioimmunoassays. In the cow, release of oxytocin was observed in response to a variety of stimuli (both tactile and conditioned) associated with milking. However, in species bred for milk production (cow and goat), milking was often successfully completed without the release of oxytocin during the process. In rats and women there is clear evidence that very little milk can be obtained from the gland without milk-ejection. Measurement of circulating oxytocin in nursing women shows that the pattern of oxytocin release closely parallels temporal characteristics of the milk ejection response. Suckling induces a rise in oxytocin concentration within 3 minutes (Johnston & Amico, 1986), and frequent blood sampling has shown that the hormone is released at approximately 1 minute intervals and that this pattern probably accounts for the wave-like contractions of the myo-epithelial cells (McNeilly *et al.*, 1983).

Growth hormone

Although primate GHs possess intrinsic PRL-like activity, as indicated by their ability to stimulate the activity of pigeon crop sac and the rodent corpus luteum as well as the rabbit and mouse mammary glands (for references see Forsyth & Folley, 1970), it is doubtful whether human GH (hGH) plays an essential role in human mammary development or lactation since both are normal in dwarfs who have a specific GH deficiency (Rimoin *et al.*, 1968). However, there is no doubt that ruminant GH plays a vital part in both the maintenance and stimulation of cow, goat and sheep lactation, and the commercial application of this knowledge has been the subject of thorough investigation and intense debate throughout the last decade.

The first indications of the importance of a pituitary factor in ruminant lactation arose in the 1920s (see Azimov & Krouze, 1937) when Russian researchers found that crude pituitary extracts increased milk production in cattle. Suffice it to say that the therapy was so effective that, during the chronic UK milk shortage during World War II, serious consideration was given to increasing milk production in this manner, but was deemed impractical in view of the vast quantities of pituitary material required to make a significant impact on the nation's milk production. In subsequent years, with the extraction and characterisation of the hormone, it was shown that GH was the galactopoietic pituitary component in cattle (see Johnsson & Hart, 1987; Peel & Bauman, 1987; Hart, 1988) and that the hormone was essential for the maintenance of lactation in goats (Fig. 20.1; Cowie & Tindal, 1971). The development of radioimmunoassays for the measurement of GH in cows' blood indicated a close correlation between circulating concentrations of GH and milk yield in cows (Hart, Bines & Morant, 1979). Furthermore, circulating levels of GH were higher in high-versus low-yielding cows (Hart et al., 1978), a difference which was closely correlated with the metabolic status of the two groups (Hart, 1983). This suggested that the difference in blood GH between genotypes differing in milk yield potential was primarily a consequence of the greater metabolic demand of the high-yielding udder rather than inherent genetic differences in the hormonal mechanisms controlling nutrient partitioning (see below).

The cloning and subsequent expression of cDNA produced from the mRNA for rat GH introduced the prospect of the commercial application of GH technology to the lactating cow. This was closely followed by the production of a hybrid hGH gene, and the molecular cloning of DNA complementary to the mRNA of bGH rapidly followed (Keshet et al., 1981). The technology was quickly utilised by animal health companies, and the subsequent production of hitherto unparalleled quantities of recombinant bGH (re bGH) led to the first demonstration of the galactopoietic properties of the recombinant hormone in cows (Bauman et al., 1982) and to a subsequent explosion of studies investigating use of re bGH under a large number of nutritional and physiological conditions (see Hart, 1988; Hart & Rehman, 1991). The majority of these have successfully sought to demonstrate the efficacy of re bGH, in terms of milk production, and its safety to both cows and humans. However, many studies have been directed towards understanding the mechanism by which the hormone stimulates milk production and these have been extensively reviewed (see Johnsson & Hart, 1987; Peel & Bauman, 1987; Hart, 1988). There is no doubt that treatment with bGH triggers a marked change in nutrient partitioning away from tissue deposition towards milk production, and this is compatible with the hormone's known diabetogenic and lipolytic/antilipogenic properties. However, Johnsson and Hart (1987) outlined the reasons why increasing nutrient availability cannot be the only factor involved in this process and reviewed the evidence for bGH increasing mammary blood flow and the number of mammary cells and suggested the possibility that the galactopoietic properties of the hormone may be mediated by IGF-I and/or other growth factors.

There are now over 1000 published studies investigating the effect of bGH on milk production (Bauman, 1991). This literature is too extensive to review here. However, there is no doubt that, when bGH becomes commercially available, it will have been the most closely reviewed, investigated and debated product on the animal health market.

Relationship between nutrition, endocrinology, mammogenesis and galactopoiesis

Driven by the economic importance of establishing the most efficient means of producing milk, the relationship between level of nutrition, content of the diet and the yield and composition of cows' milk has received close attention for many years and is now well-defined. Furthermore, there is no doubt that changes in the quality and quantity of ingested nutrients induce corresponding changes in the blood concentrations of certain hormones and their receptors on a variety of tissues. However, it is only in the last 15 years that the influence of these hormonal changes on mammary development and milk production has received close attention. There are now several reviews on this subject (Hart, 1983, 1988; Peel & Bauman, 1987; Bauman, 1991), and for the purposes of this chapter just two examples are cited in which nutrient-induced changes in hormone concentration are thought to influence mammary and lactational events.

Prepubertal nutrition and mammary development

In 1960 Swanson reported a study in which he found that the mammary parenchyma was incompletely developed at the end of the second lactation in seven Jersey cows which had been rapidly reared on a high concentrate ration as compared with their identical twin controls which had been reared on a conventional diet. Furthermore, the milk yield of the rapidly reared cows was only 85% of the controls. These and similar data relating to the phases of mammary development in growing heifers (Sinha & Tucker, 1969; Pritchard *et al.*, 1972) prompted Sejrsen (1978) to formulate a hypothesis in which he proposed that high energy intakes before puberty might affect the secretion or biological action of certain mammogenic hormones during a critical period when the gland is undergoing an important phase of mammary duct growth. Prime endocrine candidates were GH and PRL, known to be essential for later periods of mammary development, and ovarian steroids which are essential for the differentiation of mammary cells after puberty. This differentiation was postulated to trigger the cessation of allometric growth within the mammary gland and the end of the period when mammogenesis might be inhibited by high planes of nutrition.

Subsequent work in beef and dairy heifers, and also in sheep (Little & Harrison, 1981; Sejrsen *et al.*, 1982; Harrison, Reynolds & Little, 1983; Johnsson & Obst, 1984; Johnsson & Hart, 1985) supported this hypothesis and indicated that the prepubertal period of allometric mammary growth was the phase during which the gland was most sensitive to nutritional influence. Rapid rearing during this period reduced both the rate and duration of allometric mammary growth, thus resulting in poor mammary development. However, it was not until 1983 that Sejrsen and colleagues implicated GH by reporting that blood concentrations of the hormone were significantly lower in rapidly reared heifers before puberty, when high planes of nutrition depress mammogenesis, but were not affected by rearing rate after puberty. They also noted that GH concentrations and mammary development were positively correlated across treatments. Johnsson *et al.* (1985) noted similar GH differences in ewe lambs reared on different planes of nutrition and went on to demonstrate, for the first time, that the administration of exogenous GH can reverse the deleterious effect of prepubertal rapid-rearing on mammogenesis in that species (Johnsson, Hart & Turvey, 1986). Daily subcutaneous injection of 0.1 mg bGH per kg liveweight between 8 to 20 weeks of age stimulated a 50% increase in mammary parenchymal DNA, thus firmly suggesting that the reduction in circulating GH resulting from a high plane of nutrition before puberty may play a significant role in the subsequently reduced mammary development.

Relationship between diet, feeding frequency, hormonal changes and milk composition

It has been known for some years that feeding dairy cows large quantities of starchy concentrates twice daily can result in a marked reduction in the concentration of fat in milk (milk-fat depression). More recent work demonstrated that the concentration of fat in milk was restored when the same quantity of concentrates was divided into several meals throughout the day (Sutton *et al.*, 1985). Various theories were suggested to account for the phenomenon in terms of changes in the proportions of rumen volatile fatty acids, and there is no doubt that this may play a role in the process, but none of these hypotheses gained general acceptance. However, the suggestion that insulin might be closely involved in the process (McClymont & Vallance, 1962) has received considerable experimental support.

In 1986 Sutton and colleagues reported the results of an experiment in which they compared the pattern of rumen fermentation and plasma hormones and metabolites in cows fed 70% and 90% concentrates twice and six times daily. The more frequent feeding reduced the depression in milk fat caused by feeding both diets, and the data clearly suggested that the milk-fat reduction induced by feeding the 90 % concentrate diet twice daily may have been caused by an elevation in plasma insulin following a rise in rumen propionate (de Jong, 1982). High circulating levels of insulin inhibit lipolysis and increase lipogenesis in adipose tissue; thus it was reasonable to explain the reduction in milk fat in terms of insulin partitioning milk fat precursors away from milk fat synthesis towards adipose tissue deposition (Hart, 1983). Although this explanation was valid for the cows fed the 90 % concentrate ration, it did not appear to be adequate for those receiving 70 % concentrates, where increasing the frequency of feeding tended to restore milk-fat concentration, but insulin was not significantly different between cows receiving feed twice or six-times daily. However, this study only examined the causes of milk-fat depression in terms of mean daily concentrations or production rates of metabolites and hormones. In a later publication (Sutton *et al.*, 1988) the authors reanalysed the data in terms of the diurnal changes in metabolite and hormone concentrations and concluded that the partitioning of nutrients may be more critically related to the postprandial changes in circulating volatile fatty acids and insulin, and that the postprandial increase in insulin measured after feeding the 70 % concentrate ration twice daily may have been sufficient to stimulate milk-fat depression.

References

Aono, T., Shioji, T., Shoda, T. & Kurachi, K. (1977). The initiation of human lactation and prolactin response to suckling. *Journal of Clinical Endocrinology and Metabolism*, **44**, 1101–6.

Azimov, G. J. & Krouze, N. J. (1937). The lactogenic preparations from the anterior pituitary and the increase of milk yield in cows. *Journal of Dairy Science*, **20**, 289–306.

Bauman, D. E. (1991). Bovine somatotropin: review of an emerging animal technology. *Journal of Dairy Science*, in press.

Bauman, D. E., DeGeeter, M. J., Peel, C. J., Lanza, G. M., Gorewit, R. C. & Hammond, R. W. (1982). Effect of recombinantly derived bovine growth hormone (bGH) on lactational performance of high-yielding dairy cows. *Journal of Dairy Science*, **65**, (Suppl. 1), 121 (Abst.).

Bohnet, H. G. & Kato, K. (1985). Prolactin secretion during pregnancy and puerperium: response to metoclopramide and interactions with placental hormones. *Obstetrics and Gynecology*, **65**, 789–92.

Byatt, J. C. & Bremel, R. D. (1986). The lactogenic effect of bovine placental lactogen on pregnant rabbit but not pregnant heifer mammary gland explant. *Journal of Dairy Science*, **69**, 2066–71.

Cowie, A. T. (1969). General hormonal factors involved in lactogenesis. In *Lactogenesis*, Reynolds, M. & Folley, S. J., eds, pp. 157–169, Philadelphia: University of Pennsylvania Press.

Cowie, A. T., Forsyth, I. A. & Hart, I. C. (1980). *Hormonal Control of Lactation*, pp. 111–113, Berlin: Springer Verlag.

Cowie, A. T. & Tindal, J. S. (1971). *The Physiology of Lactation*. London: Edward Arnold.

Cowie, A. T., Tindal, J. S. & Yokoyama, A. (1966). The induction of mammary growth in the hypophysectomized goat. *Journal of Endocrinology*, **34**, 185–95.

Davis, A. J., Fleet, I. R., Goode, J. A., Hamon, A. H., Walker, F. M. F. & Peaker, M. (1979). Changes in mammary function at the onset of lactation in the goat: correlation with hormonal changes. *Journal of Physiology*, **288**, 33–44.

DeGezelle, H., Dhont, M., Thiery, M. & Parewyck, W. (1979). Puerperal lactation suppression and lactation. *Acta Obstetrica Gynecologica Scandinavica*, **58**, 469–72.

de Jong, A. (1982). Patterns of plasma concentrations of insulin and glucagon after intravascular and intraruminal administration of volatile fatty acids in goats. *Journal of Endocrinology*, **92**, 357–70.

del Pozo, E. & Fluckiger, E. (1973). Prolactin inhibition: experimental and clinical studies. In *Human Prolactin*, Pasteels, J. L. & Robyn, C., eds, pp. 291–301, Amsterdam: Excerpta Medica.

Dembinski, T. C. & Shiu, R. P. C. (1987). Growth factors in mammary gland development and function. In *The Mammary Gland. Development, Regulation and Function*, Neville, M. C. & Daniel, C. W. J., eds, pp. 355–381, New York: Plenum Press.

du Vigneaud, V. (1956). Hormones of the posterior pituitary gland: oxytocin and vasopressin. *Harvey Lect. Series L*, pp. 1–26.

Ely, F. & Petersen, W. (1941). Factors involved in the ejection of milk. *Journal of Dairy Science*, **24**, 211–23.

Fleet, I. R., Goode, J. A., Hamon, M. M., Laurie, M. S., Linzell, J. L. & Peaker, M. (1975). Secretory activity of goat mammary glands during pregnancy and onset of lactation. *Journal of Physiology*, **251**, 763–73.

Folley, S. J. (1952). Lactation. In *Marshalls Physiology of Reproduction* 3rd edn. Parke, A. S., ed., vol. 2, Chap. 20. London: Longmans, Green.

Folley, S. J. & Young, F. G. (1940). Further experiments on the continued treatment of lactating cows with anterior pituitary extracts. *Journal of Endocrinology*, **2**, 226–36.

Forsyth, I. A. (1974). The comparative study of placental lactogenic hormones. A review. In *Lactogenic Hormones, Fetal Nutrition and Lactation*, Josimovich, J. B., Reynolds, J. B. & Cobo, M., eds, pp. 49–67, New York: Wiley.

Forsyth, I. A. & Folley, S. J. (1970). Prolactin and growth hormone in man and other mammals. In *Ovo-implantation, Human Gonadotropins and Prolactin*, Hubinot, P. O., Leroy, F., Robyn, C. & Leleux, P., eds, pp. 266–278, Basel and New York: Kurger.

Gaines, W. L. (1915). A contribution to the physiology of lactation. *American Journal of Physiology*, **38**, 285–312.

Grosvenor, C. E. & Mena, F. (1973). Evidence for a time delay between prolactin release and the resulting rise in milk secretion in the rat. *Journal of Endocrinology*, **58**, 31–9.

Grosvenor, C. E., Whitworth, N. S. & Mena, F. (1975). Milk secretory response of the conscious lactating rat following intravenous injection of prolactin. *Journal of Dairy Science*, **58**, 1803–7.

Harrison, R. D., Reynolds, I. P. & Little, W. (1983). A quantitative analysis of mammary glands of dairy heifers reared at different rates of live-weight gain. *Journal of Dairy Research*, **50**, 405–12.

Hart, I. C. (1973). Effect of 2-bromo-α-ergocryptine on milk yield and the level of prolactin and growth hormone in the blood of the goat at milking. *Journal of Endocrinology*, **57**, 179–80.

Hart, I. C. (1975). Concentrations of prolactin in serial blood samples from goats before, during and after milking throughout lactation. *Journal of Endocrinology*, **64**, 305–12.

Hart, I. C. (1983). Endocrine control of nutrient partition in lactating ruminants. *Proceedings of the Nutrition Society*, **42**, 181–94.

Hart, I. C. (1988). Altering the efficiency of milk production of dairy cows with somatotropin. In *Nutrition and Lactation of the Dairy Cow*. Garnsworthy, P., ed., pp. 232–247, London: Butterworth.

Hart, I. C., Bines, J. A. & Morant, S. V. (1979). Endocrine control of energy metabolism in the cow: correlations of hormone and metabolites in high- and low-yielding cows for stages of lactation. *Journal of Dairy Science*, **61**, 270–7.

Hart, I. C., Bines, J. A., Morant, S. V. & Ridley, J. L. (1978). Endocrine control of energy metabolism in the cow: comparison of the levels of hormones (prolactin, growth hormone, insulin and thyroxine) and metabolites in the plasma of high- and low-yielding cattle at various stages of lactation. *Journal of Endocrinology*, **77**, 333–45.

Hart, I. C. & Rehman, J. D. (1991). Implications for the use of biotechnology to improve production performance of dairy cows by manipulation of metabolism: Research on somatotropin and its spin-offs. In *Proceedings of the XXIII International Dairy Congress*, pp. 664–678, Ottowa: Mutual Press.

Hayden, T. J., Bonney, R. C. & Forsyth, I. A. (1979). Ontogeny and control of prolactin receptors in the mammary gland and liver of virgin, pregnant and lactating rats. *Journal of Endocrinology*, **80**, 259–69.

Howie, P. W. & McNeilly, A. S. (1980). The initiation of lactation. *Midwife, Health Visitor, Community Nurse*, **16**, 142–7.

Howie, P. W., McNeilly, A. S., McArdle, T., Smart, L. & Houston, M. (1980). The relationship between suckling induced prolactin response and lactogenesis. *Journal of Clinical Endocrinology and Metabolism*, **50**, 670–3.

Johke, T. (1970). Factors affecting the plasma prolactin level in the cow and goat as determined by radioimmunoassay. *Endocrinologica Japonica*, **17**, 393–401.

Johnsson, I. D. & Hart, I. C. (1985). Pre-pubertal mammogenesis in the sheep. 1. The effects of level of nutrition on growth and mammary development in female lambs. *Animal Production*, **41**, 323–32.

Johnsson, I. D. & Hart, I. C. (1987). Manipulation of milk yield with growth hormone. In *Recent Advances in Animal Nutrition*. Haresign, W. & Cole, D. J. A., eds, pp. 105–23, London: Butterworths.

Johnsson, I. D., Hart, I. C., Simmonds, A. D. & Morant, S. V. (1985). Prepubertal mammogenesis in the sheep. 2. The effects of level of nutrition on the plasma concentrations of GH, insulin and prolactin at various ages in female lambs and their relationship with mammary development. *Animal Production*, **41**, 333–40.

Johnsson, I. D., Hart, I. C. & Turvey, A. (1986). Prepubertal mammogenesis in the sheep. 3. The effects of restricted feeding or daily administration of bovine growth hormone and bromocryptine on mammary growth and morphology. *Animal Production*, **42**, 53–63.

Johnsson, I. D. & Obst, J. M. (1984). The effects of level of nutrition before and after eight months of age on the subsequent milk production and calf yield of beef heifers over three lactations. *Animal Production*, **38**, 57–68.

Johnston, J. M. & Amico, J. A. (1986). A prospective, longitudinal study of the release of oxytocin and prolactin in response to infant suckling in long-term lactation. *Journal of Clinical Endocrinology and Metabolism*, **62**, 653–7.

Karg, H. & Schams, D. (1974). Prolactin release in cattle. *Journal of Reproduction and Fertility*, **39**, 463–72.

Karg, H., Schams, D. & Reinhardt, U. (1972). Effects of 2-Br-α-ergocryptine on plasma prolactin level and milk yields in cows. *Experientia*, **28**, 574–6.

Keshet, E., Rosner, A., Bernstein, Y., Gorecki, M. & Aviv, H. (1981). Cloning of bovine growth hormone gene and its expression in bacteria. *Nucleic Acid Research*, **9**, 19–30.

Kleinberg, D. L., Todd, J., Babitsky, G. & Greising, J. (1982). Estradiol inhibits prolactin-induced α-lactalbumin production in normal primate mammary tissue *in vitro. Endocrinology*, **110**, 279–81.

Koprowski, J. A. and Tucker, H. A. (1973). Serum prolactin during various physiological states and its relationship to milk production in the bovine. *Endocrinology*, **92**, 1480–7.

Krulich, L., Kuhn, E., Illner, P. & McCann, S. M. (1970). Blood prolactin levels in lactating rats. *Federation Proceedings*, **29**, 579 (Abstr.).

Kuhn, N. J. (1977). Lactogenesis: the search for the trigger mechanisms in different species. *Symposia of the Zoological Society London*, **41**, 156–92.

Kulski, J. K., Smith, M. & Hartmann, P. E. (1977). Perinatal concentrations of progesterone, lactose and α-lactalbumin in the mammary secretion of women. *Journal of Endocrinology*, **74**, 509–10.

Kwa, M. G. & Verhofstad, F. (1968). Studies based on radioimmunoassay of prolactin. In *Progress in Endocrinology*. Gaul, C., ed., pp. 979–83, Amsterdam: Excerpta Medica.

Little, W. & Harrison, R. D. (1981). Effects of different rates of live-weight gain during rearing on the performance of Friesian heifers in their first lactation. *Animal Production*, **32**, 362 (Abstr).

Lyons, W. R. (1958). Hormonal synergism in mammary growth. *Proceedings of the Royal Society. B.*, **149**, 303–325.

Lyons, W. R. & Dixon, J. S. (1966). The physiology and chemistry of mammotropic hormones. In *The Pituitary Gland*. Harris, G. W. & Donovan, B. T., eds, vol. 1, pp. 527–581, London: Butterworth.

Lyons, W. R., Li, C. H. & Johnson, R. E. (1953). The hormonal control of mammary growth. *Recent Progress in Hormone Research*, **14**, 219–48.

McClymont, G. L. & Vallance, S. (1962). Depression of blood glycerides and milk fat synthesis by glucose infusion. *Proceedings of the Nutrition Society*, **21**, xii (Abst.).

McNeilly, A. S., Robinson, I. C. A. F., Houston, M. J. & Howie, P. W. (1983). Release of oxytocin and prolactin in response to suckling. *British Medical Journal*, **286**, 646–7.

Markham, G. (1660). *The English House-wife*. Printed by W. Wilson for E. Brewster and G. Sawbridge, at the Bible on Ludgate-Hill, near Fleetbridge, London.

Marshall, F. H. A. (1910). *The Physiology of Lactation*, pp. 553–585, London: Longmans, Green.

Martin, C. E., Hartmann, P. E. & Gooneratne, A. (1978). Progesterone and corticosteroids in the initiation of lactation in the sow. *Australian Journal of Biological Science*, **31**, 517–26.

Nagasawa, H. & Meites, J. (1970). Suppression by ergocornine and iproniazid of carcinogen-induced mammary tumors in rats; effects on serum and pituitary prolactin levels. *Proceedings of the Society for Experimental Biology and Medicine*, **135**, 469–72.

Nandi, S. (1959). Hormonal control of mammogenesis and lactogenesis in the C3H/He Crgl mouse. *University of California Publications in Zoology*, **65**, 1–128.

Ostrom, K. M. (1990). A review of prolactin during lactation. *Progress in Food and Nutrition Science*, **14**, 1–43.

Ott, I. & Scott, J. C. (1910). The action of infundibulin upon the mammary secretion. *Proceedings of the Society for Experimental Biology and Medicine*, **8**, 48–9.

Parau, D. (1975). *Studien zur Kulturgeschüchte des Milchenzugs*. Kempten/Allgau: Volkerschwirtschaftlicher Verlag.

Peel, C. J. & Bauman, D. E. (1987). Somatrotopin and lactation. *Journal of Dairy Science*, **70**, 474–86.

Peeters, G., Massart, L. & Coussens, R. (1947). L'éjection de lais chez les bovides. *Archives Internationales de Parmacodynamie et de la Therapie*, **75**, 85–9.

Pritchard, D. E., Hafs, H. D., Tucker, H. A., Boyd, L. J., Purchas, R. W. & Huber, J. T. (1972). Growth, mammary, reproductive and pituitary hormone characteristics of Holstein heifers fed extra grain and melengesterol acetate. *Journal of Dairy Science*, **55**, 995–1004.

Rillema, J. A. (1980). Mechanism of prolactin action. *Federation Proceedings*, **39**, 2593–8.

Rimoin, D. L., Holtzman, G. B., Merimee, T. J., Rabinowitz, D., Barnes, A. C., Tyson, J. E. A. & McKusick, V. A. (1968). Lactation in the absence of human growth hormone. *Journal of Clinical Endocrinology and Metabolism*, **28**, 1183–8.

Schams, D., Reinhardt, V. & Karg, H. (1972). Effects of 2-Br-α-ergokryptine on plasma prolactin level during parturition and onset of lactation in cows. *Experientia*, **28**, 697–9.

Sejrsen, K. (1978). Mammary development and milk yield in relation to growth rate in dairy and dual-purpose heifers. *Acta Agriculturae Scandinavica*, **28**, 41–6.

Sejrsen, K., Huber, J. T. & Tucker, H. A. (1983). Influence of amount fed on hormone concentrations and their relationship to mammary growth in heifers. *Journal of Dairy Science*, **66**, 845–55.

Sejrsen, K., Huber, J. T., Tucker, H. A. & Akers, R. M. (1982). Influence of nutrition of mammary development in pre- and postpubertal heifers. *Journal of Dairy Science*, **65**, 793–800.

Shiu, R. P. C. & Friesen, H. G. (1980). Mechanism of action of prolactin in the control of mammary gland function. *Annual Review of Physiology*, **42**, 83–96.

Simpson, E. R. & MacDonald, P. C. (1981). Endocrine physiology of the placenta. *Annual Review of Physiology*, **43**, 163–88.

Sinha, Y. N. & Tucker, H. A. (1969). Mammary development – pituitary prolactin level of heifers from birth through puberty and during the oestrous cycle. *Journal of Dairy Science*, **52**, 507–12.

Stricker, P. & Grueter, F. (1928). Action due lobe anterieur de l'hypophyse sur la monte laiteuse. *Compte Rendu Seance Société Biologie*, **99**, 1978–80.

Stricker, P. & Grueter, F. (1929). Recherches experimentales sur le fonctions du lobe anterieur sur la appareil genital de la lapine et sur la montée laiteuse. *Presse Medicin*, **37**, 1268–71.

Sutton, J. D., Hart, I. C., Morant, S. V., Schuller, E. & Simmonds, A. D. (1988). Feeding frequency for lactating cows: diurnal patterns of hormones and metabolites in peripheral blood in relation to milk-fat concentration. *British Journal of Nutrition*, **60**, 265–74.

Sutton, J. D., Hart, I. C., Broster, W. H., Elliot, R. J. & Schuller, E. (1986). Feeding frequency for lactating cows: effects on rumen fermentation and blood metabolites and hormones. *British Journal of Nutrition*, **56**, 181–92.

Sutton, J. D., Broster, W. H., Napper, D. J. & Siviter, J. W. (1985). Feeding frequency for lactating cows: effects on digestion, milk production and energy utilization. *British Journal of Nutrition*, **53**, 117–30.

Swanson, E. W. (1960). Effect of rapid growth with fattening of dairy heifers on their lactational ability. *Journal of Dairy Science*, **43**, 377–87.

Talamantes, F. (1975). *In vitro* demonstration of lactogenic activity in the mammalian placenta. *American Zoologist*, **15**, 279–84.

Talamantes, F., Ogren, L., Markoff, E., Woodward, S. & Madrid, J. (1980). Phylogenetic distribution, regulation of secretion and prolactin-like effects of placental lactogens. *Federation Proceedings*, **39**, 2582–7.

Taylor, J. C. & Peaker, M. (1975). The effects of bromocryptine on milk secretion in the rabbit. *Journal of Endocrinology*, **67**, 313–14.

Tindal, J. S. & Yokoyama, A. (1960). Bioassay of milk-ejection hormone (oxytocin) in body fluids in relation to the milk ejection reflex. pp. 52–53. Report. National Institute for Research in Dairying, Reading.

Turner, C. W. & Slaughter, I. S. (1930). The physiological effect of pituitary extract (posterior lobe) on the lactating mammary gland. *Journal of Dairy Science*, **13**, 8–24.

Tyson, J. E., Friesen, H. G. & Anderson, M. S. (1972). Human milk secretion after TRH induced prolactin release. *Excerpta Medica. International Congress Series*, **263**, 396–403.

Tyson, J. E., Friesen, H. G. & Anderson, M. S. (1973). Human lactational and ovarian response to endogenous prolactin release. *Science*, **177**, 897–9.

Tyson, J. E., Khojandi, M., Huth, J. & Andreasson, B. (1975). The influence of prolactin secretion on human lactation. *Journal of Clinical Endocrinology and Metabolism*, **40**, 764–73.

Venturini, P. L., Horowski, R., Maganza, C., Morano, S., Pedretti, E., Ragni, N., Semino, F. & DeCecco, L. (1981). Effects of lisuride and bromocryptine on inhibition of lactation and serum prolactin levels: comparative double blind study. *European Journal of Obstetrics, Gynecology and Reproductive Biology*, **11**, 395–400.

Youatt, W. (1838). *Cattle, Their Breeds, Management and Diseases*. London: Baldwin and Cradock.

21

Fundamental interactions between nutrition and growth

DAVID LISTER

Prenatal development

Life begins at 40, or so the old saying goes, but for the mammalia it starts with the fertilisation of an ovum. From the earliest free living stages, the fertilised ovum and blastocyst require nutrients. Pyruvate is the prime nutrient at this stage and is supplied in the secretions of the oviduct. Later, glucose, protein and minerals become increasingly important and these are contained in uterine milk. Implantation secures the supply of oxygen and nutrients, at first by inter-cell transfer and later via the placenta and amniotic sac. Then begins a rapid phase of growth which, for the most part, is genetically and not nutritionally controlled and determines the characteristic birth weights of different species (Widdowson & Lister, 1991).

The actual weight at birth is a measure of the mother's ability to supply nutrients to the developing young and the observation holds true from mice to men, though the mechanisms whereby the control is exercised are many and varied. The position that a fetus occupies in the uterus, and the proximity of other placentae are all important in this regard, especially in rodents (Eckstein, McKeown & Record, 1955; McLaren & Michie, 1960), and probably exert their main influence through variations in blood supply. There are signs that the placenta loses its efficiency towards term which on occasion can cause fetal growth retardation. The detail for this is covered by Robinson (this volume p. 203).

Size and maturity at birth

It is well recognised that individual animals in a litter can vary enormously in weight. Appleton (1929) was one of the first to look at this aspect of growth and he chose bone development as the criterion of maturity. When food is plentiful there is rapid bone growth and development of the centres of ossification. Poor nutrition slows both. So, at the same age a larger animal will be more mature skeletally than a smaller one. At the same size, however, a more rapidly growing animal will be less mature in chemical terms than its slower growing and older counterpart.

Appleton's criterion for assessing fetal development was the amount of calcium deposited in the epiphyses and shafts of the bones. Dickerson and Widdowson (1960*a*) showed that the principles linking maturity and size also hold true for postnatal development. Moreover, there are comparable changes in the amounts and proportions of other chemical constituents of the body which long before had been identified as the body's chemical maturity (Moulton, 1923). Typical of these changes are the increase in protein and fat and the decrease in body water, attributable to the fall in the extracellular compartment. The concentration of potassium, nitrogen, phosphorus and magnesium, which are contained mainly in the cells, increases as development proceeds and the concentration of the extra-cellular ions, sodium and chloride, falls (Dickerson & Widdowson, 1960*b*). The percentage of glycogen in the tissues increases during fetal growth; cardiac glycogen may be important for the immediate survival of the newborn, for example, during periods of anoxia, and the glycogen contained in other tissues, e.g. liver and skeletal muscle, is valuable in the neonatal period before a feeding routine is established, or under en-vironmental stress (McCance & Widdowson, 1959). Some species such as the pig show great reliance on liver and muscle glycogen which fortunately they hold in abundance, for they have no fat to metabolise during early life when they are first exposed to a cold extrauterine existence. Calves and lambs carry some fat at birth which they can use for energy supply for a short period after birth. Prolonged or severe cold will eventually exhaust these reserves and without food the animals will die in hypothermia. Human babies can draw on both carbohydrate and fat but will suffer the same fate if food is not soon forthcoming. Brown fat, rich in mitochondria, is present in quantity in rabbits and guinea pigs and in smaller amounts in other species to support non-shivering thermogenesis and the maintenance of body temperature

Both water, and fat-soluble vitamins are stored by the fetus. The water-soluble vitamins are in greater concentration in fetal than maternal tissues and so their transfer from mother to fetus, across the concentration gradient, depends on active transport. In some species, though not farm animals to any degree, gamma globulins pass to the fetus to confer passive immunity on newborn animals. Farm animals receive the bulk of their immunoglobulins in colostrum shortly after birth.

Developing an appropriate level of chemical and physiological maturity is clearly of importance for survival in the perinatal period and establishing the potential for future growth. Differences between individuals of different size in a litter, for example, are, however, not very great (Widdowson, 1974a), which suggests that chronology is more important than weight in regard to biochemical development. Wallace (1948) and Palsson and Vergés (1952) amongst many others have looked at size and development at birth in relation to nutrition in pregnancy. There are effects on the internal organs and some changes in carcase composition, especially in the amount of muscle, but again, in proportional terms they are not very great. Brain development seems to progress largely unimpeded.

Nutrition of the newborn

Survival in the period immediately after birth is largely a function of the stores of nutrients with which the animal is born. Continued survival is dependent on the newborn's having access to food, usually mother's milk, within a short time after birth. For a lamb born on a bleak and wet hillside rapid access to milk is crucial despite the availability of body stores of glycogen and fat. Piglets are born with little or no fat and, though they may be housed in more sheltered accommodation, their liver and muscle glycogen is quickly metabolised and mother's milk or some equivalent must be provided. Human babies can tolerate extended periods without milk postpartum and some species, for example guinea pigs, may take solid food almost from birth, though they grow rather better if given access to their mother's milk.

Colostrum is the first food available to the young animal and it provides for protection against disease as well as nutrition in the form of milk proteins, lactose and fat. The immunoglobulin, gamma-globulin, in farm animals, is capable of absorption because the small intestine retains its permeability to macromolecules until shortly into the postnatal period. In man, 'closure', i.e. the cessation of permeability to proteins, coincides with birth whereas in other species it may not occur until 1–3 days later. The absorption and digestion of proteins is a major stimulus to the development of the digestive tract (Widdowson, Colombo & Artavanis, 1976).

Fat and carbohydrate digestion, on which early survival and con-solidation for further growth depend, are provided for by the activities of lipases and lactase in the mouth and/or digestive tract. The most important lipase is pregastric esterase which is found in the saliva of most suckling animals (Hamosh, 1979), including ruminants, whose need to digest fat is confined almost entirely to the suckling period. Lactase is found in the intestines of most young mammals, but only in man does it persist.

Early nutrition and subsequent growth

Birth is clearly a precarious time for an animal and weaning may be not much better. Small size at birth can prejudice survival and animals so affected may be less competitive during suckling. How then does such a disadvantaged individual fare subsequently?

Farmers have always viewed the runt animal with disdain, which suggests that runts may never make up the lost ground, and the scientific evidence from the classical 'runt pig', at any rate, supports this (Widdowson, 1971). But what, if any, are the general rules which regulate such interactions of food, growth and time (McCance, 1962)?

The most dramatic and, many would argue, informative experiments in this field were undertaken by McCance and his colleagues in Cambridge in the 1960s. From these experiments it was clear that there were critical periods in an animal's life when even quite short periods of undernutrition could have damaging effects on subsequent growth. Moreover, it was discovered that the earlier any growth setback occurred the greater its potential for permanent harm. Using rats, which are born small and immature after a short gestation, and pigs whose diets can be controlled for long periods from shortly after birth, it proved possible to identify key relationships between nutrition and growth which may have implications across the mammalia.

Newborn rats may be taken from their mothers shortly after birth, pooled with others and re-allocated so that some mothers are given only 3 to rear and others about 15. When the groups are weaned three weeks later, the reduced food intake of the individuals reared in groups of 15 is shown up by their small size which permanently influences their development and they become small adults. If normally reared rats are weaned at 3 weeks of age on to limited amounts of food, their growth is depressed and even when they are restored to full feeding at 6 weeks, again their final size is small. Animals which are fed less between 6 and 9 weeks of age show better recovery and rats whose growth is retarded between 9–12 weeks will recover their growth deficit completely (Widdowson & McCance, 1963).

Given the rat's immaturity at birth it may well be that any comparable critical period of growth occurs in larger mammals at a physiological stage which is confined to gestation so that the individual born small remains small. The guinea pig is born at a very mature stage of development and can be weaned to an independent life almost immediately. The size of the young at birth can be profoundly altered by varying the mother's diet and the young born small will remain so even on the best of diets (Lister & McCance, 1965).

McCance and Widdowson's research on undernourished and rehabilitated pigs (McCance, 1960) took these findings further to show that, if the period of undernutrition after birth was sufficiently severe and prolonged the final size of their experimental pigs could be very small. Provided they are kept warm and free from disease and parasites, pigs can be maintained on small amounts of a complete diet such that their weights remain within a range of 5–10 kg or so for upwards of a year. After this time restoration to *ad libitum* feeding allows them to grow and eventually to reproduce quite successfully. The growth of the pigs is, however, influenced by the particular pattern of undernutrition they experienced. Rehabilitation after 1 year's undernutrition allowed the pigs to grow quite successfully and they reached a size approximately 80 % of what control animals might reach. They stopped growing at an age similar to that at which normally fed animals reached their final size although the epiphyses of their long bones had not closed, which is the event usually responsible for the cessation of growth. The rehabilitated pigs failed to reach the size of control animals because they neither grew at a slower rate for a longer period nor grew more rapidly to compensate for the lost period of growth they had suffered. Pigs which were undernourished for 2 years reached only 70 % of their normal adult expectation for much the same reasons. Despite their being undernourished for 3 years, the usual period during which a pig reaches its adult size, this group continued to grow for a further 6 months and grew to about half the normal size (Widdowson, 1974*b*).

Poultry can be underfed and rehabilitated in a similar way and, though some may be undernourished for 6 months, the usual growth period for a fowl, they will grow satisfactorily on rehabilitation to reach sizes approximately 90 % of normal.

Thus growth in pigs and poultry may be confined within certain chronological limits, but under extreme conditions this period may be extended, though there is some cost to final size.

In man, short periods of growth restriction during illnesses or temporary undernutrition may well be followed by complete recovery unless they occur at a critical time, for example, at puberty (Morant, 1950). But mild undernutrition is known to extend the period of growth, although if full stature is not reached by the ages of 24–26 years, it never will be (Morant, 1950; Oppers, 1963). The well-known secular trends in man's adult height show the decreasing age at final height, but it may well be that people of 18 years nowadays are not as different as supposed if the comparison is made with their forebears at 26.

Growth and body composition

Kleiber (1961) chose to demonstrate the reliance of animals on the same physiological and biochemical processes for energy transduction by showing that, irrespective of differences in size and metabolism, rabbits (in number) would produce the same yield of meat as a cow given the same amount of food. Though the proposition is, no doubt, an over-simplification, the consistency of the proportionality of tissue development amongst farm animals, even those which experienced extremes of nutrition (Lister, 1980), suggests that the energetics of somatic development will not be very different. What is different is the stage of growth at which particular proportions of fat, muscle or bone are reached. So-called early maturing somatotypes will be fat at an early stage of development; others, late maturing types, will remain lean to advanced stages of growth. Chinese and Pietrain pigs are classical examples of these, but Downland and hill sheep or Hereford and Ayrshire cattle also support the notion. Changing the production characteristics of a farm animal by breeding (though nutritional manipulations can be almost as effective) relies largely on modifying its ability to deposit lean tissue, usually by adjusting mature lean body size, and by changing its maturity, i.e. the earliness or lateness of the fat depositing phase of growth (Fowler, 1976).

Another feature of maturity in relation to fat deposition, which was identified scientifically by the middle nineteenth century (Lawes & Gilbert, 1859), is the partitioning of fat in the carcass. Early maturity is associated with subcutaneous fat deposition; late maturity with internal fat development (see Lister, 1980). The genetic basis of all this may be relevant to man (Bouchard et al., 1990).

An aspect of fatness which is part of farming folk lore has stimulated much interest in recent years. The farm animal in poor/thin condition is notorious for being less fertile or fecund, and 'flushing' (a period of plentiful feed) has long been known to correct matters. Frisch (1984) has made extensive studies of the relationship between the fatness of women, and their age at menarche and maintenance of reproductive cycling. She considers that there is a threshold ratio of fat to leanness below which reproductive ability cannot be initiated or maintained and that many modern women, but especially athletes and others indulging in strenuous activities, maintain body compositions which are balanced around this threshold, and their oestrous cycling is critically influenced. Kirkwood and Aherne (1985) have reviewed the anatomical and physiological features of this in farm animal reproduction and, though the general picture is comparable, the detail differs.

Some thoughts for the future

The energetics of growth and development in farm animals have been richly researched by Blaxter, Kielanowski, Mount, Thorbek, and van Es amongst many others (see Mount, 1980). Of late, however, for a variety of reasons this area of research has fallen out of favour, yet it needs to be progressed if the potential benefits from the new biotechnologies are to be reaped. Much more still needs to be known about the ways in which, in general, the physiological and metabolic pathways are integrated to produce the variety of patterns of growth and development on which the life cycle itself depends.

Webster (1989) argues that the modification of animal growth and development may require the involvement of only a few key bioenergetic variables, and knowing how different physiological types of animal create their particular somatotypes provides the necessary information. Deer are lean largely because of their high metabolic rate; lean pigs may be so because of a reduced intake of metabolisable energy (ME). Zucker rats adjust their intake of ME to satisfy their genetic potential for lean growth; fat deposition depends more on the energy:protein ratio in their diets. Knowing this might make for a more rational approach to technological innovation in animal production. β-agonists have received wide attention on account of their effectiveness in creating lean carcasses, which is largely attributable to their ability to restrict fat deposition rather than to promote lean deposition. An improvement in diet quality could be equally effective. Porcine somatotropin, on the other hand, promotes lean and decreases fat deposition but with no change in heat production. Somatotropin would, therefore, seem to provide a logical and effective means of increasing the efficiency of production of lean meat and justifies considering novel technologies for delivering the hormone into animals whether as the exogenous hormone or, say, transgenically.

Somatotropin and β-agonists are, in many ways, a bonus for animal production from researches in other fields. Further research into the integration of nutrition and growth, and more importantly the nervous and hormonal pathways which integrate them, could provide a rich harvest. The author (Lister, 1980) looked for clues for the ways in which such integration might be recognised and the specific pathways involved. He suggested that the partition of fat in the carcase might indicate the consequences of different thresholds of sympathetic nervous sensitivity and a possible basis for the control of metabolically important, e.g. thyroid, functions. Further research into these and comparable fields could provide new opportunities for exploitation via the novel biotechnologies.

References

Appleton, A. B. (1929). The relation between the rate of growth and the rate of ossification in the foetus of the rabbit. (Preliminary communication). *Compte Rendu de l'Association des Anatomistes*, 24th Meeting, Bordeaux, pp. 3–25.

Bouchard, C., Tremblay, A., Despré, J. P., Nadeau, A., Lupien, P. J., Therianet, G., Dessault, J., Moojani, S., Pinault, S. & Fourier, G. (1990). The response to long term over-feeding in identical twins. *New England Journal of Medicine*, **322**, 1477–82.

Dickerson, J. W. T. & Widdowson, E. M. (1960*a*). Some effects of accelerating growth. II. Skeletal development. *Proceedings of the Royal Society, London*, B, **152**, 207–17.

Dickerson, J. W. T. & Widdowson, E. M. (1960*b*). Chemical changes in skeletal muscle during development. *Biochemical Journal*, **74**, 247–53.

Eckstein, P., McKeown, T. & Record, R. G. (1955). Variation in placental weight according to litter size in the guinea pig. *Journal of Endocrinology*, **12**, 108–14.

Fowler, V. R. (1976). Some aspects of energy utilization for the production of lean tissue in the pig. *Proceedings of the Nutrition Society*, **35**, 75–9.

Frisch, R. E. (1984). Body fat, puberty and fertility. *Biological Reviews*, **59**, 161–88.

Hamosh, M. (1979). The role of lingual lipase in neonatal fat digestion. In *Development of Mammalian Absorptive Processes*. CIBA Foundation Symposium, **70**, 69–98 (N.S.). Amsterdam: Excerpta Medica.

Kirkwood, R. N. & Aherne, F. X. (1985). Energy intake, body composition and reproductive performance of the gilt. *Journal of Animal Science*, **60**, 1518–29.

Kleiber, M. (1961). *The Fire of Life*. New York: Wiley.

Lawes, J. B. & Gilbert, J. H. (1859). Experimental enquiry into the composition of some of the animals fed and slaughtered as human food. *Philosophical Transactions of the Royal Society*, **149**, 493–678.

Lister, D. (1980). Hormones, metabolism and growth. *Reproduction, Nutrition et Développement*, **20**, 225–33.

Lister, D. & McCance, R. A. (1965). The effect of two diets on the growth, reproduction and ultimate size of guinea pigs. *British Journal of Nutrition*, **19**, 311–19.

McCance, R. A. (1960). Severe undernutrition in growing and adults animals. 1. Production and general effects. *British Journal of Nutrition*, **14**, 59–74.

McCance, R. A. (1962). Food, growth and time. *Lancet*, **ii**, 671–6.

McCance, R. A. & Widdowson, E. M. (1959). The effect of lowering the ambient temperature on the metabolism of the newborn pig. *Journal of Physiology*, **147**, 124–34.

McLaren, A. & Michie, D. (1960). Congenital runts. In *CIBA Foundation Symposium on Congenital Malformations*, pp. 178–194, London.

Morant, S. B. (1950). Secular changes in the heights of British people. *Proceedings of the Royal Society, London, B*, **137**, 443–52.

Moulton, C. R. (1923). Age and chemical development in mammals. *Journal of Biological Chemistry*, **57**, 79–97.

Mount, L. E. (1980). ed. *Energy metabolism*. European Association of Animal Production Publication 26. London: Butterworths.

Oppers, V. M. (1963). Analyse van de acceleratie van de menselijke lengtegroei door bepaling van het kjdstip van de groefasen. MD Thesis, University of Amsterdam.

Palsson, H. & Vergés, J. B. (1952). Effects of plane of nutrition on growth and development of carcass quality in lambs. I. The effect of high and low planes of nutrition at different ages. *Journal of Agricultural Science*, **42**, 1–92.

Wallace, L. R. (1948). The growth of lambs before and after birth in relation to the level of nutrition. Part 1. *Journal of Agricultural Science*, **38**, 93–153.

Webster, A. J. F. (1989). Bioenergetics, bioengineering and growth. *Animal Production*, **48**, 249–69.

Widdowson, E. M. (1971). Intrauterine growth in the pig. 2. Organ size and cellular development at birth and after growth to maturity. *Biology of the Neonate*, **19**, 329–40.

Widdowson, E. M. (1974*a*). Immediate and long-term consequences of being large or small at birth: a comparative approach. In *Size at Birth. CIBA Foundation Symposium*, **27**, (N.S) pp. 65–76, Amsterdam: Associated Scientific Publishers.

Widdowson, E. M. (1974*b*). Changes in pigs due to undernutrition before birth and for one, two and three years afterwards and the effects of rehabilitation. In *Advances in Experimental Medicine and Biology*. Roche, A. F. & Falkner, F. ed. vol. 49, pp. 165–181. New York: Plenum Press.

Widdowson, E. M., Colombo, V. E. & Artavanis, C. A. (1976). Changes in the organs of pigs in response to feeding for the first 24 h after birth. 2. The digestive tract. *Biology of the Neonate*, **28**, 272–81.

Widdowson, E. M. & Lister, D. (1991). Nutritional control of growth. In *Growth Regulation in Farm Animals*. vol. 7. Advances in meat research. Pearson, A. M. & Dutson, T. R., eds, pp. 67–100, London: Elsevier.

Widdowson, E. M. & McCance, R. A. (1963). The effect of finite periods of undernutrition at different ages on the composition and subsequent development of the rat. *Proceedings of the Royal Society, London, B*, **158**, 329–42.

22

Opportunities for the manipulation of nutrition and growth

PETER J. REEDS, MARTA I. FIOROTTO and
WILLIAM C. HEIRD

Approximately 20% of all the papers published in the *British Journal of Nutrition* have been indexed under growth and at least half of these investigations involve specific studies of nutrient/growth interactions. Growth (usually assessed as weight gain) has been used as an important index of dietary adequacy throughout the history of nutrition research. Indeed, the observation that growth is not sustained in the absence of an essential nutrient was a critical part of early nutrition research aimed at the identification of essential nutrients.

Once the major essential organic nutrients were identified, attention turned to quantitative studies whose aim was to define dietary allowances that would support either 'normal' or 'optimal' growth of farm and laboratory animals and that of normal (e.g. Snyderman *et al.*, 1964) and low birth weight (see Heird, 1989) infants and children recovering from protein-energy malnutrition (e.g. Ashworth *et al.*, 1968; Rutishauser & McCance, 1968). In reviewing this period, it is interesting to note that as the premise of what constituted 'optimal growth' changed (see Reeds & Fiorotto, 1990), so did the nature of nutrition recommendations. This evolution is well illustrated by the changes in the feeding recommendations for low birth weight infants (Heird, 1989).

Before 1945, low birth weight infants were generally fed human milk. However, Gordon, Levine & McNamara (1947) demonstrated that substantial increases in *weight gain* could be achieved by offering these infants cow's milk formulas which contained a higher concentration of protein than that found in human milk. Thus, feeding recommendations for the next decade tended to stress absolutely weight gain as the most important objective of feeding, and emphasised the use of high protein formulas. During this time, however, continuing research demonstrated the metabolic and functional immaturity of low birth weight infants, and

Table 22.1. *Relationships between protein (PI) and energy (EI) intake, weight gain (WG), energy (EB) and protein (PB) balance in low birth weight (LBW) infants, growing malnourished children (PEM), and growing pigs receiving different quantities of the same diet*

Group		
Weight gain		
LBW 1	WG = 3.1 (PI) + 0.026 (EI) − 6	$R^2 = 0.82$
PEM	WG = 0.7 (PI) + 0.028 (EI) − 24	$R^2 = 0.84$
Pig	WG = 0.12 (PI) + 0.041 (EI) − 14	$R^2 = 0.94$
Protein gain		
LBW 1	PB = 0.70 (PI) + 0.2	$R^2 = 0.86$
PEM	PB = 0.74 (PI) − 1.3	$R^2 = 0.91$
Pig	PB = 0.73 (PI) − 2.1	$R^2 = 0.86$
Energy gain		
LBW 1	EB = 0.69 (EI) − 130	$R^2 = 0.90$
2	EB = 0.50 (EI) − 65	$R^2 = 0.75$
Pig	EB = 0.66 (EI) − 340	$R^2 = 0.95$

Weight gain and protein balance are expressed in g and energy intake and balance in kJ. All values have been normalised to kg (body weight)$^{0.75}$.

References: LBW 1 Heird *et al.* (1987).

        2 Cauderay *et al.* (1988); Catzeflis *et al.* (1985).

    PEM   Ashworth *et al.* (1968); M. H. N. Golden (personal communication).

    Pig   Reeds & Fuller (unpublished observations).

they were no longer perceived merely as small, full-term infants. Further studies also showed that the ingestion of protein in excess of 4.5 g/kg/day conferred no additional benefit in terms of weight gain. Consideration of this finding, when taken together with concerns over the potentially deleterious effects of excessive protein intakes in infants with immature renal function (McCance, 1950), led to progressively lower recommended protein intakes.

Over this period, however, the available information on the rate and composition of human intrauterine growth increased (Widdowson & Dickerson, 1964; Widdowson, Southgate & Hey, 1979). Attention therefore turned to the nutrients needed to achieve both normal body weight and composition at 40 weeks gestational age. As it became evident that the energy and protein densities of human milk were insufficient to achieve these objectives, a variety of special formulae was developed. The investigation of the effectiveness of these artificial milks, in turn, enabled more precise definitions of appropriate intakes of protein and nonprotein energy to support any given rate of weight, protein, and lipid gain in low birth weight infants (Heird et al., 1987; Table 22.1).

The investigation of the relationships between protein intake, weight gain, and protein deposition is a surrogate for the investigation of the relationships between the intakes of specific amino acids and their incorporation into body protein. Recognition of the distinctive protein composition of human milk led to the humanisation of infant formulae by the 1970s (for discussion see Heine, Klein & Reeds, 1991) through their enrichment with bovine whey proteins. It was difficult to assess how well these formulae satisfied the obligatory amino acid needs of the growing low birth weight infant, however, until Widdowson *et al.* (1979) reported the amino acid composition of the human fetus.

Table 22.2 compares the results reported by Widdowson *et al.* (1979) with the amino acid composition of human milk. In this table the amino acids have been categorised under three headings: a) the classical essential amino acids, b) the nonessential amino acids, and c) a group of amino acids which in recent years has been termed 'conditionally essential' (Laidlaw & Kopple, 1987; Jackson, 1989, and this volume p. 92). Although the comparison suggests that the primary limitation to protein deposition is the supply of lysine, further consideration of the two amino acid patterns indicates other potential limitations of human milk to satisfy all the amino acid needs of low birth weight infants

The key feature of the conditionally essential amino acids is that their synthesis requires the provision of other amino acids as substrates, and there are circumstances in which the diet may supply insufficient quantities of these precursors. Furthermore, the immature organism may be incapable of synthesising the conditionally essential amino acids at a rate appropriate for the biological need. In either of these circumstances, there is a distinct dietary requirement for the respective 'conditionally essential' amino acids. Table 22.2 shows that human milk (and the milks of other species, see Heine *et al.*, 1991) is 'deficient' in glycine, arginine and, perhaps, cystine (cysteine). On the basis of their studies of nitrogen metabolism, Jackson *et al.* (1981) suggested that glycine supply may well be the major limiting factor in the ability of human milk-fed low birth weight infants to deposit protein.

Glycine, cysteine and arginine are not only deposited in body protein but are also precursors for the synthesis of compounds that are of substantial physiological importance. Glycine and arginine are obligatory precursors for creatine synthesis and glycine is the sole source of nitrogen for the

Table 22.2. *The amino acid pattern (mg amino acid per g total protein-bound amino acid) of foetal body protein compared with that of human milk*

	Foetus	Milk	M/F
Essential amino acids			
Lysine	70	62	0.88
Methionine	19	18	0.95
Phenylalanine	40	44	1.10
Threonine	40	46	1.15
Valine	46	60	1.30
Leucine	74	101	1.36
Tryptophan	(12)	18	1.50
Isoleucine	35	58	1.65
Non-essential amino acids			
Alanine	70	40	0.57
Aspartate	83	83	1.00
Serine	43	51	1.18
Glutamate	127	178	1.40
Conditionally essential amino acids			
Glycine	116	26	0.22
Arginine	74	40	0.54
Cystine	(17)	17	1.00
Proline	82	86	1.04
Histidine	23	26	1.13
Tyrosine	28	47	1.68

References: fetus, Widdowson *et al.* (1979); human milk; Renner (1983).

synthesis of haem. Furthermore, glycine and cysteine are the precursors for glutathione synthesis, and it is interesting to note that premature infants have low circulating glutathione concentrations (Hansen *et al.*, 1990). The low glutathione levels may reflect, in part, the restricted supply of glycine and cysteine. Metabolic considerations such as these have led to the notion that increased dietary provision of some specific amino acids (e.g. glycine and cysteine) may not only stimulate protein deposition, but also support the synthesis of important nonprotein end products of amino acid metabolism, particularly in the low birth weight infant. These biosynthetic pathways, therefore, should be considered as part of the protein requirement (Jackson, 1989; Reeds, 1990).

Growth manipulation

Although substantial alterations in the rate and composition of growth can be brought about by alterations to the diet, the relationship between energy and protein intake and the rate of protein deposition in the growing mammal is exponential in form. This is an indication of the fact that growth ultimately reaches a maximum value that is characteristic of the genotype of the individual. A considerable quantity of research has been devoted to attempts to alter this genetic potential. The earliest research concentrated on conventional breeding and one of the main effects of these breeding programmes was to produce animals with a larger body size (see Hammond, 1952; Falconer, 1973). By using the high anabolic drive of the immature mammal, progressively larger meat animals were slaughtered at progressively younger ages.

Concurrently, progress was being made in understanding the endocrinological factors responsible for the regulation of protein and lipid deposition within any genotype. This knowledge became increasingly important as the objective of growth manipulation in farm livestock switched from weight gain alone toward maximising protein deposition and manipulating the fat: protein ratio in the carcass.

In earlier work, the inherent differences in the growth and body composition of males and females of the same species led researchers to investigate the use of steroids (both oestrogenic and androgenic) to increase the rate of weight gain and protein deposition, particularly in castrates and females (e.g., Table 22.3). Volume 1 of the *British Journal of Nutrition* contained a paper from Braude (1947) on the use of synthetic steroids in altering the growth of pigs. Such attempts to manipulate the endocrinological status of animals to modify their growth also provided invaluable experimental approaches to understanding the endocrine regulation of the growth process itself.

The manipulation of the pituitary growth hormone (somatotropin) status of animals (Boyd and Bauman, 1989; Table 22.3) has proved to be the most successful practical application of the understanding of the endocrinological control of growth. Although the ability to insert mammalian genes into bacteria and hence to synthesise large quantities of 'recombinant' proteins was the key development in this area of study, developments in understanding of the mechanisms regulating growth hormone levels and actions at the cellular level also played a crucial part. Thus, while the earliest attempts to manipulate growth involved the injection of growth hormone, persistent alterations in endogenous growth

Table 22.3. *Effects of various growth promoting agents on protein and lipid accretion in farm livestock*

Agent	Protein deposition (%)	Lipid deposition (%)	
Trenbolone/estradiol	+100	−33	(Lobley *et al.*, 1985)
Growth hormone	+62	−51	(Campbell *et al.*, 1991)
Clenbuterol	+47	−50	(MacRae *et al.*, 1988)

hormone levels have also proved effective. Endogenous growth hormone levels have been manipulated both by injection of growth hormone releasing factor (Beerman *et al.*, 1990) and by immunising animals to inhibitors of growth hormone secretion such as somatostatin (Spencer, 1986). Most recently, as the key role of the insulin-like growth factors (IGF) in mediating the protein anabolic effects of growth hormone has become established, research has turned to the growth-stimulatory properties of IGF-I (Scheiwiller *et al.*, 1986; Lemmey *et al.*, 1990).

Separate from the ability to produce large quantities of potential growth stimulatory proteins, the 'new biology' of the last 15 years has been critical in the design of new methods for altering growth. Three developments in particular have proved to be of central importance: first, the ability to manipulate the genetic material of fertilised ova, resulting in the production of so-called transgenic animals; second, the appreciation of the key role of peptide growth factors that act in a paracrine manner to regulate differentiation and proliferation of specific cells (and hence regulate the potential mass of a given organ; Florini & Magri, 1989); and third, the rapidly increasing body of data on the nature of the genes that determine the differentiation of specific cells and hence the formation of specific organs and tissues (Weintraub *et al.*, 1991). Palmiter *et al.* (1982) reported that the growth of mice that bore multiple copies of the growth hormone gene was greatly increased, and this work was soon followed by successful attempts to manipulate growth hormone status by the production of animals bearing multiple copies of the growth hormone releasing factor gene (Hammer *et al.*, 1985). Most recently, transgenic animals that overproduce IGF-I have been developed (Mathews *et al.*, 1988); the animals also grew at an accelerated rate. This last attempt represents an approach that altered growth by manipulating the level of a trophic factor with a wide cellular specificity. It is now known that other peptide growth factors have highly specific sites of action and it is possible, in principle at least, to produce animals in which the allometry of growth has been altered by the introduction of multiple copies of such cell-specific factors. The muscle-specific effects of the β-adrenergic agonist growth promoting drugs (Reeds & Mersmann, 1991) show that such disruption of the tissue composition of protein accretion is possible.

One of the most exciting areas of study is the recent identification of genes whose protein products interact with the genome to determine the formation of specific tissues. The first report of a muscle determination gene, i.e. a gene whose product activates the differentiation programme of myoblasts, was in 1987 (Davis, Weintraub & Lasser, 1987). Since that time, at least six additional genes have been identified (Weintraub et al., 1991), including one that may be the key to the expression of the mature muscle phenotype (Miner & Wold, 1990). The potential of applying this knowledge to promote tissue-specific growth is exemplified in a recent paper. The authors reported that transgenic animals bearing multiple copies of a single regulatory gene (c-ski) demonstrate a most remarkable increase in type IIb muscle fibre diameter (Sutrave, Kelly & Hughes, 1990).

Space does not allow a detailed discussion of the potential influence of these various growth-promoting strategies on the nutrient requirements of the manipulated animals. However, there are some points which should be considered. First, the maximum efficiency with which any given dietary protein can be deposited is ultimately set by its amino acid composition (i.e. its biological value). It follows, therefore, that success of an intervention, designed to increase protein deposition without increasing protein intake (as was the case in the experiments summarised in Table 22.4), is achieved only if the preceding dietary protein use is less than the protein's biological value. This observation begs the question as to what underlies the lower efficiency of dietary protein utilisation in the control state.

The other major effect of these agents was to decrease the rate of fat deposition. Part of this response results from the inevitable reduction in the availability of 'surplus' amino acids to synthesise ATP. A reduced amino acid surplus in its turn demands the increased utilisation of nonprotein energy sources and hence a restriction in the carbon available for fat deposition. However, the relative degrees to which protein deposition was increased and fat deposition decreased varied amongst the three treatments (Table 22.4), which suggests that their mechanisms of action may be different. Whether or not this is true, the efficiency with which the growth hormone and clenbuterol-treated animals utilised their dietary non-protein

Table 22.4 *The relationship between the change in protein and fat carbon deposition with different growth-promoting agents*

Agent	Change in protein carbon	Change in fat carbon
	(g carbon/kg 0.75)	
Trenbolone	+0.6	−0.6
Growth hormone	+1.8	−5.3
Clenbuterol	+0.4	−1.5

References: LBW (TPN) Mitton and Garlick (personal communication).
LBW (Ent) Catzeflis *et al.* (1985); Cauderay *et al.* (1988).
PEM M. H. N. Golden (Personal communication).
Pigs Reeds *et al.* (1980).

energy was reduced and, to this extent, the energy requirements of the treated animals were increased.

We believe the impact of this variety of exogenous or genetic manipulations of growth potential on nutrient requirements remains undecided. Understanding the basis of these requirements offers new challenges to our understandings of the regulation of the efficiency of nutrient utilisation in general and of growth in particular.

Conclusion

Growth and nutrition are so closely intertwined that to separate them is, in many ways, artificial. Research in the areas of both growth and nutrition has become increasingly mechanistic. Nutrition research has moved from the identification of the essential nutrients through a period during which studies focused on quantitative aspects of the interaction between nutrient intake and growth. Throughout this time, however, a concern for the changes in metabolism that underlie the utilisation of the diet has grown stronger. For example, it is important to remember that much current knowledge on the hormonal regulation of cellular protein turnover, especially in man (Waterlow, 1984; Young, 1987 and this volume; Table 22.5) arose from nutrition questions. Research on growth regulation has followed a similar path and many studies are now concentrated on understanding the coordination of cellular differentiation and mass in the growing organism. These developments are leading to an increasing interest in the study of more subtle aspects of the interaction between the diet, cellular function, and gene expression. For example, over the last ten years there has been a continuing interest in the potential functional role of

Table 22.5 *Relationship between whole body protein synthesis and deposition in LBW infants, malnourished children (PEM) and young pigs*

Group	Slope	Intercept (g Protein/kg$^{0.75}$ per d)
LBW TPN	2.06 ± 0.20	7.4 ± 0.2
LBW Enteral	3.25 ± 0.78	1.3 ± 0.8
PEM	1.53 ± 0.15	7.4 ± 0.7
Pigs	1.90 ± 0.17	16.4 ± 1.2

References: LBW (TPN) Mitton and Garlick (personal communication).
LBW (Ent) Catzeflis *et al.* (1985); Cauderay *et al.* (1988).
PEM   M. H. N. Golden (personal communication).
Pigs   Reeds *et al.* (1980).

specific proteins and peptides in milk (e.g. Heird, 1989; Klagsbrun, 1978; Francis *et al.*, 1988; Nichols *et al.*, 1987). Our view of the make-up of nutrition is changing; diet is now being viewed, not only as a source of primary nutrients, but also as a source of more complex 'non-nutritional' factors which exert regulatory influences in their own right.

Acknowledgements

This work is a publication of the USDA/ARS Children's Nutrition Research Center, Department of Pediatrics, Baylor College of Medicine and Texas Children's Hospital, Houston, TX. This project has been funded in part with federal funds from the US Department of Agriculture, Agricultural Research Service under Cooperative Agreement number 58-6250-1-003. The contents of this publication do not necessarily reflect the views or policies of the US Department of Agriculture, nor does mention of trade names, commercial products, or organisations imply endorsement by the US Government.

References

Ashworth, A., Bell, R., James, W. P. T. & Waterlow, J. C. (1968). Calorie requirements of children recovering from protein-calorie malnutrition. *Lancet*, **ii** 600–3.
Beerman, D. J., Hogue, D. E., Fishell, V. K., Aronica, S., Dickson, H. W. & Schrikes, B. R. (1990). Exogenous human growth hormone-releasing factor and ovine somatotropin improve growth performance and composition of gain in lambs. *Journal of Animal Science*, **68**, 4122–33.
Boyd, R. D. & Bauman, D. E. (1989). Mechanisms of action for somatotrophin in growth. In *Current Concepts of Animal Growth Regulation*, Campion, D.,

Hausman, G. J. & Martin, R. J., eds, pp. 257–284, New York: Plenum Press.

Braude, R. (1947). Stimulation of growth and fattening of pigs by synthetic steroids. *British Journal of Nutrition*, **1**, iii.

Campbell, R. G., Johnson, R. J., Taverner, M. R. & King, R. H. (1991). Interrelationships between exogenous porcine somatotropin (PST) administration and dietary protein and energy intake on protein deposition capacity and energy metabolism of pigs. *Journal of Animal Science*, **69**, 1522–31.

Catzeflis, C., Schutz, Y., Micheli, J-L., Welsch, C., Arnaud, M. & Jequier, E. (1985). Whole body protein synthesis and energy expenditure in very low birth weight infants. *Pediatric Research*, **19**, 679–87.

Cauderay, M., Schutz, Y., Micheli, J-L., Calamie, A. & Jequier, E. (1988). Energy-nitrogen balances and protein turnover in small and appropriate for gestational age low birth weight infants. *European Journal of Clinical Nutrition*, **42**, 125–36.

Davis, D. L., Weintraub, H. & Lasser, A. B. (1987). Expression of a single transfected cDNA converts fibroblasts to myoblasts. *Cell*, **51**, 987–1000.

Falconer, D. S. (1973). Replicated selection for body weight in mice. *Genetic Research (Cambridge)*, **22**, 291–321.

Florini, J. R. & Magri, K. A. (1989). Effects of growth factors on myogenic differentiation. *American Journal of Physiology*, **256**, C701–11.

Francis, G. L., Upton, F. M., Ballard, F. J., McNeil, K. A. & Wallace, J. C. (1988). Insulin like growth factors I and 2 in bovine colostrum. *Biochemical Journal*, **251**, 95–103.

Gordon, H. H., Levine, S. J. & McNamara, H. (1947). Feeding of low birth weight infants: a comparison of human and cow's milk. *American Journal of the Diseases of Childhood*, **73**, 442–52.

Hammer, R. E., Brinster, R. L., Rosenfeld, M. G., Evans, R. M. & Mayo, K. E. (1985). Expression of human growth hormone-releasing factor in transgenic mice results in increased somatic growth. *Nature, London*, **315**, 413–16.

Hammond, J. (1952). Physiological limits to intensive production in animals. *British Agricultural Bulletin*, **4**, 222–4.

Hansen, T. N., Smith, C. V., Martin, N. E., Smith, H. W. & Elliot, S. J. (1990). Oxidant stress responses in ventilated newborn infants. *Pediatric Research*, **27**, 208A.

Heine, W. E., Klein, P. D. & Reeds, P. J. (1991). The importance of lactalbumin in infant nutrition. *Journal of Nutrition*, **121**, 277–83.

Heird, W. C. (1989). Advances in infant nutrition over the past quarter century. *Journal of the American College of Nutrition*, **8**, 22S–32S.

Heird, W. C., Kashyap, S., Schulze, K. F., Ramakrishnan, R., Zucker, C. L. & Dell, R. B. (1987). Nutrient utilization and growth in LBW infants. In *Human Lactation*. Goldman, A. S., Atkinson, S. A. & Hanson, L. A., eds, vol. III pp. 9–21, New York: Plenum Press.

Heird, W. C., Schwartz, S. M. & Hansen, I. H. (1984). Colostrum-induced enteric mucosal growth in beagle puppies. *Pediatric Research*, **18**, 512–15.

Jackson, A. A. (1989). Optimizing amino acid and protein supply and utilization in the newborn. *Proceedings of the Nutrition Society*, **48**, 293–301.

Jackson, A. A., Shaw, J. C. L., Barber, A. & Golden, M. H. N. (1981). Nitrogen metabolism in pre-term infants fed human donor breast milk: the possible essentiality of glycine. *Pediatric Research*, **15**, 1454–61.

Klagsbrun, M. (1978). Human milk stimulates DNA synthesis and cellular proliferation in cultured fibroblasts. *Proceedings of the National Academy of Sciences, USA*, **75**, 5057–61.

Laidlaw, S. A. & Kopple, J. D. (1987). Newer concepts of the indispensable amino acids. *American Journal of Clinical Nutrition*, **46**, 593–605.

Lemmey, A. B., Martin, A. A., Read, L. C., Tomas, F. M., Owens, P. C. and Ballard, F. J. (1990). IGF-I and the truncated analogue des-(1-3)-IGF-I enhance growth in rats after gut resection. *American Journal of Physiology*, **260**, E213–19.

Lobley, G. E., Connell, A., Mollison, G., Brewer, A., Harris, C. I., Buchan, V. & Galbraith, H. (1985) The effects of combined implant of trenbolone acetate and oestradiol-17β on protein and energy metabolism in finishing beef steers. *British Journal of Nutrition*, **54**, 681–94.

MacRae, J. C., Skene, P. A., Connel, A., Buchan, V. & Lobley, G. E. (1988). The action of the β-agonist clenbuterol on protein and energy metabolism in fattening wether lambs. *British Journal of Nutrition*, **59**, 457–65.

Mathews, L. S., Hammer, R. E., Behringer, R. R., D'Ercole, A. J., Bell, G. I., Brinster, R. L. & Palmiter, R. D. (1988). Growth enhancement of transgenic mice expressing human insulin-like growth factor-I. *Endocrinology*, **123**, 2827–33.

McCance, R. A. (1950). Renal physiology in infancy. *American Journal of Medicine*, **9**, 229–41.

Miner, J. H. & Wold, B. (1990). Herculin, a fourth member of the *MyoD* family of myogenic regulatory genes. *Proceedings of the National Academy of Sciences, USA*, **87**, 1089–93.

Nichols, B. L., McKee, K. S., Henry, J. F. & Putman, M. (1987). Human lactoferrin stimulates thymidine incorporation into DNA of rat crypt cells. *Pediatric Research*, **21**, 563–7.

Palmiter, R. D., Brinster, R. L., Hammer, R. E., Trumbauer, M. E., Rosenfeld, M. G., Birnberg, N. C. & Evans, R. M. (1982). Dramatic growth of mice that develop from eggs microinjected with metallothionine-growth hormone fusion genes. *Nature, London*, **300**, 611–15.

Reeds, P. J. (1990). Amino acid needs and protein scoring patterns. *Proceedings of the Nutrition Society*, **49**, 17–25.

Reeds, P. J., Cadenhead, A., Fuller, M. F., Lobley, G. E. & McDonald, J. D. (1980): Protein turnover in growing pigs. Effects of age and food intake. *British Journal of Nutrition*, **43**, 445–55.

Reeds, P. J. & Fiorotto, M. I. (1990). Growth in perspective. *Proceedings of the Nutrition Society*, **49**, 411–20.

Reeds, P. J. & Mersmann, H. J. (1991). Protein and energy requirements of animals treated with β-adrenergic agonists. A discussion. *Journal of Animal Science*, **69**, 1532–50.

Renner, E. (1983). *Milk and Dairy Products in Human Nutrition*. Regensburg, Germany: Friedrich Pustet.

Rutishauser, I. H. E. & McCance, R. A. (1968). Calorie requirements for growth after severe undernutrition. *Archives of Diseases in Childhood*, **43**, 252–6.

Scheiwiller, E., Guler, H-P., Merryweather, J., Scandella, C., Maerki, W., Zapf, J. & Froesch, E. R. (1986). Growth restoration of insulin-deficient diabetic rats by recombinant insulin-like growth factor I. *Nature (London)*, **323**, 169–2.

Snyderman, S. E., Boyer, A., Norton, P. M., Roitman, E. & Holt, L. E. (1964). The essential amino acid requirements of infants. *American Journal of Clinical Nutrition*, **15**, 313–30.

Spencer, G. S. G. (1986). Hormonal manipulation of animal production by immuno-neutralization. In *Control and Manipulation of Animal Growth.* Buttery, P. J., Lindsay, D. B. & Haynes, N. B., eds, pp. 279–292, London: Butterworths.

Sutrave, P., Kelly, A. M. & Hughes, S. H. (1990). *ski* can cause selective growth of skeletal muscle in transgenic mice. *Genes and Development,* **4,** 1462–72.

Waterlow, J. C. (1984). Protein turnover with special reference to man. *Quarterly Journal of Experimental Physiology,* **69,** 409–38.

Weintraub, H., Davis, R., Tapscott, S., Thayer, M., Krause, M., Benezra, R., Blackwell, T. K., Turner, D., Rupp, R., Hollenberg, S., Zhaung, Y. & Lassar, A. (1991). The *myoD* gene family; nodal point during specification of the muscle cell lineage. *Science (Washington),* **251,** 761–6.

Widdowson, E. M. & Dickerson, J. W. T. (1964). Chemical composition of the body. In *Mineral metabolism: an advanced treatise.* Comar, C. L. & Bronner, F., eds, vol. IIA, pp. 2–247, New York: Academic Press.

Widdowson, E. M., Southgate, D. A. T. & Hey, E. N. (1979). Body composition of the fetus and infant. In *Nutrition and Metabolism of the Fetus and Infant.* Visser, H. K. A., ed., pp. 169–177, The Hague: Martinus Nijhoff.

Young, V. R. (1987). Kinetics of human amino acid metabolism: Nutritional implications and some lessons. *American Journal of Clinical Nutrition,* **46,** 709–25.

23

Nutrition and human pregnancy

J. V. G. A. DURNIN

In the present context 'nutrition' is such a broad term, encompassing macro and micronutrients, that little pretence could be made to deal with the diversity of topics in any particularly enlightening way. Therefore, a very restricted critique will be essayed here of 'nutrition and human pregnancy' dealing mainly with energy and protein requirements and with some of the implications of these to the iron and calcium needs of the pregnant mother.

Energy

Superficially, the extra energy needs of pregnancy ought to be a problem of little complexity. Additions of many kinds are being made to the mother's body during pregnancy: the fetus is growing, the uterus increases in size, the placenta has to be formed, there is a considerable increase in body fluids including the blood, the breasts grow larger, and a variable amount of fat is deposited, primarily as an energy store for lactation and, possibly, for late pregnancy. All of these changes involve an energy cost and this has bene quantified for the various components by Hytten & Leitch (1971) and subsequently by Hytten & Chamberlain (1980), with more or less general acceptance of their calculations.

One large and highly variable constituent in this array is the amount of adipose tissue added to the mother's body. There is a certain amount of misuse of terms here, with a relatively small potential for calculation error since the extra weight of fat is deposited as adipose tissue (i.e. as chemical lipid together with the increase in cell membranes, connective tissue, and extracellular fluid), but if it is actually measured this measurement is of only the fat or chemical lipid. The energy cost of depositing these differs by 10–20 % – adipose tissue 'costing' about 8000–9000 kcal (33.5–37.7 MJ)/ kg whereas fat or lipid deposition has an equivalent value of 10000–11000 kcal (41.8–46.0 MJ)/kg. Since any attempt to measure the increase

Table 23.1. *Mean energy cost of pregnancy* (*kcal*)

	W (kg)	kcal
Fetus	3.5	8 300
Placenta	0.6	700
Uterus, fluids, breasts	5.0	3 000
Maternal fat	2.0	22 000
	(alternative 5.0)	(55 000)
Total		34 000 (67 000)
BMR		31 000 (31 000)
Grand total		65 000 (98 000)

Adapted from Hytten & Leitch (1971).

in maternal body *fat* involves procedures which do not estimate adipose tissue but only the lipid portion of the adipose tissue, then the energy cost of this is taken as 10 000–11 000 kcal (41.8–46.0 MJ)/kg.

Clearly large differences in the amount of fat added to the body during pregnancy will result in very different requirements of energy. Hytten & Chamberlain (1980) suggested 3.5 kg of fat as a reasonable average. At the present time, much obstetric advice recommends (indirectly) a fat gain of about 2–2.5 kg. On the other hand, in the USA a weight gain of 16–18 kg is advised (in order to reduce the likelihood of low birth weight babies) and this would almost certainly involve an addition of 5 kg of fat or more to the prepregnant body stores, with an energy cost of perhaps 60 000 kcal (251 MJ) upwards. The energy needed for these increases in fetal and maternal tissues thus involves a quantity varying from about 35 000 to 70 000 kcal (146–293 MJ).

In addition to this, the progressive increase in tissue mass results in a rise in BMR of about 31 000 kcal (130 MJ) over the whole of pregnancy, giving a grand total of increased energy of from 65 000 kcal (272 MJ) to almost 100 000 kcal (418 MJ) (Table 23.1). In fact, the increase might be more than this because the greater mass of the mother means that any movement or activity she undertakes will require a greater expenditure of energy.

The simple conclusion which might be made from the data is that, depending on whether 2 or 5 kg of fat have been added to the mother's body, she should need an extra 240 to 360 kcal (10–15 MJ)/d throughout the whole of pregnancy.

These simple calculations generate enormous emotional reactions without these reactions necessarily being based on more than hypothetical real-life situations, because the basic assumption often made is that the mother does not alter her behaviour markedly throughout pregnancy compared to the prepregnant state; and, it is postulated, even if sometimes she does, the allowances for pregnancy should be sufficient to cater for mothers who actually continue their normal prepregnant behaviour pattern. Therefore, many of the national and international recommendations about energy requirements for pregnancy suggest increments in energy intake large enough to cater for these energy costs.

One of the reasons why these recommendations have persisted so long is the difficulty and comparative scarcity of properly controlled scientific observations of the alterations in energy intake occasioned by pregnancy. Until recently, almost all such studies have been largely cross-sectional so that the same women have not been followed at different stages of pregnancy, the methodology has often not been of much precision, the numbers have been statistically inadequate to demonstrate reliable findings, and the first set of measurements of food intake has been done late in the first trimester instead of, ideally, in the prepregnant state.

Prepregnant measurements are necessary to provide a reliable baseline; food intake often falls from between gestational week 6–8 to week 12–14, presumably owing to morning sickness, so that any comparisons between intakes at that period and intakes in the second and third trimester may give misleading information.

However, in spite of that qualification, of the comparatively few studies which have been published where values are quoted for energy intakes at differing stages of pregnancy, only a minority seem to show any consistent augmentation. Table 23.2 gives a few illustrations of such data, and the overall impression is of little or no increase in energy intake.

This poses a conundrum which is difficult to solve. It might legitimately be supposed that in our industrialised society, where most people – men and women – lead a relatively sedentary existence, there would be little scope for the significant and considerable reduction in physical activity which would be necessary to effect the energy saving to allow the energy costs of pregnancy to proceed without an equivalent increase in energy intake. Even more persuasive, in many developing countries with a mainly rural economy, most women might be supposed to carry on working in the fields and tending their household with little apparent possibility to change activity right up to near delivery of the baby. Their energy costs, although probably consistently lower because of the smaller fat gain, would seem necessarily to be met either by an increased food intake or by an actual reduction in maternal body stores – muscle as well as fat. How is it, then,

Table 23.2. *Energy intakes during pregnancy*

Source	'n'		Gestation stage	Energy intake (Kcal/d)	
Grafe (1983)	89		5th month	2753	
			8th month	2755	
van der Rijst	499		1st trimester	2620	
(1962)			2nd trimester	2720	
			3rd trimester	2620	
English &	26		2nd trimester	2150	
Hitchcock (1968)			3rd trimester	2030	
Lunell, Persson & Sterky	58		1st trimester	2035	
(1969)			2nd trimester	2185	
			3rd trimester	2137	
Blackburn &	21		24 weeks	2065	
Calloway (1976)			33 weeks	1801	
			39 weeks	2000	
Doyle *et al.*	68		1st trimester	1613	
(1982)			2nd trimester	1723	
			3rd trimester	1772	
Whitehead *et al.*	25		2nd trimester	1950	
(1981)			3rd trimester	2005	
	Edin	*Lon*		*Edin*	*Lon*
Schofield, Wheeler &	85	53	1st trimester	2028	1953
Stewart	38	84	2nd trimester	2059	2199
(1987)	107	110	3rd trimester	1913	2172
Haste *et al.*		206	28 weeks	2017	
(1990)		178	36 weeks	1923	

that food intakes of pregnant women in the developing countries also do not demonstrate much change? The problem lies partly in deciding whether it is practically and physiologically possible for them to go through a normal pregnancy without markedly increasing food intake, and partly in the unsatisfactory available data. There has not been, until recently, reliable information either about the actual food intakes of an adequately sized sample of normal healthy women measured initially in the prepregnant state and then followed by serial measurements throughout pregnancy, or of their activity pattern to see whether energy savings occur.

An attempt was made to mount a study to fulfil all these requirements and almost 250 women participated in Scotland and Holland (Durnin, 1987; Van Raai *et al.*, 1987). A coordinated project using the same basic methodology was also done in The Gambia, Thailand and The Philippines. The detailed results of the Scottish study, with a brief summary of the

Energy increments (kcal) thoughout pregnancy

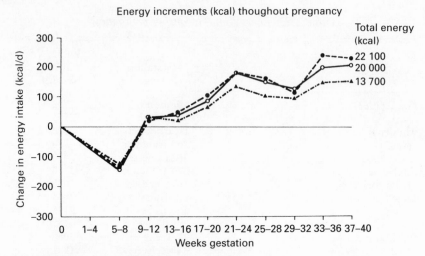

Fig. 23.1 ▲–·–·–·▲ Whole group of Scottish women ($n = 162$); O———O excluding those with low intakes ($n = 131$); ●————● group of women measured initially in the prepregnant state and excluding low intakes ($n = 101$).

Dutch data, has been published recently (Durnin, 1991). In Scotland, on 162 women, measurements were made of food intake, weight and fat gain, basal metabolic rate, oxygen consumption while walking at a standardised rate on the treadmill, normal daily activity pattern, and (in the first 26 women only) total daily energy expenditure. Measurements of these variables were repeated throughout the whole of pregnancy, most of them at 2- to 4-weekly intervals, and 100 of the women were studied initially on three different occasions in the prepregnant state. A reliable prepregnant baseline was thus available for comparison.

The women were all healthy and produced normal healthy babies. The increase in body weight coincided almost exactly with Hytten & Chamberlain's (1980) projection. Yet the detailed data on energy intake showed very small increases, occurring mostly near the end of pregnancy and considerably less than the supposed requirements. Figure 23.1 illustrates the pattern of energy increments. This figure shows three different ways of representing these alterations. The lowest line includes all of the data obtained on the whole group of 162 women. However, some of the intakes which were measured are low enough to raise some doubts as to whether or not they represent the mean normal intake of energy by these women: the actual measurements may have been correct but extraneous influences might have resulted in the measured values being less than the real normal

Table 23.3. *Possible energy savings during pregnancy related to changed activity pattern*

	Energy saving (kcal/d)
1 h 'standing' replaced by 'sitting'	42
$\frac{1}{2}$ h 'housework' replaced by 'sitting'	45
1 h 'sitting' replaced by 'lying-down'	30
$\frac{1}{2}$ h 'walking' replaced by 'sitting'	48
Total	165

value. An alternative presentation of the data is given as the middle line in the figure where the values which were considered to be possibly too low to be genuinely representative have been excluded. There were 31 of these women, so this middle line refers to 131 women. The exclusion of these 31 women was based on an assumption that intakes equivalent to $1.2 \times BMR$ (about 1800 kcal (7.6 MJ)/d in this case) or less, represent the energy expenditure of someone who is almost completely inactive for the whole 24 h of the day (Durnin 1990), and such values are probably not realistic as the norm. Finally, to reduce any possible bias even further, a line was plotted for only the women whose initial measurements were made in the prepregnant period (101 of them), also with those who had very low intakes being excluded. It can be seen that the resultant three different levels differ by very little – at a maximum about 8400 kcal (35 MJ), which is equal to about only 30 kcal (125 kJ) per day.

The only way to marry these findings with the actual energy cost of pregnancy is to postulate that energy savings have occurred; these could have been in three different forms: 1) in BMR, 2) in the efficiency of movement, and 3) by a reduction in physical activity. No evidence was found for savings in BMR or in mechanical efficiency and, although there was only limited evidence to suggest reduced activity, in fact, as Table 23.3 shows, these reductions could be effective in causing the requisite energy saving and yet be small enough to make detection virtually impossible with any equipment presently available.

On the basis of these comprehensive findings in Scotland, together with the similar data from Holland, the conclusion seems to be that an extra energy intake of 100–150 kcal (418–628 kJ)/d during the second and third trimesters ought to be a more than adequate reflection of the energy requirements.

Table 23.4. *Mean protein intakes throughout pregnancy*

Weeks	g/d (incl. low intakes)	g/d (excl. low intakes)
pre-pregnant	70	72
5–8	67	69
21–24	74	78
33–36	75	78

Similar findings have been reported in Thailand and the Philippines (Thongprasert *et al.*, 1987; Tuazon *et al.*, 1987), and indeed an earlier study in Papua New Guinea (Greenfield & Clark, 1975) also demonstrated reduction in physical activity which almost compensated for the extra energy cost of both pregnancy and lactation.

Protein

The protein requirements of pregnancy are not an area of nutrition where the conclusions are clear cut. The average gain in protein in the maternal and fetal tissues can be reasonably calculated, in a similar fashion to that for energy – perhaps even with greater precision. The average gain is about 925 g protein plus 30 % (to cover plus 2 SD). There then needs to be an adjustment for the efficiency with which dietary protein is converted to fetal and maternal tissues; there is no direct evidence on this and an efficiency factor of 0.70, derived from growth data in children, is used. Obviously, the extra protein required will vary with the stage of gestation, being greatest in the third trimester, but evidence from animal studies suggests that the actual deposition of protein does not proceed on this simple basis and is comparatively greater early on in pregnancy and less in the late stages. Thus, protein requirements are recommended as a uniform addition throughout the whole of pregnancy, the amount suggested being 6 g/d. A further correction for the digestibility of the protein fraction of the diet should also be made, although this will add no more than about 1 g/d to the 6 g/d. For a woman weighing about 62 kg in the prepregnant state, her requirements for dietary protein during pregnancy will be about 53 g/d.

A possible area of concern is whether the fact that the real *energy* requirements of pregnancy are of such apparently small magnitude may give rise to a danger of protein deficiency occurring because the virtual

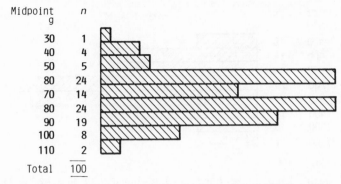

Midpoint g	n
30	1
40	4
50	5
80	24
70	14
80	24
90	19
100	8
110	2
Total	100

Fig. 23.2 Mean protein intakes (g/d) of 100 women at 29–40 weeks' gestation.

absence of any need for extra food to provide energy might mean that the extra protein requirements are not covered. Table 23.4 and Fig. 23.2 illustrate clearly that this is unlikely to occur for other than a tiny percentage of the group.

The situation is different with pregnant women in developing countries because it might be anticipated that their normal intakes of protein might not be in excess of requirements and their ability to obtain even the small extra amount of protein might be limited. If the situation is such that populations are poorly nourished with low energy and protein intakes, then there may well be a need to provide for extra protein.

Calcium

Calcium is such an important mineral in the diet, especially perhaps for women, that it might naturally be assumed that there is an additional requirement during pregnancy, with the formation of the fetal skeleton being an obvious focus. However, there is no evidence that calcium intake in the diet is related to bone health in pregnant women, and multiple pregnancies also seem unconnected to this. Mobilisation of maternal calcium stores seems to be the appropriate source for the additional calcium needs of pregnancy rather than a dietary increment; bone density diminishes in the first 3 months of both pregnancy and lactation to provide a calcium reservoir which is replenished by 6 months post-partum. The efficiency of calcium absorption is also greater in pregnancy than in the prepregnant state.

The recommended intake for calcium is therefore the same in pregnancy as for the non-pregnant women and is about 700 mg/d (Department of Health, 1991). As shown in Fig. 23.3, the vast majority of the Scottish

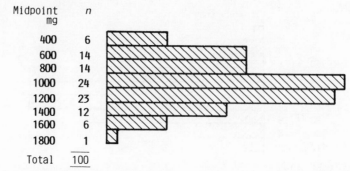

Fig. 23.3 Mean calcium intakes (mg/d) of 100 women at 29–40 weeks' gestation.

women described above had intakes well above this value, although the picture would have been quite different had the standard been that recommended in the USA, 1200 mg/d. (NRC 1989).

Iron

It is estimated that the amount of iron needed for the formation of the maternal and fetal tissues in pregnancy is about 680 mg. However, this should not usually need to be supplied from dietary sources since normal women of child-bearing age should have adequate stores to cope with the demands of pregnancy. The fact that menstruation has ceased and the efficiency of iron absorption increases, will also result in extra supplies being available for the pregnant woman.

The requisite intake during pregnancy is therefore supposed to be 14.8 mg/d. If that level is accepted, Fig. 23.4 shows that about two-thirds of the Scottish group of women would have inadequate intakes. It is perhaps surprising that the human organism, in such an important function as providing sufficient iron for the mother and the developing fetus, has organised itself so badly that it requires amounts of iron in the diet which probably about 90% of the world's population of women are unable to obtain. This is probably more a criticism of the supposed amounts of iron needed in the diet of a non-pregnant woman than of the requirements of pregnancy. It may also be that there is little physiological importance if a women is moderately anaemic through iron deficiency. Certainly, if iron status is equated to blood haemoglobin, there are few disadvantages in having 70 to 80% of the normal quantity. Even at that reduced level, physical activity is the only function which will be affected and then only to the extent that participating in competitive athletics, or some such comparable exercise, would be significantly impaired. Perhaps iron

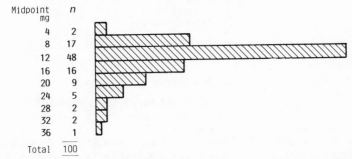

Fig. 23.4 Mean iron intakes (mg/d) of 100 women at 29–40 weeks' gestation.

requirements could equally well be set at somewhat lower levels, which would be highly unlikely to exert an influence on any function involving iron, other than in the formation of haemoglobin, and would modify this to an extent which would barely be detected in an otherwise healthy woman. However, such views, although more realistic than the setting of targets which can only be attained by the use of pharmacological agents, would not be popular.

Conclusion

Giving nutritional advice to women who are, or intend to become, pregnant is something requiring unusual care and solicitude. Concern for the welfare of the mother and fetus predisposes towards making any possible error on the generous side. On the other hand, advice which is likely to lead to an excessive intake, particularly of energy, may have its own inherent disadvantages and dangers. Many women blame the onset of their obesity on the excessive fat gain they acquired during pregnancy.

Both aspects of this nutritional advice therefore need to be carefully weighed up – the dangers of too little or of too much. Avoiding these dangers when good experimental data are scarce is difficult. Nevertheless, the majority of the published work indicates quite definitely that only a small increase in energy intake in the later stages of pregnancy should be nutritionally adequate, and this is compatible with the provision of sufficient protein, calcium and, probably, iron as well. It has been believed for a very long time that the fetus is well protected against maternal malnutrition – that indeed it behaves like a parasite oblivious to the health of its host. However, the long-term health of the mother is of great importance, not only to the mother but also to the future welfare of the fetus itself. The recommendations discussed here should pose no threat to the health of either mother or fetus.

Acknowledgements

The work described here was funded by a research grant from the Nestlé Foundation.

References

Blackburn, M. W. & Calloway, D. H. (1976). Energy expenditure and consumption of mature, pregnant and lactating women. *Journal of the American Dietetic Association*, **69**, 29–36.

Department of Health. (1991). *Dietary Reference Values for Food Energy and Nutrients for the United Kingdom*. London: HMSO.

Doyle, W., Crawford, M. A., Laurance, E. M. & Drury, P. (1982). Dietary survey during pregnancy in a low socio-economic group. *Human Nutrition: Applied Nutrition*, **36A**, 95–106.

Durnin, J. V. G. A. (1987). Energy requirements of pregnancy: An integration of the longitudinal data from the five-country study. *Lancet*, **ii**, 1131–3.

Durnin, J. V. G. A., McKillop, F. M., Grant, S. & Fitzgerald, G. (1987). Energy requirements of pregnancy in Scotland. *Lancet*, **ii**, 897–900.

Durnin, J. V. G. A. (1990). Low energy expenditures in free-living populations. *European Journal of Clinical Nutrition*, **44**, Suppl. 1, 95–102.

Durnin, J. V. G. A. (1991). Energy requirements of pregnancy. *Diabetes*, **40** (2) in press.

English, R. M. & Hitchcock, N. E. (1968). Nutrient intakes during pregnancy, lactation and after the cessation of lactation in a group of Australian women. *British Journal of Nutrition*, **22**, 615–24.

Grafe, H. K. (1983). Dietary intake during pregnancy. In *On the Role of Nutrition in Normal Human Pregnancy*. van den Berg, H. & Bruinse, H. W., eds, pp. 175–178, University of Utrecht Press.

Greenfield, H. & Clark, J. (1975). Energy compensation in childbearing in young Lufa women. *Papua New Guinea Medical Journal*.

Haste, F. M., Brooke, O. G., Anderson, H. R., Bland, J. M., Shaw, A., Griffin, J. & Peacock, J. L. (1990). Nutrient intakes during pregnancy: observations on the influence of smoking and social class. *American Journal of Clinical Nutrition*, **51**, 29–36.

Hytten, F. E. & Leitch, I. (1971). *The Physiology of Human Pregnancy*. 2nd edn. Oxford: Blackwell Scientific Publications.

Hytten, F. E. & Chamberlain, G. V. P. (1980). *Clinical Physiology in Obstetrics*. Oxford: Blackwell Scientific Publications.

Lunell, N. O., Persson, B. & Sterky, G. (1983). Energy and nutrient intake according to parity, smoking behaviour, season and pregnancy outcome. In *On the Role of Nutrition in Normal Human Pregnancy*. van den Berg, H. & Bruinse, H. W., eds, pp. 179–180, University of Utrecht Press.

National Research Council (1989). *Recommended Dietary Allowances*. Food and Nutrition Board. Washington: National Academy Press.

Schofield, C., Wheeler, E. & Stewart, J. (1987). The diets of pregnant and post-pregnant women in different social groups in London and Edinburgh: energy, protein, fat and fibre. *British Journal of Nutrition*, **58**, 369–81.

Thongprasert, K., Tanphaichitre, V., Valyasevi, A., Kittigool, J. & Durnin, J. V. G. A. (1987). Energy requirements of pregnancy in rural Thailand. *Lancet*, **ii**, 1010–12.

Tuazon, M. A. G., van Raaij, J. M. A., Hautvast, J. G. A. J. & Barba, C. V. C.

(1987). Energy requirements of pregnancy in the Philippines. *Lancet*, **ii**, 1129–31.

Van Raaij, J. M. A., Vermatt-Miedema, S. H., Schonk, C. M., Peek, M. E. M. & Hautvast, J. G. A. J. (1987). Energy requirements of pregnancy in The Netherlands. *Lancet*, **ii**, 953–5.

Van den Rijst, M. P. J. (1983). Nutrient intake relative to recommended daily allowances. In *On the Role of Nutrition in Normal Human Pregnancy*. van den Berg, H. & Bruinse, H. W., eds, pp. 181–185, University of Utrecht Press.

Whitehead, R. G., Paul, A. A., Black, A. E. & Wiles, S. J. (1981). Recommended Dietary Amounts of Energy for Pregnancy and Lactation in the United Kingdom. *UNU Food and Nutrition Bulletin, Supplement* 5, 259–64.

24

Early nutrition and later outcome

ALAN LUCAS

Over the past 50 years more research has been conducted in infant nutrition than in virtually any other field of paediatrics, yet uncertainty persists over nearly every major area of practice. A key factor in this uncertainty has been a lack of knowledge on whether diet or nutritional status in early life has a long-term or permanent influence on health, function or achievement. Until such information is established, the most appropriate nutritional management of sick children in hospital and the most prudent advice for healthy infant feeding practice will remain speculative and prone to changing fashion.

The concept that nutrition in infancy could have long-term significance, however, raises issues of fundamental biological importance. Is it plausible or, arguing teleologically, evolutionarily likely that such a brief period of life could be a critical one for nutrition? What could be the nature of the triggering mechanisms for these events? If the consequences of early nutrition are expressed in later life, how and where is the 'memory' of the early event stored, whilst the cells of the body are constantly replicating or being replaced? And are there indeed convincing data showing that early nutrition influences long-term outcome in animals or man? This brief chapter gives consideration to these important issues.

The concept of early biological programming

There are many ways in which an early event (nutritional or otherwise) could have permanent or long-term consequences (see Lucas, 1991):

1. direct damage (for example, loss of limb due to vascular accident or trauma);
2. induction, deletion, or impaired development of a permanent somatic structure as the result of stimulus or insult operating at a 'critical' or 'sensitive' period;

3. physiological 'setting' by an early stimulus or insult at a 'critical' or 'sensitive' period, resulting in long-term consequences for function; the effects could be immediate or deferred.

The second and third of these three processes will be referred to as 'programming', though others might use the term in a more limited sense. As a working definition, then, 'programming' occurs when an early stimulus or insult, operating at a critical or sensitive period, results in a permanent or long-term change in the structure or function of the organism. An essential component of this concept is the notion of a 'sensitive' or 'critical' period – a critical window in time – when an early event may operate.

Programming as a general biological process

The idea that events occurring at 'critical' or 'sensitive' periods could have lifelong significance was first observed in relation to imprinting in birds. Smart (1986) points out that Pliny described 'a goose that followed Lacydes as faithfully as a dog', and in the nineteenth century Spalding (1873) defined the critical period during which ducks hatched in the absence of their mother will follow the first moving object.

Since the 1920s it has been recognised that drugs acting at critical periods in early fetal life could induce developmental abnormalities of life-long consequence. Thalidomide is a good example of an otherwise safe drug that can cause devastating teratogenic effects in man during a relatively brief period of early development.

Programming may be seen as a normal part of biological development or it may occur in response to unphysiological events. It may be affected by genetically determined internal triggers, or by exogenous stimuli, sometimes operating over very short periods. For example, at a critical period in male fetal rats, the brain is programmed for male sexual behaviour by the endogenous release of testosterone from the developing testis. At this stage, a single exogenous dose of testosterone administered experimentally to a female fetal rat will permanently reorientate sexual behaviour (Angelbeck and DuBrul, 1983).

Hormones indeed have a well-established role as programming agents (for review see Lucas, 1991). Thyroxine is critical for early brain development, with transient deficiency resulting in permanent changes that would not be seen later in life. Conversely, excess thyroxine in the neonatal period in experimental animals will reset the pituitary–hypothalamic axis with respect to thyroid stimulating hormone response in later life. The substantial evidence that a wide variety of hormones and growth factors operate at critical periods raises the possibility, discussed below, that an intermediary role of hormones could explain some long-term effects of early nutrition.

Other agents which have a known programming influence include sensory stimuli, for example, in the development of the visual pathway, and antigens in immunological development. Drugs may have programming effects in postnatal life. For instance, a single dose of phenobarbitone given to a newborn rat will programme a life-long change in cytochrome P450-dependent mono-oxygenase activity (Bagley & Hayes, 1983), highlighting the exquisite sensitivity that may exist to early programming stimuli.

Nutritional programming in animals

Animal studies have shown that nutrition may programme long-term outcome. Hahn (1984) manipulated litter size in rats to produce litters of 4 or 14 pups. In small litters the pups were overfed during the short suckling period. In adulthood, the previously overfed rats developed permanently raised plasma cholesterol and insulin concentrations. Rats weaned on to a high carbohydrate diet also showed lifelong increases in activities of two key enzymes in lipid biosynthetic pathways: fatty acid synthetase and HMG CoA reductase (important in fat and cholesterol synthesis).

Rats are born immature, and might be especially sensitive to early programming and would not be a good model for man (though it is pertinent that human infants may now survive extreme prematurity). Nevertheless, long-term programming has also been demonstrated in primates. In a study by Lewis and co-workers (1986), infant baboons were randomly assigned to one of three formulae for the first 4 months. The formulae provided low, normal and high energy intakes. After the 4-month period all the animals were fed in the same way. The excess weight gained during infancy in the animals with high energy intakes was soon lost. In female baboons, especially, early overfeeding resulted in a dramatic increase in body weight and fat mass during adolescence and early adult life. In this instance, the effects of the initial 'programming' event were not manifested until a much later stage in life, raising the important question as to how the 'memory' had been stored in the meantime.

The influence of breast versus formula feeding on later lipid metabolism and vascular disease has also been explored in a series of studies by Mott,

Lewis and co-workers (1991) using the baboon model. In these studies random assignments were made to breast or formula feeding during infancy (first 4 months): beyond that the animals were fed in the same way. Compared with the breast-fed group, those who were formula-fed in infancy had, in adult life, increased cholesterol absorption, reduced cholesterol turnover and, when placed on a high saturated fat, western-style diet, developed higher plasma levels of LDL and VLDL cholesterol and lower levels of potentially protective HDL cholesterol. These lipid abnormalities would be expected to result in an increased risk of atherosclerosis, and indeed the animals showed, at post-mortem, a significantly greater area of atherosclerotic plaque if they had been breast-fed in infancy.

By using formulae with different cholesterol content, the investigators established that cholesterol intake itself did not account for their findings, which remain unexplained. The significance of these data for man is not known, and indeed it could be argued that in humans, morbidity from vascular disease may be more related to thrombotic events than to atherosclerosis *per se*. Nevertheless these data emphasise the importance of long-term studies on human nutrition.

In addition to the work on early diet and later metabolism and morbidity, a large body of animal data, principally from studies on rats, have indicated that the quality of nutrition at a vulnerable period of early brain development could have permanent consequences for brain size, brain cell number and performance (Dobbing, 1981). Smart (1986) has reviewed the extensive literature on whether early undernutrition influences later learning and memory. In this review of 165 animal experiments, the number of studies in which undernourished animals fared significantly worse than controls ($n = 80$) outweighed studies coming to the opposite conclusion ($n = 12$). Whilst there may be a reporting bias for positive studies, it is likely that these data reflect long-term consequences of early underfeeding. The relevance of these studies to man requires further work.

These, and other animal studies, provide convincing evidence that nutrition in early life may influence a wide variety of metabolic, developmental and pathological processes in adulthood.

Dietary programming in man: previous studies

Unfortunately the great majority of investigations on the consequences of early nutrition in man have been retrospective and flawed by problems with study design.

There has been major interest in the relation of early protein-calorie malnutrition to later achievement (Grantham-McGregor, 1987). Given the enormous investment in these studies, it is disappointing that firm conclusions cannot yet be made. These largely retrospective studies are seriously confounded by the poverty, poor social circumstances and lack of stimulation that generally accompany malnutrition.

The effects of individual nutrients, however, on later brain development is receiving increasing attention (for overview see Lucas, 1991). Iron deficiency in infancy, common both in the West and developing countries, has been shown to relate to poor developmental performance. Some evidence suggests that subsequent iron supplementation may not prevent later poor cognitive ability at 5 years and that a brief period of relatively mild deficiency could have long lasting consequences for behaviour and school performance. Irreversible long-term consequences of early iron deficiency have also been demonstrated in rats.

The possibility that inadequate long chain n-3 fatty acids in the diets of formula-fed preterm infants might impair cerebral and retinal development has caused concern. Developing brain (notably cerebral cortex) and retina accumulate large quantities of docosahexaenoic acids ($22:6n3$). Such long-chain lipids are not present in significant amounts in many formulae, which frequently have low contents of the precursor, linolenic acid ($18:3n3$). Compelling primate data (Neuringer *et al.*, 1986) now show that insufficiency of these fatty acids at a critical stage of retinal development results in long-term, irreversible impairment of retinal function.

A number of investigations have focused on early diet in relation to diseases found in affluent countries. Whether early lipid intake in man influences later lipid status or atherosclerosis has not been established. Early salt intake has not been convincingly related to later blood pressure, despite earlier concerns.

The long-term consequences of early excessive food intake is an important issue needing further study. Many groups have examined the relationship between infant obesity and later obesity, which, in general, are weakly correlated (Poskitt & Cole, 1977). However, this may not be the best approach. Using the doubly labelled water method to explore energy metabolism in free-living infants (Lucas *et al.*, 1987), unpublished data have indicated that additional energy in the diet may be expended and not necessarily deposited in body stores. If so, it is early energy intake and not just fatness that needs to be correlated with later fatness and morbidity. Preliminary investigations show that energy intake at 3 months of age does not correlate with skinfold thickness at that age, but is significantly related to skinfold thickness at two years. These findings are consistent with those of Kramer (1981) who found that, compared with bottle-fed babies, those breast-fed in infancy received some protection against obesity in later childhood and adolescence, even after adjusting for confounding factors. It is likely that bottle-fed infants at that time consumed more energy than breast-fed babies. Conversely, mothers who were undernourished in the third trimester during the Dutch Hunger Winter had children who grew up to be of normal height and intelligence, but were thinner than their peers (Stein *et al.*, 1975).

The preterm infant as a model for programming studies

The lack of prospective long-term outcome studies on diet in man has related to the unattractiveness of this type of work to many investigators, unwillingness of funding bodies to support it, disbelief that early influences could have lasting effects and the inherent difficulties in mounting formal randomised longitudinal studies. One circumstance in man where it is practical and ethical to assign infants randomly to diet and follow them up long term is following preterm birth.

Between 1982 and 1985 nearly 1000 preterm infants were assigned to different diets, studied intensively in the newborn period and are now being followed up indefinitely (Lucas *et al.*, 1984). The babies were randomised at birth, in four parallel trials, either to a preterm formula (enriched in protein, energy, macrominerals and trace nutrients to meet the calculated increased requirements of preterm infants) versus donor breast milk; or to preterm formula versus a standard formula; for each comparison these feeds were used as sole diets or as supplements to mother's own milk. The infants remained on the assigned diets for an average of one month; after that there was no influence on dietary management. Follow-up data are available to 18 months corrected age; a 7–8 year follow-up is in progress.

Whilst the trials are providing essential outcome data that will guide clinical management of preterm infants, the study offers a unique opportunity to test, in a human model, whether early diet could influence long-term outcome in man. The principal medium-term outcome response chosen was neurodevelopment, but a number of other key outcomes have been explored. In this chapter, three examples of outcome data have been selected that support the concept of programming.

Table 24.1. *Family history of atopy, neonatal diet and allergic reactions at 18 months in infants born preterm*

Allergic reaction	Family history of atopy			No family history			Interaction between family history and diet (P value)
	Human milk (n = 38)	Preterm formula (n = 37)	Odds ratio (95% CI)	Human milk (n = 189)	Preterm formula (n = 182)	Odds ratio (95% CI)	
Eczema	16% (6)	41% (15)	3.6* (1.2, 11)	21% (40)	16% (29)	0.7 (0.4, 1.2)	< 0.01
Reactions to:							
cows' milk	3% (1)	5% (2)	2.1 (0.2, 25)	5% (9)	3% (5)	0.6 (0.2, 1.7)	
all foods	11% (4)	22% (8)	2.3 (0.6, 8.3)	10% (18)	9% (16)	0.9 (0.5, 1.9)	
drugs	3% (1)	16% (6)	7.1 (0.8, 50)	7% (14)	5% (10)	0.7 (0.3, 1.7)	
Wheezing or asthma	21% (8)	30% (11)	1.6 (0.6, 1.4)	24% (40)	22% (40)	0.9 (0.6, 1.5)	
Any of above	34% (13)	65% (24)	3.6* (1.4, 9.1)	46% (86)	42% (76)	0.9 (0.6, 1.3)	< 0.001

Infants were divided into two groups according to whether or not there was a family history of atopy. Within each group the percentage incidence of allergic reactions (number of subjects) is compared in infants randomly assigned to donor milk or preterm formula as sole diets or supplements to mother's milk (thus the donor milk-fed group received only human milk). The odds ratio (95% confidence interval, CI) is recorded for the incidence of allergy on preterm formula versus human milk. Corresponding odds ratios in the two family history groups are also compared, to test for an interaction between family history and diet.

* *P* < 0.05.

Early diet and later allergic reactions

The effect of early diet on later allergy has been much debated. A major problem in the interpretation of results from many studies arises from the lack of random assignment to diet. Clearly, random assignment to breast feeding versus formula feeding would be unethical in healthy infants, and yet social and demographic differences found between these two groups confound comparative analyses. In preterm infants random allocation to human milk or formula is ethical and feasible. In one limb of our trial we compared infants randomly assigned to banked donor breast milk as sole diet or supplement to mother's milk (i.e. all received only human milk) versus those fed a preterm formula as sole diet or supplement (i.e. all exposed to cows' milk formula). Beyond 1 month, on average, trial diets were discontinued and there was no significant difference in dietary management between groups. At 18 months the pattern of response depended on whether or not the child had a family history of allergy (Lucas *et al.*, 1990). In infants with no such history, interestingly, those fed previously on cows' milk formula had a small (non-significant) reduction in the incidence of reactions to cows' milk, other food or drugs, and in eczema and wheezing. In contrast, in the smaller subgroup with a positive family history of allergy, babies given cows' milk formula rather than breast milk in the neonatal period had a dramatic increase in these allergic responses, notably in eczema and reaction to food or drugs. Data, shown in Table 24.1, demonstrate that, in genetically susceptible individuals, a brief period of dietary manipulation 'programmes' the infants' propensity for developing a wide range of allergic or atopic manifestations.

Early diet and later linear growth

Using multiple regression analysis on our cohort of infants (Lucas *et al.*, 1989), out of a large number of clinical and demographic factors analysed (over 50), apart from sex, four perinatal factors with a significant independent relationship to body length at 18 months were identified. Being a twin or triplet was associated with a 1 cm shorter length at 18 months; infants fed exclusively on human milk were also on average 1 cm shorter; being born small for gestation was associated with a 1.3 cm shorter length and those having biochemical evidence of severe metabolic bone disease in the newborn period (plasma alkaline phosphatase over 1200 IU/1) had a 1.6 cm shorter length. The latter condition, most common in preterm infants fed unsupplemented breast milk, reflects inadequate phosphorus and calcium intake to meet the rapid bone mineralisation that would have occurred *in utero* in the third trimester. The additive effect of the adverse factors for body length described would be to displace the infant's body length from the fiftieth centile to the third.

It is pertinent that, of all the factors analysed, those few that were related to reduced long-term linear growth were all factors associated with a period of reduced linear growth in the perinatal period due to impaired fetal or neonatal nutrition – in the case of bone disease, due specifically to impaired mineral supply.

It seems reasonable to suggest that early nutrition has a programming effect on long-term linear growth, and preliminary studies later in childhood continue to support that view. One could speculate, teleologically, that it makes good sense from an evolutionary point of view for an infant to monitor its environment after birth and set growth projections according to nutrient availability. In an environment with poor nutrient supply, for instance, it would be advantageous to be small. Babies born after placental insufficiency or impaired postnatal nutrition due to prematurity might 'interpret' their environment as 'nutrient poor' and, perhaps irreversibly, set themselves up for shorter stature.

Early diet and later mental and motor development

Our preterm infant feeding trial has provided the first opportunity to study the effect of a brief period of dietary manipulation on later brain development in a large, strictly randomised prospective trial in man. Studies at the 18 months follow-up, for example (Lucas *et al.*, 1990), show that infants randomly assigned to a standard term formula rather than a nutrient-enriched 'preterm' formula for, on average, the first 4 weeks, subsequently had a major deficit in developmental scores. This was particularly marked for motor development, where the deficit was of the order of one standard deviation. As in animal studies, the greatest effects of diet were seen in infants born small for gestation, who were already born nutritionally deprived: such infants fed term formula had deficits in mental and motor development of 16 and 23 points (see Fig. 24.1).

Whether these long-term dietary effects on development relate to the early differences in brain growth observed between diet groups (Lucas *et al.*, 1984), or to the lack of a specific critical nutrient or signal for cerebral development now requires intensive investigation. Our cohort is currently being assessed at 7–8 years.

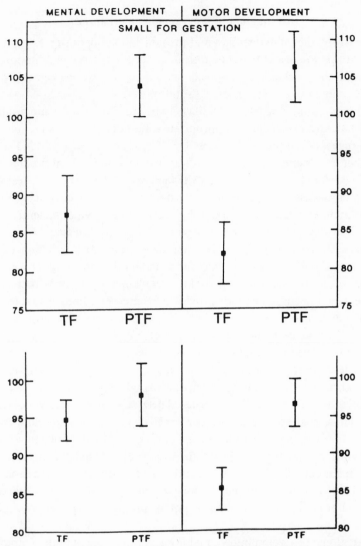

Fig. 24.1. Mental and motor development indices (Bayley Scales) at 18 months in infants randomly assigned to a standard 'term' formula (TF) or a special nutrient-enriched 'preterm' formula (PTF) during the early weeks *post partum*, in babies born small (*above*) and appropriately sized for gestation (*below*). Bars represent mean (SE) neurodevelopmental scores. (Adapted from Lucas *et al.*, 1990.)

Investigation of programming mechanisms

Collectively, the animal studies and the new human data suggest that the newborn period is a critical one for nutrition. If so, it becomes important to define the mechanisms involved since these may prove central to an understanding of a major route to adult disease.

Some programming effects are likely to be immediate. An acute insult or lack of a critical signal at the appropriate stage could irreversibly interrupt or change a developmental process.

Other programming effects, as indicated in some animal studies, are deferred. Here the question is how the memory of the early event is stored and later expressed. Three cellular mechanisms might be envisaged. First, the nutrient environment of a developing cell line may permanently alter gene expression, so that cellular progeny will have the 'message' passed on to them. Alternatively, as in the immune system, early nutrition might affect clonal selection. For instance, animal data showing long-term effects of diet on nutrient absorption could be explained if the early pattern of nutrients in the gut lumen influenced which enterocyte lines were selected. Finally, as has been hypothesised for the programming of adiposity, early nutrition could permanently influence cell number. These mechanisms need to be explored, initially in animal models.

Nutrients may not always act directly, but through an intermediary mechanism. Previously, it has been speculated that gut hormones are a potential set of intermediary agents. Their pattern of release is highly related to the pattern of nutrients consumed (for instance major differences in gut hormone release between breast- and formula-fed infants have been reported); gut peptide receptors are widely distributed throughout the body; it has been shown that gut peptide release is dramatic in the neonatal period, perhaps implying that they have a unique role in early life, and finally, hormones are known to be potent programming agents in other contexts.

Nutritional programming is a major unexplored area of human biology, with broader implications for understanding the legacy of childhood experience for adult disease and achievement.

References

Angelbeck, J. H. & DuBrul, E. F. (1983). The effect of neonatal testosterone on specific male and female patterns of phosphorylated cytosolic proteins in the rat pre-optic hypothalamus, cortex and amygdala. *Brain Research*, **264**, 277–83.

Bagley, D. M. & Hayes, J. R. (1983). Neonatal phenobarbital administration results in increased cytochrome P450-dependent mono-oxygenase activity in adult male and female rats. *Biochemical and Biophysical Research Communications*, **114**, 1132–7.

Dobbing, J. (1981). Nutritional growth restriction and the nervous system. In *The Molecular Basis of Neuropathology*, Davison, A. N. & Thompson, R. H. S., eds, pp. 221–33, London: Edward Arnold.

Grantham-McGregor, S. (1987). Field studies in early nutrition and later achievement. In *Early Nutrition and Later Achievement*, Dobbing, J., ed., pp. 128–74, London: Academic Press.

Hahn, P. (1984). Effect of litter size on plasma cholesterol and insulin and some liver and adipose tissue enzymes in adult rodents. *Journal of Nutrition* **114**, 1231–4.

Kramer, M. S. (1981). Do breastfeeding and delayed introductions of solid food protect against subsequent obesity? *Journal of Pediatrics*, **98**, 883–7.

Lewis, D. S., Bertrand, H. A., McMahon, C. A., McGill, H. C. Jr, Carey, K. D. & Masoro, E. F. (1986). Preweaning food intake influences adiposity of young adult baboons. *Journal of Clinical Investigation*, **78**, 899–905.

Lucas, A. (1991). Programming by early nutrition in man. In *The Childhood Environment and Adult Disease*. Ciba Foundation Symposium 156, pp. 38–55, Chichester: Wiley.

Lucas, A., Gore, S., Cole, T. J. *et al.* (1984). A multicentre trial on the feeding of low birthweight infants: effects of diet on early growth. *Archives of Diseases of Childhood*, **59**, 722–30.

Lucas, A., Ewing, G., Roberts, S. B. & Coward, W. A. (1987). How much energy does the breast-fed infant consume and expend? *British Medical Journal*, **295**, 75–7.

Lucas, A., Brooke, O. G., Baker, B. A., Bishop, N. & Morley, R. (1989). High alkaline phosphatase activity and growth in preterm neonates. *Archives of Diseases of Childhood*, **64**, 902–9.

Lucas, A., Brooke, O. G., Morley, R., Cole, T. J. & Bamford, M. F. (1990). Early diet of preterm infants and development of allergic or atopic disease. *British Medical Journal* **300**, 837–40.

Mott, G. E., Lewis, D. S. & McGill, C. C. Jr. (1991). Programming by early nutrition in man. In *The Childhood Environment and Adult Disease*. Ciba Foundation Symposium 156, pp. 56–76, Chichester: Wiley.

Neuringer, M., Conner, W. E., Lin, D. S., Barstad, L. & Luck, S. (1986). Biochemical and functional effects of prenatal and postnatal n3 deficiency on retina and brain of rhesus monkey. *Proceedings of the National Academy of Sciences*, **83**, 4021–5.

Poskitt, E. M. E. & Cole, T. J. (1977). Do fat babies stay fat? *British Medical Journal*, **i**, 7–9.

Smart, J. (1986). Undernutrition, learning and memory: review of experimental studies. In *Proceedings of the XIII International Congress of Nutrition*, Taylor, T. G. & Jenkins, N. K., eds, pp. 74–8, London: John Libbey.

Spalding, D. A. (1873). Instinct with original observations on young animals. *MacMillan's Magazine*, **27**, 282–93; reprinted 1954 *British Journal of Animal Behaviour*, **2**, 2–11.

Stein, Z., Susser, M., Saenger, G. & Marolla, F. (1975). *Famine and human development: the Dutch hunger winter of 1944–45*, New York: Oxford University Press.

25

Nutrition and growth in tropical environments: the use of anthropometry

ERICA F. WHEELER

Introduction

What hope is there for children whose growth process has been interfered with by inadequate nutrition?

(Gangulee 1939, p. 88)

The Nutrition Society was established in 1941, by which time several major studies of child growth had been carried out in Europe and North America (Tanner, 1981); many of them anticipated the reasons for the tropical studies which will be reviewed here. For example, de Villermé and Quetelet, working in France and Belgium respectively, laid the foundations of anthropometry as a means of identifying the effects of public health problems. Rowntree (1913), in his York study, documented the differences in height between the children of 'utterly poor' and artisan families. Paton and Findlay (1926) showed that there was a 6 cm difference between the average heights of rural and urban Scottish preschool children. 'In North America, a powerful child welfare movement ... provided the soil for a crop of longitudinal studies' (Tanner, 1981, p. 299) from which were derived the Harvard and Fels growth standards. These surveys show the growing awareness among public health workers, clinicians and educationalists that measurements of children provided invaluable objective data to support statements about inequalities in income, health and welfare.

By 1941 some studies of children's heights and weights had also been made in tropical countries as part of studies of health and nutrition. Aykroyd and Rajagopal at the Indian Nutrition Research Laboratories in Coonoor, and Wilson and colleagues at the All-India Institute of Public Health in Calcutta used anthropometry in investigations of the nutritional state of schoolboys in Bengal, the Punjab, and Tamil Nadu (Aykroyd & Rajagopal, 1936; Wilson, Ahmad & Mitra, 1937). This work, carried out by well-established scientific research institutes in India, showed clear differences between economic and ethnic groups. The Nyasaland Nutrition Survey, made by B. S. Platt and his team in 1938–39, is the first example of a nutritional study to be commissioned in a tropical country by HM Government, just 3 years before the Nutrition Society was founded. The measures of children's heights and weights clearly show seasonality differences between ecological zones in Nyasaland (now Malawi) and differences between the Nyasaland data and measurements on London school children (Grant, 1951). The outcome of the survey was the formation of a Nutrition Development Unit, an early example of the use of nutritional data to support the establishment of a multi-sectorial group with the objective of improving food production and intake in a then colonial tropical country (Berry & Petty, 1992).

Since the 1930s the applications of child anthropometry in the tropics have developed, at least in part, to meet two specific demands. One is the succession of food-related crises, mainly in 'developing' countries, which have occurred in parallel with the production of food surpluses in industrialised countries, creating a demand for criteria and mechanisms for distributing the bulk of the latter to the sites of the former (Beaton *et al.*, 1990). The other arises from the growth of the concept of planned economic and social development, with its demand for indicators to be used in planning and evaluation (Payne, 1975; Hakim & Solimano, 1976). In this chapter, after a brief discussion of some technical aspects of anthropometric indicators, their use for *assessment*, *advocacy*, *planning*, and *evaluation* will be reviewed, taking examples from the 1930s to the present time. Although 'anthropometry' correctly includes the measurement of any bodily dimensions, height (length), and weight, in children aged 5 y and less will be mainly referred to.

Developing anthropometric indicators

The measurement of a child's height and weight provides both a summary of its past and a prediction of its future. It is therefore possible to use grouped data on children's height and weight to expose and comment on elements of their past experience, and to evaluate interventions which may be intended to alter the course of their development (Fig. 25.1).

Those who intend to use anthropometric measurements for such purposes need first to distinguish among the *causes of variation*, and secondly to agree on *limits of acceptable adaptation* to varying environ-

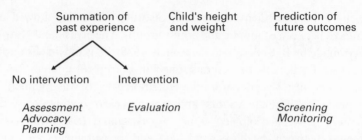

Fig. 25.1. The uses of anthropometry.

ments. Both of these stages must be passed before it is possible to reach consensus on *standardisation* and *cut-off points* for the definition of at-risk groups. Clearly, if groups of children are measured and their heights and weights are found to differ significantly, explanations for this include expected normal variation due to genetic diversity, age and sex, which must be allowed for before any deductions are made about the effect of other factors such as food intake and health status. Figure 25.2 summarises the

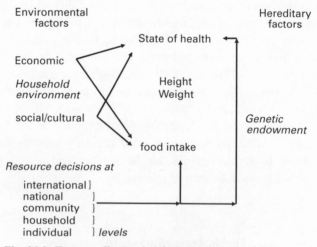

Fig. 25.2. Factors affecting height and weight in children.

factors which result in variation in height and weight. The extent of 'normal' biological variation is such that the coefficient of variation in healthy children of the same age and sex is 4% for height and 10% for weight at age 18 months (USDHEW, 1976). Age and sex-related differences can be allowed for by the use of standard values, but debate continues as to the need to develop sets of national standards for different countries in the light of ethnic differences, especially in height (as shown in Eveleth &

Tanner, 1976). Ongoing secular trends make the fixing of any national standard a difficult matter, and one solution is to use a common 'international' standard (Habicht *et al.*, 1974), recognising that acceptable mean values for different ethnic groups will be found at different centile or z-score positions and will shift over time, especially in countries undergoing economic and social change, or in immigrant groups (Davies & Wheeler, 1989).

Standardisation is needed because anthropometric measurements by themselves are not particularly useful. It is the comparison of a child's height or weight with 'normal' standard values which indicates the presence or absence of some growth-retarding factor(s). Indices such as height-for-age or weight-for-height identify a child's placing in relation to the range of normal values. Such an index, in combination with cut-off points defining levels of risk, provide indicators which can then be used in establishing prevalences of smallness and shortness ('wasting' and 'stunting') which fall below the limits of healthy 'normality' (Waterlow, 1972). Such indicators can provide objective evidence of the impact of planned, and indeed of unplanned, economic and social change (Dowler *et al.*, 1982). One important difference between modern studies and those of the 1930s, cited above, is that Aykroyd and Platt and their colleagues simply compared the mean heights and weights of the children they measured with mean values from the UK. There were no tools at that time for examining the variance of the data or calculating the percentage of small or short children that would be expected within a normal distribution. Hence prevalences of malnutrition could not be established. The survey anthropometrist in Nyasaland struggled to analyse the growth data which had been recorded (Grant, 1951). She had no recourse to the wealth of centile curves and standard values which have now been developed, or to the enormous theoretical and practical literature on the uses of anthropometry which now exists. Much of this literature is now associated with the work of UN agencies which were finding their feet in the post-war period (for example, Beaton *et al.*, 1990). The Indian workers saw the need for such analysis: 'It should, however, be possible by statistical treatment of abundant data to devise a table of measurements...so that a maximum of children showing signs of deficiency disease would be selected' (i.e. identified by anthropometry) (Aykroyd & Rajagopal, 1936).

It is now possible to classify children according to accepted anthropometric indices, but discussion continues as to the meaning of observed differences. On the one hand, the risk of death associated with a given weight deficit has been quantified, but these indicators have limited predictive value (Heywood, 1986). On the other hand, it is strongly argued that for a child to grow at a rate less than that of a standard healthy population is not necessarily a disadvantage, and that smallness may confer benefit, or at least not lead to disadvantage, in adult life (Payne, 1990). Here it is important to distinguish between weight and height indices. It is now argued (Lutter *et al.*, 1990) that it is only until the age of 2–3 years that a height deficit relative to standards reflects an *ongoing* failure to grow, which is unlikely to be compensated by an improved environment. Weight deficit, on the other hand, can always be regarded as reflecting the current situation, since the weight-for-height index can catch up at most ages. With regard to height, a UN document states that 'it is the factors associated with the *process* of becoming small, not the *state* of being small, that are of real concern ... it is not considered that "being small" – as opposed to becoming small – is in itself harmful to the individual' (Beaton *et al.*, 1990).

Assessment and advocacy

Anthropometry may be used in all the processes shown in Fig. 25.1: problem assessment, advocacy, screening, monitoring, planning and evaluation. *Assessment* simply means arriving at an objective statement about the extent of a problem. How many children fall within certain categories of risk? what kind of families do they come from? what is their age/sex distribution? Large numbers of nutritional surveys provide a problem assessment of this kind. *Advocacy* goes further, for it means speaking on someone's behalf. The term 'nutritional advocacy' has been coined to describe the process wherein information about individuals' nutritional state is used to influence policy decisions in directions intended to benefit disadvantaged groups of people: 'the use of nutrition indicators and nutrition-focused analysis to improve planning, targeting, monitoring and evaluation of policy activities' (E. A. Dowler, personal communication). Anthropometric data need not be presented only in an epidemiological sense, showing the factors associated with retarded growth. They may be used especially to emphasise those differences between children which arise from socio-economic, health, ecological and other factors affecting their families. In other words, child anthropometry can be used to define and highlight problems affecting children, following which a case can be made for policies and interventions on their behalf. It may also be used to sensitise planners, officials and bureaucrats to the fact that economic and social policies may have a direct physical effect on children (and by extension, on their families) (Dowler *et al.*, 1982). Some development agencies are increasingly using anthropometric surveys in this manner. Others take the opposing view, that productivity rather than 'welfare' should be the main criterion in project and programme planning. (Payne & Wheeler, in preparation.)

Anthropometric measurements of children and teenagers have been used since the beginning of the nineteenth century to demonstrate and quantify the physical effects of poverty. In 1829 de Villermé commented that 'the circumstances which accompany poverty delay the age at which complete stature is reached, and stunt adult height' (quoted in Tanner, 1981, p. 162). He backed his statement with measurements of French conscripts which showed an association for *arrondissements* of Paris between the mean height of young men and the numbers of people owning their own homes. Both in the UK and in France, measurements of the height of children were included in the investigations of health and working conditions; in the UK these contributed to the Factory Acts of the 1830s and 1840s, and among other things highlighted the extensive abuse of existing legal limits on the ages and working hours of children employed in factories and mines (Tanner, 1981).

In the twentieth century, in many parts of the world including the Tropics, child anthropometry has been used to quantify the effects of a wide range of environmental, social and economic problems affecting poor households. The Indian studies, cited above, provide assessments of the nutritional state of schoolboys and clearly demonstrate social, economic and ecological differences in size. The authors used the data to back up their assertions that many Indian households were receiving inadequate diets. Another example, from the late 1940s, is Culwick's study of families in an area of the Sudan which benefited from a large irrigation scheme. As well as measuring diets, Culwick measured children, and showed that considerable seasonal fluctuations in their weight and height gains occurred, even in an area where food production had been increased by agricultural modernisation. She used these data, in a process of advocacy, to argue for better distribution of food within the family, opposing the conventional wisdom that the most appropriate nutritional intervention would take the form of education to mothers (Culwick, 1951, p. 156).

Through the 1970s and 1980s studies from South Asia and Latin America in particular have demonstrated the uses of anthropometry in identifying adverse effects on child growth which go far beyond general statements of the 'Malnutrition is due to poverty and ignorance' type. Table 25.1 summarises the findings of some of these studies. For example,

Table 25.1. *Some studies showing factors which contribute to retarding the height and weight gain of children*

Country	Reference	Factors
India	1	Poor housing, low income
India	2	Food price inflation
Sri Lanka	3	Women having restricted opportunity to influence household resource allocation
Guatemala	4	Landlessness, or very small landholding
Guatemala	5	Parasitic infestation (*Giardia* and *Ascaris*)
The Gambia	6	Infections (diarrhoea and lower respiratory tract infection

References:
1. Hanumantha Rao & Satyanarayana (1976).
2. Thimmayamma *et al.* (1976).
3. Wandel & Homhoe-Offersen (1988).
4. Valverde *et al.* (1977).
5. Gupta & Urrutia (1982).
6. Rowland, Cole & Whitehead (1977).

anthropometric measurements have been used to demonstrate the interacting effects of family size and family assets on the growth of Bangladeshi children (Becker *et al.*, 1986), the consequences to a family of having little or no access to land (Valverde *et al.*, 1977), and the growth-retarding effects of infections and parasites (Mata, Urrutia & Lechtig, 1971; Farthing *et al.*, 1986). One study of particular interest separates out the interacting effects of the type of work a Guatemalan mother is able to do, and the age of her preschool child, in determining whether her working status has a positive or negative effect on that child's height and weight (Engle & Pedersen, 1989). The principle established by the early anthropometrists, that child measurement may be used as a means of highlighting inequalities and disadvantage, has been continued up to the present time.

It is not, however, always easy to disentangle causalities. Sen and Sengupta (1983) documented greater relative growth deficits of preschool girls than of boys in two Indian villages, and concluded that there was a 'systematic sex bias' in the allotment of food to girls. They had no data either on food intake, or food supply, or on access to health care, and it was therefore counter-argued that differentials in health care, rather than food, might lead to the differences between girls' and boys' growth rates (Harriss & Watson, 1987). Although other studies have documented smaller amounts of food being allotted to young girls (Abdullah & Wheeler, 1985), this problem illustrates the reason for one major criticism that is made of the use of anthropometry in assessment and advocacy. There are always likely to be multiple causes of variation in children's heights and weights when anthropometric indicators are being used as a means of assessing the welfare of children. For example, two groups of children may have mean weights below two standard deviations for their age, or height. In one group the outstanding explanation may be a contaminated environment, leading to extensive diarrhoea; in another, seasonal food shortage exacerbated by civil war. Those using anthropometry as a tool must have the capability and the information necessary to provide explanations for observed differences. This information may itself consist of other indicators such as family income or access to clean water. The question then arises: why should height and weight be measured, simply in order to demonstrate that families with low standards of living have small children?

There can be no fixed answer to this problem, and the question again becomes one of advocacy. In some circumstances an effective way of mobilising resources in favour of poor communities may be to demonstrate that their health is poor; or that their children are growing slowly and thus more likely to be ill and underperforming; or that their environment is polluted. In many cases anthropometry is effective *because* it shows the combined effect of several causes. Data on child growth have been so used, for example, in a series of analyses of the situation of women and children in African countries (e.g. UNICEF, 1984).

The question that must be asked, is 'Why anthropometry at all?' If advocacy (and indeed evaluation, as will be shown) requires information on social, environmental and economic factors to be added to anthropometry, in order that the results should be interpreted, then are not the anthropometric indices themselves redundant information? Is it not sufficient to demonstrate that children and their families live in poor conditions, for action to be planned and taken? In many circumstances this is not enough. In order to stimulate politicians and planners to act, it is necessary to demonstrate that the poor environments do indeed have an adverse effect on their inhabitants. Even to demonstrate a high incidence of disease may not be enough. Anthropometry can show that the combined effects of the factors making up a poor environment are holding back the development of children, and contributing to high death rates. In the

context of advocacy and evaluation, anthropometric indicators make the
point that children are growing poorly, and the other data point up the
interlocking causes which may be addressed through both health and
agriculture and food policies.

Evaluation

Since the early days of what Tanner (1981) called 'auxological epidemiology', heights and weights of children have been used to follow the
effects of changes in welfare, the environment, health and nutrition. It is
now accepted that such measurements may be used to evaluate the effects
not just of nutritional, or even of health, programmes and projects, but of
a wide range of interventions intended to improve human welfare and/or
productivity. The argument for doing so is that if a development project
(whether cash crop production, forestry, a co-operative, or anything else)
does not result in an increase in the growth rates of the children of the poor
families involved, then it can hardly be deemed a success in human welfare
terms. There is a debate as to whether such projects should be evaluated in
terms of human welfare or human capital, but development of a 'human
capital' argument logically requires information about the physical state
of both present and future workers.

Two studies of considerable interest attempted to discover whether
changes over time in the economic activity of a community would
necessarily benefit its members, using child anthropometry as the index
measurement. Studies of the same community in India in 1961 and in 1974
showed little or no change in anthropometric indices of preschool children,
although employment opportunities had widened, facilities such as housing
had improved and average incomes had risen by a factor of 2.5. The
explanation was that, in the same period, food prices had trebled
(Thimmayamma et al., 1976). In a study in Mexico it was shown that an
agricultural development programme, although it had resulted in large
increases in food production, and had been accompanied by considerable
improvements in vital statistics and civil amenities, had brought about no
change in the percentage of malnourished children in the area (Hernandez
et al., 1974). The main change was an increase in the mean weights of
'normal' (non-malnourished) children. Indeed, since the population of the
region increased (mainly due to immigration) it can be argued that the
numbers of malnourished children increased in the wake of the agricultural
development. Anthropometric measurements go a step beyond indicators
of production and consumption, measuring the state of individuals and

stimulating questions about the mechanisms by which economic, social and health factors are interlinked. Indeed, studies such as that of Hernandez *et al.* (1974) have been influential in promoting examination of the possible *disbenefits* of development programmes to the poorer classes of the community.

The multiple usefulness of child anthropometry is well illustrated by a study from Indonesia, an evaluation of a programme where child weighing itself was the main activity in an attempt to improve the care and nutritional state of village children. The author recounts how children were regularly weighed, and how a small increase in anthropometric indices resulted. After a time, there was no further improvement, and this plateauing of the growth indices stimulated the project workers to investigate further the reasons for poor growth. They successfully identified low incomes, frequent illness, lack of appreciation of the high energy needs of children, and mothers' lack of time, as factors holding back the further improvement in weight and height indices (Priyosusilo, 1988). This work shows clearly how measurements of children's weights prevented complacency, by demonstrating that in spite of attendance at group meetings, and acceptance of new ideas, mothers were unable to implement changes in their children's diets to an extent which would affect their growth. This contrasts with reports of education and other projects where knowledge and attitude alone are taken as indicators of success, and illustrates another of the uses of anthropometry.

Conclusions

What then are the uses of anthropometry? At the simplest level, it provides measures which enable the physical development of children to be monitored over time, and compared with healthy peers. In combination with other indicators of health, environment and welfare, anthropometric indicators provide clear assessments of the conditions in deprived communities, and a powerful means of evaluating a wide range of developments, by no means exclusively nutritional or health related. They can well be used in the process of advocacy, of presenting the case of the underprivileged for a share of national resources.

It is, however, the case that many reports of anthropometric studies stop short at problem description and give no hint of advocacy. Advocacy goes on from objective reporting and points out why, where and on whose behalf changes should be sought and action should occur. Some scientists have difficulty in accepting this role, especially when working in tropical countries as expatriates. The contrast between the concluding statements, below, of two papers published consecutively in the same issue of one scientific journal, and both documenting the adverse effects of poverty on child growth, illustrate how similar conclusions may, or may not, lead to advocacy on behalf of the subjects of the investigation.

As found in other parts of the world, the children in rural Bangladesh with richer or more educated parents are more likely to consume a greater variety of foods, especially animal foods, and are less likely to be ill, and will have better than average growth

(*Becker* et al., *1986*)

It is unlikely that substantial improvements with a reduction of the differentials described above will take place unless profound social change is brought about. In terms of agricultural policy, these changes must necessarily imply a more equitable distribution of land

(*Victora* et al., *1986*).

The uses of anthropometry, as with any tool or method, are determined by the standpoint of the user.

References

Abdullah, M. & Wheeler, E. F. (1985). Seasonal variations and the distribution of food in a Bangladeshi village. *American Journal of Clinical Nutrition*, **41**, 1305–13.

Aykroyd, W. R. & Rajagopal, K. (1936). The state of nutrition of school children in South India. *Indian Journal of Medical Research*, **24**, 419–37.

Beaton, G., Kelly, A., Kevany, J., Martorell, R. & Mason, J. (1990). *Appropriate Uses of Anthropometric Indices in Children, Nutrition Policy Discussion Paper no 7*, Geneva: ACC/SCN.

Becker, S., Black, R. E., Brown, K. H. & Nahar, S. (1986). The relationship between socioeconomic status and morbidity, food intake and growth in young children in two villages in Bangladesh. *Ecology of Food and Nutrition*, **18**, 251–64.

Berry, V. & Petty, C., eds. (1992). *The Nyasaland Nutrition Survey Papers 1938–1943. Agriculture, Food and Health*. London: Academy Books.

Culwick, G. (1951). *Diet in the Gezira Irrigated Area*, Sudan. Khartoum: Sudan Survey Department.

Davies, A. G. & Wheeler, E. F. (1989). Analysis of the weights of children of Bangladeshi origin attending two clinics in Tower Hamlets, *Child Care, Health and Development*, **15**, 167–74.

Dowler, E. A., Payne, P. R., Seo, Y., Thomson, A. M. & Wheeler, E. F. (1982). *Food Policy*, **7**, 99–112.

Engle, P. L. & Pedersen, M. E. (1989). Maternal work for earnings and child nutritional status in urban Guatemala. *Ecology of Food and Nutrition*, **22**, 211–23.

Eveleth, P. & Tanner, J. M. (1976). *Worldwide Variation in Human Growth*, Cambridge: The University Press.

Farthing, M. J. G., Mata, L., Urrutia, J. J. & Kronmal, R. A. (1986). Natural history of *Giardia* infection of infants and children in rural Guatemala and its impact on physical growth. *American Journal of Clinical Nutrition*, **43**, 395–405.

Gangulee, N. (1939). *Health and Nutrition in India*. London: Faber and Faber.

Grant, M. (1951). *Techniques for the Analysis of Height and Weight Data in Tropical Countries*, Mimeo, Human Nutrition Unit, London School of Hygiene and Tropical Medicine.

Gupta, M. C. & Urrutia, J. J. (1982). Effect of periodic antiascaris and antigiardia treatment on nutritional status in preschool children. *American Journal of Clinical Nutrition*, **36**, 79–86.

Habicht, J. P., Martorell, R., Yarbrough, C., Malina, R. M. & Klein, R. E. (1974). Height and weight standards for preschool children. *Lancet*, **i**, 611–14.

Hakim, P. & Solimano, G. (1976). Nutrition and National development: establishing the connection. *Food Policy*, **1**, 249–59.

Hanumantha Rao, D. & Satyananarayana, K. (1976). Nutritional status of people of different socio-economic groups in a rural area, with special reference to pre-school children. *Ecology of Food and Nutrition*, **4**, 237–42.

Harriss, B. & Watson, E. (1987). The sex ratio in South Asia. In *Geography of Gender*. Momsen, J. H. & Townsend, J., eds, London: Hutchinson.

Hernandez, M., Hidalgo, C. P., Hernandez, J. R., Madrigal, H. & Chavez, A. (1974). Effect of economic growth on nutrition in a tropical community. *Ecology of Food and Nutrition*, **3**, 283–91.

Heywood, P. F. (1986). Nutritional status as a risk factor for mortality in children in the highlands of Papua New Guinea. In *Proceedings of the XIII International Congress of Nutrition*, Taylor, T. G. & Jenkins, N. K., eds, p. 103, London: John Libbey.

Lutter, C. K., Mora, J. O., Habicht, J-P., Rasmussen, K. M., Robson, D. S. & Herrera, M. G. (1990). Age-specific responsiveness of weight and length to nutritional supplementation. *American Journal of Clinical Nutrition*, **51**, 359–64.

Mata, L. J., Urrutia, J. J. & Lechtig, A. (1971). Infection and nutrition of children of a low socio-economic rural community. *American Journal of Clinical Nutrition*, **24**, 249–59.

Paton, D. N. & Findlay, L. (1926). *Poverty, Nutrition and Growth*. Medical Research Council Special Report Series no 101. London: HMSO.

Payne, P. R. (1975). The assessment of needs and priorities. *Food and Nutrition* (FAO) **1(4)**, 6–10.

Payne, P. R. (1990). Themes in food security: measuring malnutrition. *Bulletin of the Institute of Development Studies*, **21**, 56–70.

Priyosusilo, A. (1988). Health in the balance: the under-fives weighing program. *Indian Journal of Paediatrics*, (Suppl.), **55**, S88–99.

Rowland, M. G. M., Cole, T. J. & Whitehead, R. G. (1977). A quantitative study into the role of infection in determining nutritional status in a Gambian village. *British Journal of Nutrition*, **37**, 441–50.

Rowntree, S. (1913). *Poverty: A Study of Town Life*, London: Nelson.

Sen, A. & Sengupta, S. (1983). Malnutrition of Indian children and the sex bias. *Economic and Political Weekly*, **18**, 855–64.

Tanner, J. M. (1981). *A History of the Study of Human Growth*, Cambridge: The University Press.

Thimmayamma, B. V. S., Rau, P., Desai, V. K. & Jayaprakesh, B. N. (1976). A study of changes in socio-economic conditions, dietary intake and nutritional status of Indian rural families over a decade. *Ecology of Food and Nutrition*, **5**, 235–60.

United Nations Children's Fund (UNICEF) (1984). *Situation Analysis of Children and Women in Kenya*. Republic of Kenya Central Bureau of Statistics, Nairobi.

US Department of Health Education and Welfare (USDHEW) (1976). *NCHS Growth Charts*, HRA 76-1120, 25, 3: Rockville, Md.

Valverde, V., Martorell, R., Meija-Pivaral, V., Delgado, H., Lechtig, A., Teller, C. & Klein, R. E. (1977). Relationship between family land value and nutritional status. *Ecology of Food and Nutrition*, **6**, 1–7.

Victora, C. G., Vaughan, J. P., Kirkwood, B., Martines, J. C. & Barcelos, L. B. (1986). Child malnutrition and land ownership in Southern Brazil. *Ecology of Food and Nutrition*, **18**, 265–75.

Wandel, M. & Homhoe-Offersen, G. (1988). Women as nutrition mediators: a case study from Sri Lanka. *Ecology of Food and Nutrition*, **21**, 117–30.

Waterlow, J. C. (1972). Classification and definition of protein-calorie malnutrition. *British Medical Journal*, **2**, 566–9.

Wilson, H. E. C., Ahmad, B. & Mitra, D. D. (1937). Nutritional survey of schoolboys in Calcutta and the Punjab. *Indian Journal of Medical Research*, **24**, 817–38.

Part five
Deficiencies of energy and protein

26

Undernutrition in Germany in the post-war period

ELSIE M. WIDDOWSON

Studies on undernutrition during and immediately after the war

When the war ended in May 1945 and the terrible situation in the concentration camps was exposed, several groups of investigators went to Europe to make what tests they could on the surviving inmates (Lipscomb, 1945; Murray, 1947; Hottinger *et al.*, 1948). However, the plight of the prisoners, their overcrowding and state of starvation and disease made it impossible for the investigators to do all that they had planned, for relief had to take precedence over research. Some valuable information was collected during the period of rehabilitation, particularly the large amount of food that was consumed (Murray, 1947). Seven Danish doctors were among those deported to Germany and imprisoned in Neuengamme concentration camp, and they were able to make some clinical studies and to record their observations on their fellow prisoners. They also followed up over 1000 of them after liberation (Helweg-Larsen *et al.*, 1952).

Between September 1944 and May 1945 the transport system in Holland was paralysed by a strike, and for these 8 months there was a severe shortage of food and consequent hunger and undernutrition. Beattie and his colleagues went to Holland soon after the war ended and made studies of the effect of undernutrition for eight months on oxygen consumption and nitrogen balance (Beattie & Herbert, 1947a, b; Beattie, Herbert & Bell, 1947, 1948). Smith (1947a, b) also went to Holland and examined records of weights of infants born at two hospitals during the period of food shortage. He found that infants born between October 1944 and February 1945 weighed on average 240 g less than those born before the period of food shortage. The birth weights rose again as food became plentiful. Antonov (1947) made similar observations in Leningrad during the siege. Between September 1941 and February 1942 very little food was available, and babies born during that time were on average 540 g lighter than those born in times of plenty.

In the United States, Keys and his colleagues devoted much time and effort to making an experimental study of 'semistarvation' and rehabilitation on 32 young men. The results, and an extensive review of the literature on starvation and undernutrition, were published in two large volumes (Keys *et al.*, 1950).

The food situation in Germany in the postwar period and the background to our studies

The food supply for the German population during the war was reasonably adequate, though the important principle adopted in the United Kingdom that bread and potatoes should remain unrationed was not part of the German rationing scheme, and all foods were rationed. When the war ended food became scarce. All foods were still rationed, but by June 1946 the rations provided the normal consumer with only 1052 kcal (4.4 MJ) a day. Professor McCance saw the opportunity of making studies of the effects of undernutrition on the human body in a way that had not been possible in the atmosphere of crisis and emotion that prevailed just after the war. Sir Edward Mellanby, then Secretary of the Medical Research Council, supported him, and in March 1946 he and I, with Wing-Commander (Dr) Smart, seconded from the Air Force to act as our escort, travelled around Germany in a Volkswagen in search of a base from which we might work. After visiting Hamburg, Hannover and Düsseldorf, we came to Wuppertal. This was spread along the valley of the river Wupper and was the fusion of Elberfeld and Barmen. Before the war it had derived its fame and wealth from the textile industry, particularly lace, ribbons and elastic goods. It was now in ruins after several severe bombing raids and housing was at a premium. It had two great advantages from our point of view. First there were the I.G. Farben Laboratories where we could have laboratory accommodation, and secondly there was a large municipal hospital, and more important, Dr Dorothy Rosenbaum, who had been in charge of the hospital during the war years while the men were away, and was now a senior physician. She had a German father and English mother, she spoke colloquial English, and she was a great anglophile. She proved to be of immense value to us, and it is doubtful whether we could have done our work without her.

We came back to England in April. The MRC agreed to finance our project and we began to get our team together. We persuaded doctors and scientists with expertise in various aspects of medicine and physiology to come to Wuppertal for several months and use their skills to investigate the effects of undernutrition on some aspect of function or structure of the human body. We returned to Wuppertal in June 1946, and with the co-operation and goodwill of the Control Commission for Germany who arranged for our accommodation, food and transport, we started work. We organised an outpatient clinic which all those applying for extra rations for hunger oedema had to attend before the rations were granted, and it was from this source that all the subjects taking part in our investigations came. We had three wards at our disposal to which they were admitted.

As the months went by the energy value of the rations for the normal consumer remained at 1000 to 1500 kcal (4.2 to 6.3 MJ) a day. There were long bread queues, and those at the end of the queue often did not get their allocation. There were many scales of extra rations for children, expectant and nursing mothers, heavy workers, and for those certified as having hunger oedema, which provided 480 kcal (2 MJ) a day. There were also unofficial ways of obtaining extra food, the most important of which was 'hamstering'. People in the towns went by very crowded trains, sometimes on the roof, into the surrounding countryside with whatever goods they had available. They went from farm to farm in the hope of exchanging their goods for food – often a sack of potatoes. The farmers were supposed to sell all they grew to the authorities, but of course they did not; for money was of little use to them! There was nothing to buy with it. It was only the young and strong who could make these hamstering expeditions, and old people living alone, and those living in institutions had nothing but their rations. Consequently they tended to be the most undernourished section of the population. Others severely undernourished were men who had been taken as prisoners of war to Russia and who were now being repatriated. More men than women attended our hunger oedema clinic, and of these nearly half were over 60 years old. Because men were more severely undernourished than women, most of our detailed investigations were made on them.

Investigations on adults

One of Professor McCance's interests was hunger oedema. There was a large literature on this manifestation of undernutrition (McCance, 1951*a*), but the fundamental reason for the oedema, particularly round the legs and ankles, so often described among populations who were short of food, had never been satisfactorily explained. The oedema was more common in men than in women, and in older men than younger ones. If it was not too severe it disappeared while the person was lying down at night and reappeared during the day. There was generally a diuresis during the night. The concentration of proteins in the serum was low, and this was undoubtedly one reason for the oedema, but it was not the whole story. We measured total body water by urea dilution (isotopes were not available to us then) and extracellular fluid volume with sodium thiocyanate. We found that all the undernourished men we studied, whether they had oedema or not, had an excess of extracellular fluid in their bodies (Widdowson & McCance, 1951). The oedema that could be seen and felt in the legs represented only a small fraction of the excess extracellular fluid in the body, and whether it appeared as oedema or not depended on posture and the state of the capillaries.

In 1946 liver punctures and heart catheterisation had just come in as techniques that could safely be applied to patients to assess the function of the liver and heart. Sheila Sherlock and Sheila Howarth came to Germany as experts in these two fields. The results showed that the function of the liver was normal in undernutrition (Sherlock & Walshe, 1951), and the heart also functioned normally, though the pulse rate was slow and the arterial blood pressure low (Howarth, 1951). Radiological examination showed that the size of the heart appeared more appropriate to the person's height and his weight when well nourished than to his weight at the time of the examination (Berridge, 1951a), which suggests that the heart muscle is preferentially preserved.

The renal function of undernourished men was found to be normal (McCance, 1951b), indicating that renal failure was not a cause of the oedema. Radiological examination of the alimentary tract showed that stomach emptying and intestinal transit times were significantly longer than normal (Berridge, 1951b), and there were no complaints of diarrhoea. Radiological measurements of the bones were difficult to interpret because the marrow cavity had lost its marrow and become filled with extracellular fluid which was more opaque to X-rays than fat (Berridge & Prior, 1951).

Undernutrition, therefore, brought about structural changes in the body, particularly loss of fat, and an inevitable loss of protein, and an increase in the volume of extracellular fluid. In spite of this the functions of the organs remained normal. There were, however, behavioural changes and emotional disturbances, but it was concluded that these were not caused by the undernutrition directly, but were due to the anxiety that accompanied it (Russell-Davis, 1951).

Towards the end of the 6 months of investigations I made a study of the response of 20 undernourished men aged 26 to 80 to unlimited food

(Widdowson, 1951*a*). All the men had lost weight (mean 17%) and they all had hunger oedema. They were admitted to hospital and for the first week they had only the hospital diet, which provided 1900 kcal (7.9 MJ) a day. All the preliminary tests were made during this time. Then we provided extra food, cheese, tinned meat and fish, dried milk and cocoa sufficient to supply another 1500 kcal (6.3 MJ) a day. In addition to this, there were unlimited amounts of bread, margarine and sugar. When the men sat down to eat their first breakfast they all took enough to provide 2000 kcal (8.4 MJ), and four of them 3000 kcal (12.6 MJ) at one meal. One of these was 80 years old. There were no ill effects. The rehabilitation continued for six weeks, and the mean energy intake over this time was 6000 kcal (25.1 MJ) a day. The six men who were 60–80 years old ate a little less food than the under-60s, 5600 kcal (23.4 MJ) a day. The body weight increased from 59 to 69 kg over the six weeks, and the older men gained almost as much weight as the younger ones. There was a significant rise in serum protein concentration and a reduction in extracellular fluid volume, both in absolute terms and as a percentage of the body weight. However, the oedema did not entirely disappear, which disappointed the men. We tried giving them less salt, but this had no effect. Apart from this there was a great improvement in physical and mental condition. At first the men were apathetic and miserable. At the end they were bright and cheerful, and proud to have taken part in such a pleasant experiment.

Although the studies so far described were made on men, some investigations were made on women, in particular on the size of their babies at birth and the yield of breast milk (Dean, 1951), and on milk composition (Gunther & Stanier, 1951). The Landesfrauenklinik in Wuppertal provided facilities for this work. Meticulous records had been kept at the hospital for many years of the weights of infants born there and of the amounts of breast milk they took, and these records were made available to us. Records of 22000 births between 1937 and 1948 were analysed. Food was plentiful in 1937, and the average birthweight was 185 g more than in 1945 when food became scarce. In 1937 the infants took 25% more breast milk, measured by test weighing from the fifth to the ninth day, than they did in 1945. The composition of milk secreted by German women in 1946 was similar in respect of protein, fat, calcium and vitamins to that reported for English women during the war.

Studies in infants and children

During a period of food shortage in Italy in 1944, mixtures of soya flour and malted cereals had been used as a supplement for children's diets. Dame Harriette Chick was asked by the United Nations Relief and Rehabilitation Administration (UNRRA) to investigate this further. She paid several visits to us while we were in Germany, accompanied by Dr Hume, and she arranged with Rex Dean that he should carry out controlled trials to see whether young children would thrive when such mixtures made up a large part of their diet. He made several studies on infants, and on children up to 11 years. There were problems, partly because of illness unconnected with the diet, and partly because at the beginning we knew nothing about the presence of a trypsin inhibitor in soya and so did nothing to remove it. We learned about it after the trials began. However, after many troubles and setbacks some satisfactory trials were completed which showed that adequate substitutes for milk could probably be made from plant sources (Dean, 1953). The importance of this work lies, not so much in the results of these particular trials, but because as a consequence of them Rex Dean was asked by Sir Harold Himsworth, Secretary of the MRC in the early 1950s, to go to Uganda where infantile malnutrition was known to be prevalent, as leader of a small research group, to investigate the use of plant proteins for infant feeding. Dr Whitehead describes what arose from this in his chapter (p. 303).

During our first six months in Germany we weighed and measured some hundreds of children living in various orphanages, and they were examined clinically. It is probable that these children were typical to a greater or lesser degree of all children living on the German rations. They were short and light for their ages when compared with British and American standards. The older children were worse than the younger ones and the boys were worse than the girls. In other respects the children seemed normal and lively though in rather poor physical condition. I have described in my *Recollections* (Widdowson, 1991) how, just as we thought we should be coming home from Germany at the beginning of 1947, Sir Edward Mellanby commissioned me to set up a study on undernourished children to compare the nutritive value of breads made from flours of different extraction rates to provide information which would help in the decision about the 'Postwar loaf'. We found a children's home in Duisburg where we made the investigations and they took us 2 years. The end of it all was that under the conditions of the experiment, unlimited amounts of bread made from 100%, 85% and 72% extraction flours, and 72%

extraction flour enriched with B vitamins and iron, all promoted excellent growth and improvement in physical condition in undernourished children, even though bread accounted for 75% of the total energy intake. The rest of the diet was made up of the German rations of vegetables, which were all made into soups, and small amounts of milk and other animal foods which contributed only 4% of the total energy, and 8 grams of animal protein a day. Total protein provided 13% of the energy, fat 11% and carbohydrate 76%. All the flours were fortified with calcium carbonate. The children were underweight and underheight at the outset. They all grew at a rapid rate and improved in physical condition whatever bread they were eating. Growth was not further improved by the addition of 500 ml of milk a day.

I will finish with one other observation we made, quite unplanned and almost by accident (Widdowson, 1951*b*). While the bread experiment was going on in Duisburg we weighed and measured all the children every fortnight in two smaller homes in Wuppertal where they were getting nothing but their German rations. We planned, after 6 months, to give extra bread to one home and not to the other. As the first 6 months went by we realised that the children were gaining weight at very different rates at the two homes, although their ages and sex distribution were similar, they were equally underweight and they were receiving the same German rations. We had promised the extra bread to the home where the children were growing more rapidly, but to our astonishment when we did this the children stopped gaining weight so fast, and they gained considerably less than they had done in the first 6 months although we knew they were now eating more food. Simultaneously, in the other home where the children were getting no extra food they started to gain weight faster. There was clearly something else going on that outweighed the benefit of the extra food we were providing. This something else was a most unpleasant housemother who was in charge of the children at the home where they gained weight slowly during the first 6 months, and who was moved by the authorities to the other home just at the time when we began to supply the extra bread. The children were in constant fear of her and she chose mealtimes to scold them publicly. They had to sit in silence while this was going on with their bowls of soup getting cold in front of them. By this time they were in a state of agitation and some of them were in tears.

We recorded the amount of food the children ate at both homes, and during the second 6 months those children who were provided with extra bread had an energy intake 20% higher than it had been during the first six months, and yet they failed to put on so much weight. The most likely explanation seems to be that the unhappiness and nervous tension raised the metabolic rate and consequently the energy expenditure.

Conclusions

I have found it an interesting exercise going over the investigations we made in Germany 45 years ago. What we did may seem dull and out of date today in this country of affluence and plenty, where the problem is over- rather than undernutrition. But millions are still undernourished and starving in Africa and other parts of the world, and again relief takes precedence over research. We took an opportunity of studying the effects of undernutrition on individuals who had previously been well nourished, but for a period of about two years had insufficient food to meet their requirements. The degree of undernutrition was not life-threatening, so we were able to make our investigations without feeling that we must at all costs provide extra food.

If I were asked which of our observations I regard as having the most relevance today I would select four. The first is that, in spite of the changes in the composition of the body that accompany the loss of weight in undernourished individuals, the functions of the organs and systems of the body remain normal. The second is the very large amount of food and of energy that undernourished adults and children need and will take in order to bring their weights back to normal. The third is the high nutritive value of wheaten bread, whatever the extraction rate, so long as the rest of the diet provides the minerals and vitamins that the cereal lacks. For the fourth I will quote from a new Danish publication entitled *The Child in Focus. A Manual for Staff at Children's Institutions in Romania.* It refers to my observations and concludes 'Children need love in order to grow and develop'.

References

Antonov, A. N. (1947). Children born during the siege of Leningrad in 1942. *Journal of Pediatrics*, **30**, 250–9.

Beattie, J. & Herbert, P. H. (1947*a*). The estimation of the metabolic rate in the starvation state. *British Journal of Nutrition*, **1**, 185–91.

Beattie, J. & Herbert, P. H. (1947*b*). Basal metabolism during recovery from severe undernutrition. *British Journal of Nutrition*, **1**, 192–202.

Beattie, J., Herbert, P. H. & Bell, D. J. (1947). Nitrogen balances during recovery from severe undernutrition. *British Journal of Nutrition*, **1**, 202–16.

Beattie, J., Herbert, P. H. & Bell, D. J. (1948). Famine oedema. *British Journal of Nutrition*, **2**, 47–65.

Berridge, F. R. (1951*a*). Radiological observations on the heart. In *Studies of Undernutrition, Wuppertal 1946–9*, pp. 260–272. Special Report Series. Medical Research Council No. 275, London: HMSO.

Berridge, F. R. (1951b). Radiological observations on the alimentary tract. In *Studies of Undernutrition, Wuppertal 1946–9*, pp. 97–110. Special Report Series. Medical Research Council No. 275, London: HMSO.

Berridge, F. R. & Prior, K. M. (1951). Radiological observations on the bones. In *Studies of Undernutrition, Wuppertal 1946–9*, pp. 289–295. Special Report Series. Medical Research Council No. 275, London: HMSO.

Dean, R. F. A. (1951). The size of the baby at birth and the yield of breast milk. In *Studies of Undernutrition, Wuppertal 1946–9*, pp. 346–378. Special Report Series. Medical Research Council No. 275, London: HMSO.

Dean, R. F. A. (1953). *Plant Proteins in Infant Feeding*. Special Report Series. Medical Research Council No. 279, London: HMSO.

Gunther, M. & Stanier, J. E. (1951). The volume and composition of human milk. In *Studies of Undernutrition, Wuppertal 1946–9*, pp. 379–400. Special Report Series. Medical Research Council No. 275, London: HMSO.

Helweg-Larsen, P., Hoffmeyer, H., Kieler, J., Hess Thaysen, E., Hess Thaysen, J., Thygesen, P. & Wulff, M. H. (1952). Famine disease in German concentration camps. Complications and sequelae. Copenhagen: Ejnar Munksgaard.

Hottinger, A., Gsell, O., Uhlinger, E., Salzmann, C. & Labhert, A. (1948). *Hungerkrenkheit, Hungerödem, Hungertuberculose*. Basal: Benno Schwabe & Co.

Howarth, S. (1951). Cardiac output and the peripheral circulation. In *Studies of Undernutrition, Wuppertal, 1946–9*. Special Report Series. Medical Research Council, No. 275, pp. 238–259, London: HMSO.

Keys, A., Brozek, J., Henschel, A., Mickelesen, O. & Taylor, H. L. (1950). *The Biology of Human Starvation*, Vols I and II. Minneapolis: The University of Minnesota Press.

Lipscomb, F. M. (1945). Medical aspects of Belsen concentration camp. *Lancet* ii, 313–15.

McCance, R. A. (1951a). The history, significance and aetiology of hunger oedema. In *Studies of Undernutrition, Wuppertal 1946–9*. Special Report Series. Medical Research Council No. 275, London: HMSO.

McCance, R. A. (1951b). Aspects of renal function and water metabolism. In *Studies of Undernutrition, Wuppertal 1946–9*, pp. 175–192. Special Report Series. Medical Council No. 275, London: HMSO.

Murray, R. O. (1947). Recovery from starvation. *Lancet* i, 507–11.

Russell-Davis, D. (1951). Emotional disturbances and behavioural reactions. In *Studies of Undernutrition, Wuppertal 1946–9*, pp. 147–164. Special Report Series. Medical Research Council No. 275, London: HMSO.

Sherlock, S. and Walshe, V. M. (1951). Hepatic structure and function. In *Studies of Undernutrition, Wuppertal 1946–9*, pp. 111–134. Special Report Series. Medical Research Council No. 275, London: HMSO.

Smith, C. A. (1947a). Effects of maternal undernutrition upon the new-born infant in Holland (1944–45). *Journal of Pediatrics*, **30**, 229–43.

Smith, C. A. (1947b). The effect of wartime starvation in Holland upon pregnancy and its product. *American Journal of Obstetrics and Gynecology*, **53**, 599–606.

Widdowson, E. M. (1951a). The response to unlimited food. In *Studies of Undernutrition, Wuppertal, 1946–9*, pp. 313–345. Special Report Series. Medical Research Council No. 275, London: HMSO.

Widdowson, E. M. (1951b). Mental contentment and physical growth. *Lancet*, **i**, 1316–8.

Widdowson, E. M. (1991). In *The Nutrition Society 1941–1991. Presidents and Honorary Members. Their stories and recollections*, pp. 79–86. Compiled by E. M. Widdowson. CAB International Wallingford, Oxon.

Widdowson, E. M. & McCance, R. A. (1951). The effect of undernutrition and of posture on the volume and composition of the body fluids. In *Studies of Undernutrition, Wuppertal 1946–9,* pp. 165–174. Special Report Series. Medical Research Council No. 275, London: HMSO.

Widdowson, E. M. & McCance, R. A. (1954). *Studies on the nutritive value of bread and on the effect of variation in the extraction rate of flour on the growth of undernourished children.* Special Report Series. Medical Research Council No. 287, London: HMSO.

27

Kwashiorkor in Uganda

R. G. WHITEHEAD

The invaluable role that working in the old colonial territories, and now the third world, has played as a training ground for British nutritional science has been stressed many times. In some ways this was only to be expected because the more extreme forms of nutritional disorder encountered were bound to stimulate both interest in the subject as well as the consciences of bright young doctors and scientists. What was not anticipated when they were first encouraged to conduct nutritional research in the tropics was the extent to which this experience would be priceless for the development of diet-orientated health programmes in the United Kingdom. It was, after all, not until the late 1970s that it became widely recognised that we too still have nutritional problems, albeit arising primarily from affluence rather than poverty. This chapter describes the contribution made by Uganda. As the title implies, the main theme will be kwashiorkor, but I will also be emphasising the evolution of basic investigative philosophies that have become central to nutritional science in general.

It is always invidious to single out key figures in science, especially when a venture has been essentially a corporate effort, but in terms of my own personal scientific development there were really three people in Uganda who influenced me the most, Dr Hugh Trowell, Prof 'Rex' Dean and Prof 'Dick' Jelliffe. Each was very different from the other both in terms of personality as well as professional interest. In many ways there was little direct scientific interaction between them. Then, as now, it was largely necessary for young investigators to integrate the wisdom of wise men for themselves!

Hugh Trowell

Hugh Trowell was the first of this triumvirate to arrive in East Africa. He was very much one of the old school of colonial physicians, with strong missionary leanings. As with the rest of his colleagues his patients definitely came first and science second. But in spite of this order of priorities, in a remarkably short period of time they had set up a medical school at Mulago hospital that was to become second to none in 'Black Africa'. Ultimately it was integrated within Makerere University College.

In the 1930s, when Hugh Trowell arrived, the child with gross oedema was all too common a sight. There was, however, much debate as to its cause. Perhaps because of a preoccupation with infectious diseases and parasitology it is not surprising that round-worm or hook-worm infestations were considered the prime culprits by most physicians. It was easy to justify this point of view as virtually every child treated would be afflicted by one or both of these two parasites.

In Uganda there was another striking clinical feature which intrigued the pathologists and this was the presence of extensive skin lesions. In many ways these lesions resembled those of pellagra, with the notable exception that they did not predominate in the exposed parts of the skin, but in areas like the groin where there was mechanical friction. Nevertheless, pellagra became one of the accepted alternative explanations but, because of the atypical features, the term 'infantile pellagra' was coined. In so far as Uganda was concerned, this was the beginning of the diet versus infection controversy, something that was to go on for many years.

A greater issue was to emerge, however. Hugh Trowell started to speculate on the possibility that the disease could have a much more basic nutritional aetiology and be due to a deficiency of weaning foods containing adequate amounts of protein.

It is not as widely recognised as it should be that at exactly the same time as Cicely Williams was carrying out her pioneering work in West Africa, Hugh Trowell was having very similar ideas in Uganda. In those days, however, there was little or no contact across Africa. Cicely Williams and Hugh Trowell never met until the conclusion of the Second World War and after she had transferred to the Malaya service and been a prisoner of war. Medical and scientific literature was also difficult to find in Africa. I am always intrigued by the apology at the end of Cicely Williams' first paper on kwashiorkor for the lack of any references (Williams, 1933). She explains that there was no library for her to obtain any! I wonder if any journal editor would be so farsighted nowadays as to publish a paper with such an omission, however valid the excuse?

On 'leave' in the United Kingdom Hugh Trowell was given little encouragement for his protein deficiency hypothesis. The experts he consulted were convinced that if the Uganda disease were a nutritional one it was pellagra. Not a man to be easily put off, Trowell continued with his beliefs, but a new and quite bizarre episode was about to begin which was to hold up the development of nutritional science in Uganda for some time.

The concept of protein deficiency in a British Protectorate was deemed politically objectionable. Infections were unavoidable, they were always with us; vitamin deficiencies were new and thus not having planned for them was defendable; but something as basic as a lack of protein was quite unacceptable. This was not the whole saga, there was worse to come! Trowell heard, quite incorrectly, from a visiting academic, that the literal meaning of Cicely Williams' term 'kwashiorkor' was 'red boy' (Trowell and Dean, 1952). This was not too implausible as some cases did tend to develop reddish hair, but when Trowell started to use this interpretation in his lectures the colonial authorities decided there were political overtones and he became virtually ostracised!

Understandably this sort of treatment had a profound effect on Trowell from which he never really recovered. Certainly he retained a narrowness of vision about the causes of kwashiorkor. Even a couple of weeks before his death in 1989 when he came to see me in Cambridge, he expressed his concern about my own suggestions that infection could play a major exacerbatory role in the development of oedema via loss of albumin into the gut resulting from diseases such as diarrhoea (Lunn, Whitehead & Coward, 1979). He was also upset by comments that micronutrient deficiencies might also be important after all. I fear he felt that even his friends were beginning to stab him in the back.

I have gone into this strange and somewhat sad story because, not only does Trowell deserve recognition along with Cicely Williams for their joint pioneering work, it sets the scene for the later, more scientific work from Uganda. Furthermore, being told this story as a young postdoctoral scientist warned me about what can happen when the results of scientific research are incompatible with current political sensitivities. This was to stand me in good stead on many occasions, both in Uganda and after returning to the UK!

Rex Dean

Dean was a quite different sort of person from Trowell. He was from the McCance and Widdowson school of nutrition and could be quite tough and ruthless. His first task was to persuade the Medical Research Council that the high prevalence of oedematous malnutrition in Uganda made

Kampala an ideal place for them to set up a research unit. The case that eventually appealed to the Council was that it provided an excellent opportunity to settle once and for all that this exotic disease truly was caused by primary protein malnutrition.

Most of the work that Dean did in the early 50s was directed to this end (Dean & Schwartz, 1953). In retrospect, much of it now seems rather indefinite. By demonstrating that kwashiorkor was associated with low plasma albumin concentrations as well as widespread enzyme deficiencies, which were protein in nature, and by showing that the clinical and biochemical signs could be readily reversed by therapies using diets high in protein, the primary role of protein deficiency was deemed proven. It is easy to be critical of such reasoning now, but at the time the techniques used were very much state of the art, especially in the heart of Africa.

It was into this intellectual climate that I myself arrived in 1959. It was made clear that research into vitamins and minerals was quite unnecessary as was invoking infection into any hypothesis. It was mainly for these reasons that my own initial work centred on amino acid metabolism, and the inability of the fat-infiltrated liver to catabolise histidine, phenyl-alanine, tyrosine and lysine, for example. Later I was to concentrate on plasma imbalances in the relative concentrations of various essential amino acids vis-a-vis the non-essential ones (Whitehead, 1969). Because of the infection 'embargo', however, any cases I investigated in whom an intercurrent infection was diagnosed had to be removed from the data set! This presented difficulties to a young scientist trying to build up enough information for his first papers! But it had a more serious significance. It meant that my published data ran the risk of becoming atypical of the great majority of cases of kwashiorkor as seen in Uganda.

Relating this story perhaps suggests an implied criticism of my predecessor. This is not my intention. Scientific interpretation is inevitably influenced by the scientific dogma of the time, but we must allow new concepts to emerge as relevant information becomes available, painful though this may be to those who have fought hard to establish conflicting concepts.

Rex Dean was one of the great pioneers of nutritional research into kwashiorkor. He was as crucial to the development of the 'Uganda school' of nutritional thought as John Waterlow was for the 'Jamaican' one. It is a sad fact, however, that few remember Dean. His active life in research was essentially limited, cut short by an incurable disease that he contracted whilst on a consultation for the United Nations in the Far East. He struggled on in great pain and fortitude for a number of years, sufficient to give a number of young people, including myself, their scientific chance in life and for this we are all grateful. It is not easy to look back and assess objectively someone whom you have known only during a traumatic phase of his life. Although essentially a physiologist by inclination, he had great breadth of vision and encouraged individual young scientists to tackle many different aspects of the topic. These covered not only an understanding of the intricacies of the pathophysiology of kwashiorkor, but also the associated sociology and anthropology of its causation.

On arrival in Uganda one clinical issue that disturbed Dean greatly was the high mortality in cases of kwashiorkor and marasmus that seemed to be acceptable in the hospital wards. Indeed his uncompromising and frequently caustic comments to this effect made him many enemies. To Dean the dietary therapy seemed all too haphazard. Often the children were given little more than the standard hospital food in spite of the fact that the children's physiological ability to digest, absorb and assimilate such food was grossly impaired. Ultimately he developed a liquid mixture based on dried skimmed milk which was to prove much more effective. Dried skimmed milk was readily available as an aid food, but in the 1950s few really knew how the high-quality protein could best be used. It was often left dumped in stores until it was beyond any value. Incredible though it may seem to us now, it was not realised that the protein in the dried skimmed milk could not be utilised by the body unless supported by sufficient dietary energy. The aid food supplied was essentially a waste product and had had much of its energy removed during the manufacturing of butter! Dean solved this problem by adding two local products, cotton seed oil and sugar. Interestingly he found that the final product still remained a powder after dry mixing, as the oil became coated around the milk protein particles. In keeping with the philosophy of the time he also added calcium caseinate, not only for its mineral content but also to increase still further the total protein. Whether or not this could be totally justified in the light of modern knowledge is very much open to doubt, but there can be no disputing the fact that the children certainly recovered much more rapidly and with a marked reduction in mortality on this therapeutic mixture than they had done on previous ward food (Dean, 1960).

It is arguable that this success was equally due to a second of Dean's nutritional innovations. Dean forcefully introduced into the Ugandan paediatric world the concept of 'dietary discipline'. Coining this term was his way of emphasising that prescribing a precise number of calories and amount of protein, and stating the exact times of the day when they should be given, was just as important as for drug therapy with which the ward staff were more familiar. His observations had led him to the conclusion that insufficient attention to such details had resulted in critically ill children not receiving the quantities of nutrients necessary for them to stand any chance of restoring their anabolic processes. It was essential, in his view, that not only should the prescribed amount of therapeutic formula per 4 hourly feed be systematically recorded, but also the amount actually consumed. When this was significantly less than 4 g protein/kg/d and 150 kcal/kg/d the child was immediately switched to intragastric tube feeding.

The type of discipline he insisted upon reminds me of that which I encounter in present-day intensive baby care units where the basic dietary problems of feeding very low birthweight babies are similar. The degree of technological sophistication one now sees is different from what we had over 30 years ago in the middle of Africa, but the same attention to detail is familiar. Dean indeed was a pioneer. His clinical and nutritional methods for the therapy of kwashiorkor and marasmus have had an impact throughout the third world. As a product of the McCance/Widdowson fold, however, Dean was primarily driven by scientific curiosity. It is sad he was unable to witness the products of his scientific inspiration that were to bear fruit at the Dunn in Cambridge and at Keneba in The Gambia.

Dick Jelliffe

In the same way that Dean was very different from Trowell, Jelliffe was totally unlike Dean. With Jelliffe the main driving force was the prevention of kwashiorkor and marasmus via the introduction of simple public health and nutritional measures. Jelliffe was always keen to emphasise the 'multifactorial' causation of malnutrition. For him a lack of food or a lack of a specific nutrient such as protein was but one component causing what, by the late 1960s, was becoming known as protein-calorie malnutrition. Under his overall leadership as professor of paediatrics there were two further notable innovations in Uganda.

One of these was 'Mwanamugimu'. This was a rehabilitation centre housed in a relatively primitive building close to the brand new and architecturally splendid Mulago hospital. The difference in appearance and philosophy could not have been greater! Mwanamugimu's main purpose was to demonstrate to the mothers of malnourished children that they could rehabilitate even very severely wasted children themselves using local foods grown in their own gardens or 'shambas'. Once the child was out of the acute phase of malnutrition and no longer needed to be tubefed, the mothers were shown how to prepare nutritious foods which enabled their offspring to put on weight again at an astonishing rate. Cost realism was a major consideration for Jelliffe and his colleagues. They were able to point out that whilst *2 weeks* in the paediatric wards of Mulago hospital cost \$117.60, a *6 weeks stay* at Mwanamugimu for both mother and child required only \$77.

The medical care provided was kept within a carefully regulated perspective. As the cure proceeded the emphasis on strictly medical matters was replaced by 'lay care' of a much more broadly based nature. The aim was to fight the ignorance and superstition that had often contributed to the child's illness. It was also of crucial importance to obviate any sense of dependency on the part of the mother whose child had been treated. Success was measured by a lack of readmissions either of that particular child or of any subsequent sibling from the family. Jelliffe firmly believed that the health awareness of the community was adversely affected by the conventional hospital operating along curative doctor-dominated lines (Jelliffe & Jelliffe, 1973). In leading the child back to health, the emphasis had to be moved from the hospital environment, in which the mother was a passive recipient and mere observer of the wonders of medical care and cure, to a home type environment.

There was inevitably a strong element of 'evangelism' in the running of 'Mwanamugimu' and I have to admit to being critical of some of the scientifically unsubstantiated components of the associated educational programmes. There are, however, two lasting accolades that Mwanamugimu justly deserves. It inspired the setting up of similar organisations in many other parts of Africa and indeed throughout the third world. Even more importantly, it survived the political upheavals that wrecked rather more scientifically ambitious bodies such as the one I myself directed. Mwanamugimu continues to be an inspiration as to how malnourished children can be rehabilitated using simple, inexpensive low technology approaches.

The other development I would like to mention made an even deeper impression on me, perhaps, than Mwanamugimu. This was a health demonstration facility set up at a village called Lutete. Here the subjects at whom the advice was directed were not just mothers of children already malnourished, but the community in general. This was an attempt at true preventive medicine.

It was at Lutete that the broadly based philosophies of Jelliffe and his colleagues really came to the fore. The target for improvement was not just producing more nutritious foods, although these did get their due share of attention, but the whole environment of the family. Adjacent to the health clinic in Lutete were a multiplicity of improvement demonstrations. Some were rather obvious such as gardens in which could be grown and harvested the local foods which formed the basis of the more traditional nutritional education. There were also improved kitchen designs built in such a way that they could be reproduced in any traditional home. At a more adventurous agricultural level the villagers were shown, for example, how to clear and drain previously unusable swampy land. The resultant 'fields' could then be used, not only for growing food for home consumption, but the production of cash crops was also encouraged in order to take advantage of the lucrative tourist hotel market that was just beginning to develop. Jelliffe and his colleagues recognised that poverty was often an underlying factor in the development of malnutrition, and thus generating wealth amongst the poor was a valid component of preventive medicine. Such comments may seem rather commonplace in the 1990s, but in the 60s many eyebrows were raised at the sight of fruits like pineapples and paw-paws being encouraged by a nutrition education and health orientated team! Naturally this breadth of effort could not be handled by health workers operating in isolation. This was a multidisciplinary team effort involving Ministries of Agriculture and Community Development as well as Health, cooperating with various religious and charitable bodies.

The fact that infection, particularly diarrhoeal disease, but also a whole plethora of other communicable diseases, could no longer be ignored in nutrition education programmes was also becoming generally accepted. We began to use phrases such as protein-calorie malnutrition being a product of the 'nutrition-infection complex': 'tropical failure-to-thrive' was another useful term. Around this time I produced a simple graph (Fig. 27.1), showing that not only growth faltering, but also low plasma albumin concentrations ultimately leading to oedema, occurred in association with batches of different infections (Frood, Whitehead & Coward, 1971). I have received more requests for this graph to be reproduced in textbooks and reviews than anything else I have had published! This astonishing interest in a relatively minor piece of work reflected, I judge, a wish by the public health workers to reconsider nutritional issues such as the deficiency hypothesis in the light of their association with other causal factors.

In so far as nutritional education at Lutete was concerned, this broader approach towards the aetiology of kwashiorkor and marasmus expressed itself in an increased emphasis on topics such as hygienic latrines, improved

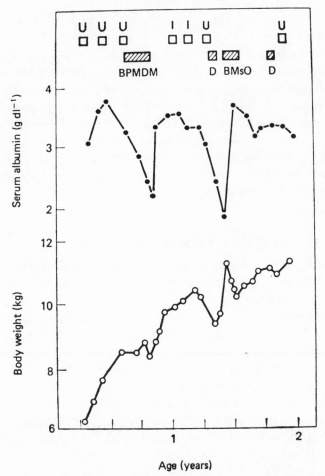

Fig. 27.1 Relationships between pattern of infection, weight faltering and episodes of hypoalbuminaemia in a Ugandan child (Frood, Whitehead & Coward, 1971). U: upper respiratory tract infections. O: suppurative otitis media; B: bronchitis; P: pneumonia; D: diarrhoea; Ms: measles; M: malaria; I: Impetigo.

water supplies, water conservation and insect protection, etc, but always with a firm accent on simple technologies that could be built and operated at a 'self-help' level. Perhaps the most unusual feature at Lutete was the brick-making machine. It was recognised that unless families had basic and decently constructed houses in which to live there was always the probability of poor hygiene. These brick-making machines were supplied by the Uganda Government so that self-help groups could get together and build better homes. The involvement of Lutete in such an enterprise was irresistible!

Writing these comments after so many years has made me realise that the East Africa of the 1950s and 1960s was quite different from that of today. This had been an era of optimism. Our thoughts were not as dominated by crisis situations as they are now. In our planning, the target was to maintain the momentum of improvement, not just to achieve survival. The main discussion points concerned the *appropriateness* of the changes we were trying to introduce. Development still is a key issue, but I fear that the young health worker of today cannot free himself as easily as we could from dealing with the emotion-sapping demands of a never ending succession of crises. Inescapably, the latter now play the dominant role in most sets of nutritional priorities.

Trowell, Dean, Jelliffe and current research

All of us reflect to a greater or lesser extent a range of influences arising from the characters of the people with whom we have been closely associated. I have always been firmly a member of the fundamental research camp originated by McCance/Widdowson and loyally continued in Uganda by Dean. Nevertheless, the influences of clinicians like Trowell and community paediatric specialists such as Jelliffe have been strong. After returning from Uganda in 1973 I was determined to try and blend the 'pure' and 'applied' aspects of nutritional science within the UK as my predecessors have done in Uganda. I may have encouraged a much more '*High-Technology*' approach, but this was because it is often the only way one can get at the basic level of understanding required. Surely it is not fanciful to conclude, however, that the underlying *motivation* behind many of the approaches we at the Dunn now follow were preconditioned by events which were occurring in Uganda between 1930–70.

References

Dean, R. F. A. (1960). Treatment of kwashiorkor with moderate amounts of protein. *Journal of Paediatrics*, **56**, 675–89.

Dean, R. F. A. & Schwartz, R. (1953). The serum chemistry in uncomplicated kwashiorkor. *British Journal of Nutrition*, **7**, 131–47.

Frood, J. D. L., Whitehead, R. G. & Coward, W. A. (1971). A relationship between the pattern of infection and the development of hypoalbuminaemia and hypo-B-lipoproteinaemia in rural Ugandan children. *Lancet*, **ii**, 1047–9.

Jelliffe, E. F. P. & Jelliffe, D. B. (1973). In *Nutrition Programmes for Pre-school Children*. Jelliffe, D. B. & Jelliffe, E. F. P., eds, Zagreb: Institute of Public Health of Croatia.

Lunn, P. G., Whitehead, R. G. & Coward, W. A. (1979). Two pathways to kwashiorkor? *Transactions of the Royal Society for Tropical Medicine and Hygiene*, **73**, 438–44.
Trowell, H. C. & Dean, R. F. A. (1952). Kwashiorkor. *British Encyclopaedia of Medical Practice*, **Suppl 113**, 2–5.
Whitehead, R. G. (1969). The assessment of nutritional status in protein-malnourished children. *Proceedings of the Nutrition Society*, **28**, 1–16.
Williams, C. D. (1933). A nutritional disease of childhood associated with a maize diet. *Archives of Diseases of Childhood*, **8**, 423–33.

28

Protein-energy malnutrition in Jamaica

J. C. WATERLOW

Background of the Tropical Metabolism Research Unit

I first went to the West Indies in 1945, just after the end of the European War. The Colonial Office was very much concerned about the state of nutrition in that region; then, as now, the people of the Caribbean relied heavily on imported food, and they were in a bad situation because so many of the food ships had been sunk by German submarines. B. S. Platt, under whom I was working at that time, was Nutrition Adviser to the Colonial Office, and had made a short visit to the West Indies in 1943. My task, the first I ever had in nutrition, was to follow up this visit and specifically to find out why so many children were dying.

I went first to Trinidad, next to British Guiana as it then was, finally to Jamaica, working in the paediatric wards and the hospital laboratories on severely malnourished children, a great many of whom died. Oedema was prominent and attributed by the local doctors to various causes, such as nephrosis and worms. I was convinced that it was nutritional, but I knew nothing of the literature and it was not until I returned after nearly a year to the UK that I made the connection with kwashiorkor, as described by Cicely Williams in the Gold Coast (Williams, 1935). I was particularly impressed by the enormous fatty liver, which often seemed to be a cause of death, and I called the condition 'fatty liver disease' (Waterlow, 1948). At the same time I tried to make a distinction from the general malnutrition which nowadays we call marasmus.

At that time, in the winter of 1945, a commission from the UK was visiting Jamaica to plan the setting up of a West Indian university and medical school. I decided to join that new school as soon as I could, but 5 years had to pass, including a spell of 18 months in the Gambia, before that became possible. At the end of 1950 I was able to go back to Jamaica with the double job of part-time lecturer in physiology and part-time MRC staff, continuing research on malnutrition. However, I gradually realised that it was going to be very difficult to make much progress in understanding the pathophysiology of kwashiorkor and the reasons for the high mortality rate without a substantial increase in effort. Therefore, after 3 years I put a proposal to the MRC for a small unit to be set up with its own ward and laboratories under one roof. To my surprise Sir Harold Himsworth and the MRC accepted what seemed to me a very ambitious proposal, and the Tropical Metabolism Research Unit (TMRU), with four scientific staff, was approved in 1954 and came into operation in 1955. It was at about the same time that the Unit under Rex Dean was established at Kampala, as described by Whitehead in the preceding chapter (p. 303). I have written elsewhere in more detail of the early background in Jamaica (Waterlow, 1974).

Although our aims were very similar, with virtually the whole emphasis on childhood malnutrition, there were certain differences between the two units. Because of my previous connection with the University, the TMRU, although financed and administered from London, operated *de facto* as a department of the Faculty of Medicine and of the University hospital. This relationship with the UWI had important implications for the future.

A second difference was in the name. 'Tropical Metabolism' was chosen to emphasise the metabolic aspects of nutrition and to make the terms of reference wide, so that we could work on any metabolic problems which seemed of interest in that environment. Certainly until very recently by far the greatest part of the TMRU's effort has been devoted to research on severe protein-energy malnutrition (PEM). Now, however, that condition is becoming quite rare in the Caribbean, and the Unit can, without distortion of its role, move into different areas of medicine, such as eclampsia, diabetes and hypertension, which in that region present many features of special interest.

The third difference between the TMRU and the Kampala Unit is, from the scientific point of view, the most important. Particularly in the early days we regarded PEM strictly from the medical point of view, as a disease which presented a clinical challenge – to reduce the appallingly high mortality that was running at 20–30%. We made virtually no effort to investigate the nutritional and social circumstances under which this 'disease' arose or to study its natural history in the community. It was otherwise with the Uganda Unit; their studies on the biochemical and endocrine changes at different stages in the development of malnutrition and in different communities represented a kind of biochemical epidemiology which was, and I think still is, unique. It seems to me that the importance of those contributions is insufficiently appreciated nowadays.

In the 1960s we began to recruit to the scientific staff of the TMRU graduates of the UWI, some of whom I had myself taught in their preclinical years. The earliest and most senior were David Picou, who succeeded me as Director, and George Alleyne (now Sir George) who became Professor of Medicine at UWI and is now Assistant Director of the Pan American Health Organisation, the Western hemisphere regional office of WHO. After a few years, as was the usual practice, I recommended that these members of staff should be given permanent appointments by the MRC, but that was turned down on administrative, not scientific, grounds. It was clear that, as a result, the Unit would have two categories of senior scientific staff with different conditions of service and career structures, and that was not a tolerable prospect. Negotiations were therefore set on foot which resulted, in 1970, in the University accepting responsibility for the TMRU, which became *de jure* as well as *de facto* one of its departments, with financial support for a limited period from the British government (ODA). At that time I withdrew as Director and returned to the UK.

I have recounted these facts about the background and history of the TMRU because they are important for understanding the scientific development of the Unit and the continuity of its existence.

Scientific work

There were two principal and related aims of our work: to reduce the mortality and to get a better understanding of the processes that were occurring or were breaking down in severe PEM. Cicely Williams, who visited us from time to time, told us that this research was unnecessary; all that was needed was food and tender loving care. I think this was an oversimplification, but all the same her words did plant a seed which later grew, as I shall recount later. Undoubtedly at that time we paid too little attention to the psychological and emotional damage inflicted on children who became severely malnourished.

As far as concerns the first aim, the reduction of deaths, we did succeed in reducing the mortality from 16% in the early 1960s to about 2% 10 years later. In Table 28.1 I have listed the main lines of research, particularly in the early days, which may have contributed to this result. A fuller account is given in a number of reviews, e.g. Waterlow, Cravioto and Stephen (1960) and Waterlow and Alleyne (1971). The book by Alleyne *et al.* (1977) brings together the work of the Jamaican and Ugandan units. I

Table 28.1. *Some aspects of PEM on which research was done at TMRU,*
1954–89

Electrolyte disturbances
Body composition
Composition of liver and muscle
Muscle mass
Cardiac function
Renal function
Gut function
Fatty liver
Basal metabolism
Energy expenditure
Temperature regulation
Fat metabolism
Carbohydrate metabolism
Endocrine changes (insulin, cortisol, thyroxine,
  growth hormone, somatomedin)
Enzyme adaptations
Nitrogen absorption and retention
Iron absorption
Nutritional value of leaf protein
Nutritional requirements for growth during
  recovery
Folic acid deficiency
Albumin turnover
Protein turnover
Urea metabolism
Zinc deficiency
Other trace element deficiencies
Membrane damage
Free radicals
Malnutrition and mental development
School meals

do not want to give the impression that the TMRU was unique, except in longer continuity of clinical research. Sadly, almost all the metabolic wards around the world which were active in the 1960s and 1970s are now defunct either for political reasons, as in Uganda and Lebanon, or because emphasis has shifted to prevention and primary health care.

The Wellcome classification (1970) was born at a meeting in Jamaica in 1969. We did not in my time make much distinction between kwashiorkor (K) and marasmus (M), but it has received more emphasis in recent years in the work of Golden and Jackson (see below). Cases of marasmic kwashiorkor (MK) were common and certainly the most difficult to treat; in spite of my earlier attempt at a distinction (Waterlow, 1948), there was obviously much overlap between K and M. The two conditions seemed to be interconvertible, the presence of oedema, the distinguishing criterion, being determined at least in part by the state of fluid balance. On the theory that was current in the 1960s, that the clinical picture depended on the balance between energy and protein in the preceding diet, any hard and fast distinction would be unrealistic. I shall return to this question later. As far as concerns many of the changes that we studied, e.g. cardiac and renal function, it was seldom possible to show any clear difference between kwashiorkor and marasmus.

In the following sections I shall describe very briefly a few of the lines of research listed in Table 28.1, with rather more emphasis on the earlier than the later work.

Body composition

It was considered ethical to use ^3H_2O for determining body water, although before liquid scintillation counters became available the measurement of specific radioactivity was very difficult. Large increases in total body water were found; the evidence suggested that the increase was mainly extracellular, although it was and still is very difficult to rule out the possibility of an increase in intracellular water (see below).

A corollary of the excess of water in the body was a massive decrease in body cell mass. We were particularly interested in muscle, as the largest mass of protein in the normal body. Measurements by the classical method of 24-hour creatinine output supported the idea that muscle acted as a reserve, which was much more depleted than the body as a whole. This was confirmed in later studies in which muscle mass and its rate of repletion were measured with ^{15}N-creatine (Reeds *et al.*, 1978).

Garrow's analyses of the bodies of children who died more than doubled the number of analyses of cadavers of children that have been published in the world literature (Garrow, Fletcher & Halliday, 1965). This work showed, among other things, how the brain is relatively well preserved. At the chemical level collagen is preserved while cellular protein is lost (Picou, Halliday & Garrow, 1966). These studies enabled us to build up a picture of changes in both body composition and organ pattern which is very important for the interpretation of functional measurements, e.g. of BMR and protein turnover.

Electrolytes

Hansen in Cape Town had shown by balance studies the extent of potassium loss in PEM. We were able to follow this up with a 40 π whole body counter, which made possible serial measurements of total body K on large numbers of children. It became clear that supplementary K must be a mandatory part of treatment; however, rectifying the K deficit unmasked a concurrent deficit of magnesium, so that Mg supplements also have to be given routinely.

The physiological consequences of depletion of K and Mg have been little investigated although Garrow (1967), in a paper that has received surprisingly little attention, showed that in children with a low total body K, the K content of the head, which in effect means the brain, was reduced by about 30 per cent.

I believe that K deficit is an important cause of oedema, although the distortions of body composition to which I have referred above made it impossible to show conclusively that oedematous children were more deficient in K than those without oedema. The retention of water is accompanied by retention of sodium and, as mentioned above, the question remains whether excess Na and water have entered cells, which would be a very serious breakdown in homeostasis. Studies on membrane function and the sodium pump in leucocytes have provided some evidence that this may occur (Patrick & Golden, 1977).

Metabolic rate

Our early measurements of BMR (Montgomery, 1962) showed that in some children with PEM the BMR per kg body weight was higher than normal, as was observed by Talbot as long ago as 1921. This is to be explained by the distortion of body composition, in which brain, with a high metabolic rate, is preserved and muscle, with a low rate, is lost. I believe that the best way of expressing functions such as BMR is to relate them to total body K as a measure of active cell mass, once specific K deficiency has been overcome. When the BMR is expressed in this way, it is undoubtedly depressed (Brooke & Cocks, 1974), showing that the flame of life must be flickering very low in these malnourished children. One consequence of the low metabolic rate is inability to maintain body temperature and to prevent hypothermia, which is a serious hazard to life if adequate precautions are not taken.

Fatty liver

The extent of the fatty infiltration in kwashiorkor, up to 50 % of the wet weight, is greater than in any other condition I know, and is far greater than the modest increase produced by starvation, infections or poisons. Since it was often the cause of death from liver failure, it seemed justifiable to investigate the extent of the fatty change and the rate of clearance of fat by serial liver biopsies (Waterlow, 1975). There were no harmful effects from this procedure. Some evidence was obtained that the rate of clearance of fat was greater on a high protein diet. Truswell in S. Africa had shown that the fatty liver is accompanied by a reduction in serum β-lipoprotein concentration. Moreover, as the fat begins to disappear, serum triglyceride levels rise to a peak. These findings suggest that the reason for the accumulation of fat is decreased synthesis of the apolipoproteins that are the carriers for transporting fat out of the liver. Impairment of the synthesis of these proteins would be in line with the reduction in albumin synthesis that occurred very rapidly when children were put on a low protein diet (James & Hay, 1968).

Protein turnover and nitrogen metabolism

The hypothesis was proposed that perhaps some children died, even when electrolyte disturbances and infections had been overcome, because the ability to synthesise protein was impaired. Since the machinery for synthesising protein itself consists of proteins, such an impairment might well be irreversible. To test the hypothesis it was necessary to devise a way of measuring whole body protein turnover. For this purpose we used ^{15}N-glycine, the only amino acid labelled with ^{15}N that was then available (Picou & Taylor-Roberts, 1969). The hypothesis was partially confirmed; in children with PEM whole body protein turnover per kg was reduced by about $\frac{1}{3}$ compared with normal children (Golden, Waterlow & Picou, 1977). As in the case of BMR, even a modest reduction in the rate of protein turnover in vital organs must, one may suppose, have serious functional consequences. Since these early studies the ^{15}N-glycine method has been modified to make it theoretically more sound and practically more useful, and it is now quite widely used in various clinical situations.

The availability of ^{15}N-labelled compounds made it possible to study urea metabolism in these children (Picou & Phillips, 1972). It appears that when N supply is limited in relation to demand, there is a mechanism by which a larger proportion of the urea produced in the liver is metabolised in the colon, the ammonia derived by bacterial urease being then available for amino acid synthesis (Jackson et al., 1990). This clearly represents an important means of economising nitrogen.

In an attempt to enlarge our attack on the problem of measuring whole body protein turnover in man we made some preliminary studies in adults with ^{14}C-lysine. It would not have been ethical to use this radioactive isotope in children. In those days we did not have an amino acid analyser sensitive enough for measuring free lysine in plasma. We therefore adapted the Cartesian diver technique, which I had developed for measurements of enzymes in tissue biopsies, so that lysine could be determined from the CO_2 produced by lysine decarboxylase (Waterlow & Stephen, 1967). I think it is fair to claim that this work did something to stimulate the numerous studies of protein turnover with labelled amino acids that have been made since then in the UK and the USA.

Recovery from PEM

Even after the initial disturbances in electrolytes and infections had been overcome, some children still died a week or so after admission. It was found that this mortality could be reduced by putting the children for some days on a diet which provided only maintenance amounts of protein and energy. Presumably this is because many functions, as described above, are profoundly disturbed and cannot be instantly restored. For example, the enzymes of the urea cycle are reduced (Das & Waterlow, 1974; Stephen & Waterlow, 1968), and overloading with amino acids which cannot be disposed of either into urea or into protein could have toxic effects.

The first sign that the child is ready for more generous feeding is a return of appetite. We soon realised that in practice the factor that limits the rate of growth in this phase of recovery is not protein, which can easily be supplied as dried milk, but energy. To meet the energy needs some form of fat had to be added, such as coconut or groundnut oil. Detailed feeding schedules were worked out, which were applied in the regional hospitals of Jamaica and which formed the basis of a WHO manual on the treatment of malnutrition (Picou *et al.*, 1975). During the period of very rapid weight gain trace elements such as zinc may become limiting, and unless a full quota of these essential nutrients is supplied the tissue laid down may contain too little lean and too much fat (Jackson & Golden, 1987). It is a remarkable thing that most children, when they have regained their expected weight for height, show a spontaneous reduction in appetite and slowing in the rate of growth (Ashworth, 1969). We have no idea how this comes about, but it is clearly important for a better understanding of appetite control. Another interesting observation is that catch-up in height tends to follow catch-up in weight, rather than the two going forward hand in hand (Walker & Golden, 1988).

Studies of endocrine function during the various phases of recovery have shown a rapid restoration to normal of the initially low plasma levels of insulin, thyroid hormones and somatomedin C (Robinson *et al.*, 1980). The stimuli for growth are therefore in place. The important problem that remains is the cause at the nutritional/metabolic/biochemical level of the stunting in linear growth that is so common in third world children.

Free radical damage

In the last few years Golden has opened up a whole new field of work at TMRU, focused on the effect of malnutrition and of the infections that so often accompany it, on the production of free radicals and the capacity to dispose of them. This work will not be discussed in any detail here because it has been described in a number of recent reviews, e.g. Golden and Ramdath (1987). The underlying hypothesis represents a departure from our earlier line, that the differences between kwashiorkor and marasmus are ones of degree rather than kind. According to the new hypothesis, the specific features of kwashiorkor result from the effects of free radicals, perhaps through lipid peroxidation of cell membranes. Some of the systems responsible for scavenging free radicals, many of which are dependent on trace elements, are more reduced in kwashiorkor than in marasmus, the most striking example being in the levels of red cell glutathione (Jackson, 1986). Whether or not the theory succeeds in explaining the pathogenesis of the particular characteristics of kwashiorkor, it has a great deal to tell us about why some children die and others survive.

Mental development

I have left this subject to the last because the body of work directed by S. McGregor brought the Unit for the first time into close and continuous connection with the community. It began in 1970 when at long last, under the stimulus of the late Professor Jack Tizard, we began to take seriously the mental as well as the physical development of the children in the ward. The first step was to show the effect of stimulation in counteracting the very severe depression of mental development that the children show on admission. Later it was found that the reduction in developmental quotient (DQ) was associated with stunting rather than with an acute episode of malnutrition with oedema and wasting. Intervention in the home, with a combination of stimulation and supplementary feeding, has been successful in restoring the DQ to something approaching normal levels (Grantham-McGregor, Powell & Walker, 1989). Other studies by McGregor and her group have been concerned with the determinants of failure in school and with the importance of school meals.

Over the years this work on child development has become one of the main thrusts of the TMRU's activities. It is opportune that this should be so, because severe clinical PEM is becoming rather rare in Jamaica; on the other hand, marginal malnutrition, particularly in the form of stunting, continues to present a challenge both to research and to public health policy.

Conclusion

Some general points about the work of the TMRU remain to be made.

First, in many of the areas of our research parallel animal experiments have made an important contribution. They were particularly valuable in relation to studies of tissue composition and tissue enzymes and as models for establishing methods of measuring protein turnover (e.g. Waterlow & Stephen, 1967).

Secondly, in recent years there has been a great increase in interest in the developed countries in the nutritional state of patients hospitalised for trauma, chronic infections, neoplasms, etc. The studies on PEM in the third world are relevant to these problems, although the relevance has often not been recognised.

Thirdly, I hope that this condensed account of the TMRU's research illustrates how apparently unrelated subjects may come together and how one thing leads to another. This requires continuity of work over many years, and institutional arrangements that make continuity possible. That is why I began this story with some account of the history and structure of the TMRU.

Lastly, work on childhood malnutrition in Africa and the West Indies has been an important stimulus to nutritional research in Britain, as is evident from the contributors to this volume.

What of the future? One immediate aim must be better application of the knowledge that has been gained. In many countries the case-fatality rate of children with severe protein-energy malnutrition, even if the children reach hospital, is still very high, and most of these deaths are preventible. It is probable, however, that there will be reduced opportunities for basic clinical research on PEM because the good news is that it is becoming less common. For example, even in Calcutta, one of the poorest cities in the world, kwashiorkor is now seldom seen (A. K. Bhatacharriyya, personal communication). Where it does persist it is likely to be in situations where no more than observational studies are possible. Such studies, however, are still important because our knowledge of the epidemiology is still scanty.

In recent times the tendency has quite rightly been to concentrate on the community and public health aspects of malnutrition. However, the fact that it is at bottom a social and political problem should not blind us to the many scientific questions that remain. For example, there is much difference of opinion on the relative importance of nutrition and infection in the spectrum of morbidity and mortality in young children, a question that has obvious implications for the use of scarce resources. Our estimates of the energy and protein requirements of young children are still not securely based, and virtually nothing is known at the biological level of the processes leading to the stunting in linear growth that is so common in third world children. It will be fruitful to apply to these problems the experience and disciplines of the research that I have described in this chapter.

References

Alleyne, G. A. O., Hay, R. W., Picou, D. I., Stanfield, J. P. & Whitehead, R. G. (1977). *Protein-energy Malnutrition.* Arnold, London.

Ashworth, A. (1969). Growth rates in children recovering from protein-energy malnutrition. *British Journal of Nutrition*, **23**, 835–45.

Brooke, O. G. & Cocks, T. (1974). Resting metabolic rate in malnourished babies in relation to total body potassium. *Acta Paediatrica Scandinavica*, **63**, 817–25.

Das, T. K. & Waterlow, J. C. (1974). The rate of adaptation of urea cycle enzymes, amino transferases and glutamate dehydrogenase to changes in dietary protein intake. *British Journal of Nutrition*, **32**, 353–73.

Garrow, J. S. (1967). Loss of brain potassium in kwashiorkor. *Lancet*, **ii**, 643–5.

Garrow, J. S., Fletcher, K. & Halliday, D. (1965). Body composition in severe infantile malnutrition. *Journal of Clinical Investigation*, **41**, 1928–35.

Golden, M. H. N. & Ramdath, D. (1987). Free radicals in the pathogenesis of kwashiorkor. *Proceedings of the Nutrition Society*, **46**, 53–68.

Golden, M. H. N., Waterlow, J. C. & Picou, D. (1977). Protein turnover, synthesis and breakdown before and after recovery from protein-energy malnutrition. *Clinical Science and Molecular Medicine*, **53**, 473–7.

Grantham-McGregor, S., Powell, C. & Walker, S. (1989). Nutritional supplements, stunting and child development. *Lancet*, **ii**, 809–10.

Jackson, A. A. (1986). Blood glutathione in severe malnutrition in childhood. *Transactions of the Royal Society of Tropical Medicine and Hygiene*, **80**, 911–13.

Jackson, A. A., Doherty, J., de Benoist, M-H., Hibbert, J. & Persaud, C. (1990). The effect of the level of dietary protein, carbohydrate and fat on urea kinetics in young children during rapid catch-up weight gain. *British Journal of Nutrition*, **64**, 371–85.

Jackson, A. A. & Golden, M. H. N. (1987). Severe malnutrition. In *Oxford Textbook of Medicine*, Weatherall, D. J., Ledingham, J. G. G. & Warrell, D. A., eds., 2nd Edn. 8.12–8.28. Oxford University Press.

James, W. P. T. & Hay, A. M. (1968). Albumin metabolism: effect of the nutritional state and the dietary protein intake. *Journal of Clinical Investigation*, **47**, 1958–72.

Montgomery, R. D. (1962). Changes in the basal metabolic rate of the malnourished infant and their relation to body composition. *Journal of Clinical Investigation*, **41**, 1653–63.

Patrick, J. & Golden, M. (1977). Leucocyte electrolytes and sodium transport in protein energy malnutrition. *American Journal of Clinical Nutrition*, **30**, 1478–81.

Picou, D., Alleyne, G. A. O., Kerr, D. S., Miller, C., Jackson, A., Hill, A., Bogues, J. & Patrick, J. (1975). *Malnutrition and Gastroenteritis in Children. A Manual for Hospital Treatment and Management.* Caribbean Food and Nutrition Institute. PO Box 140, Kingston, Jamaica.

Picou, D., Halliday, D. & Garrow, J. S. (1966). Total body protein, collagen and non-collagen protein in infantile protein malnutrition. *Clinical Science*, **30**, 345–51.

Picou, D. & Phillips, M. (1972). Urea metabolism in malnourished and recovered children receiving a high or low protein diet. *American Journal of Clinical Nutrition*, **25**, 1261–6.

Picou, D. & Taylor-Roberts, T. (1969). The measurement of total protein synthesis and catabolism and nitrogen turnover in infants in different nutritional states and receiving different amounts of dietary protein. *Clinical Science*, **36**, 283–96.

Reeds, P. J., Jackson, A. A., Picou, D. & Poulter, N. (1978). Muscle mass and composition in malnourished infants and children and changes seen after recovery. *Pediatric Research*, **12**, 613–18.

Robinson, H. M. P., Cocks, T., Kerr, D. & Picou, D. (1980). Hormonal control of weight gain in infants recovering from protein-energy malnutrition. *Pediatric Research*, **14**, 28–33.

Stephen, J. M. L. & Waterlow, J. C. (1968). Effect of malnutrition on activity of two enzymes concerned with amino acid metabolism in human liver. *Lancet*, **i**, 118–19.

Walker, S. P. & Golden, M. H. N. (1988). Growth in length of children recovering from severe malnutrition. *European Journal of Clinical Nutrition*, **42**, 395–404.

Waterlow, J. C. (1948). *Fatty liver disease in infants in the British West Indies.* Medical Research Council Special Reports Series no. 263. London: HMSO.

Waterlow, J. C. (1974). The history of the Tropical Metabolism Research Unit, U.W.I. *West Indian Medical Journal*, **23**, 151–9.

Waterlow, J. C. (1975). Amount and rate of disappearance of liver fat in malnourished infants in Jamaica. *American Journal of Clinical Nutrition*, **28**, 1330–6.

Waterlow, J. C. & Alleyne, G. A. O. (1971). Protein malnutrition in children: advances in knowledge in the last ten years. *Advances in Protein Chemistry*, **25**, 117–235.

Waterlow, J. C., Cravioto, J. & Stephen, J. M. L. (1960). Protein malnutrition in man. *Advances in Protein Chemistry*, **15**, 131–238.

Waterlow, J. C. & Stephen, J. M. L. (1967). The measurement of total lysine turnover in the rat by infusion of L-(U-^{14}C)-lysine. *Clinical Science*, **33**, 489–506.

Wellcome Trust Working Party (1970). Classification of infantile malnutrition. *Lancet*, **ii**, 302–3.

Williams, C. D. (1935). Kwashiorkor: a nutritional disease of children associated with a maize diet. *Lancet*, **ii**, 1151–2.

Part six

Policies for food, nutrition and health

29

Food and nutrition policies in wartime

DOROTHY F. HOLLINGSWORTH

The American Public Health Association presented the Lasker Group Award of 1947 to the British Ministries of Food and Health 'For the unprecedented program of food distribution in Great Britain, with resulting improvement in the health of the people'. The award was made for scientific and administrative achievement to the two Ministries and 'to the four great leaders in this historic enterprise, Lord Woolton, Sir Jack Drummond, Sir Wilson Jameson and Sir John Boyd Orr' for 'the greatest demonstration in public health administration that the world has ever seen'. (The quotations are taken from the award citation.) How was this achieved?

Historical introduction

Experience in the First World War had shown how important it would be, in the event of another war, to plan food supplies for the British people. It could be foreseen that there would be shortages of shipping, labour and packing materials as well as of food; that, unless controlled, prices would rise; that catering would be difficult unless advice was given on the optimal use of available foods, and that campaigns to prevent waste of food would be needed. Such problems led to the development of wartime food policy.

At the time of the 1914–1918 war, nutritional science was at an early stage, and the nutritional value of food supplies and the nutritional needs of people were not taken into consideration by the Government until it was almost too late. In 1939, when the Second World War broke out, the situation was different. Nutritional science had developed rapidly in the 1920s and 1930s, and concern grew about the nutritional condition of the people, particularly during the economic depression of the 1930s. There was general anxiety about the national diet, which arose partly because the total supply of foods was calculated to be nutritionally inadequate in some respects and partly because there was great inequality in food distribution. It was thought that the supply would have been satisfactory if distribution had been according to physiological need, but it was known that it was not. Gross inequality of distribution was demonstrated by Orr (1936) and confirmed by Crawford & Broadley (1938).

Such was the unease about the nutritional condition of the public that committees were instituted to consider nutritional problems.

Pre-war committees

The first of these, composed mainly of physiologists, was appointed in 1931 'to advise the Minister of Health on the practical application of modern advances in the knowledge of nutrition'. It led to the appointment by the Minister of Health and the Secretary of State for Scotland in 1935 of the Advisory Committee on Nutrition with the following terms of reference: 'To inquire into the facts, quantitative and qualitative, in relation to the diet of the people, and to report as to any changes therein which appear desirable in the light of modern advances in the knowledge of nutrition'. This Committee reported in 1937 (Ministry of Health, 1937). In 1933 the British Medical Association set up a Nutrition Committee of which the terms of reference were 'To determine the minimum weekly expenditure on foodstuffs which must be incurred by families of varying size if health and working capacity are to be maintained and to construct specimen diets' (British Medical Association, 1933).

Internationally, the League of Nations Mixed Committee on the Relation of Nutrition to Health, Agriculture and Economic Policy began its work. It is still worthwhile to study its final report (League of Nations, 1937).

Pre-war plans

These Committees and Orr (1936) produced a fund of information on which the Food (Defence Plans) Department of the Board of Trade, established in 1936, could base its First Report (Board of Trade, 1938) 'to explain in broad outline a part of the preparations that are being made...for feeding the population in the event of war'. One of the aims was to ensure that 'supplies of essential foodstuffs at controlled prices are available to meet the requirements of all types of consumers and in all parts of the country, if, and when, an emergency arises'. The Report states that to secure this food control, the organisation of supplies and the regulation of consumers' demands were essential, and that food control has three aspects in which the consumer is vitally concerned: guarantee of regular supplies; limitation of prices and profits; and equality of sacrifice in the event of shortage. Initially, there was great emphasis on the need to control inflation in wartime because high food prices and industrial unrest rather than actual shortage of food had been primarily responsible for the appointment of the first Food Controller in 1916 (Hammond, 1951).

Ministry of Food policies

Plans for food rationing and distribution based on ensuring regular supplies, limiting prices and profits, and imposing equality were made by the Board of Trade. These plans were adopted by the Ministry of Food, instituted in September 1939 immediately after the outbreak of war. Legally and politically the Ministry was brought into existence overnight. The growth of its administrative machine was rapid, and by the summer of 1940 it had achieved a settled form that was to survive well into the post-war years (Hammond, 1951).

The control of prices and distribution of foods extended beyond what might be regarded as essential foodstuffs, and the Ministry's responsibilities towards the nutritionally vulnerable groups, infants, children, expectant and nursing mothers and invalids also went beyond what was originally foreseen. Probably because of this, nutritional considerations became more important than they were when the initial plans were made.

The Ministry's objectives were to ensure equal shares of the more scarce foods to all consumers; to make special provision of milk and other foods for the nutritionally vulnerable groups; to leave unrationed for as long as possible certain major sources of energy, particularly bread and flour but also potatoes; and to provide communal eating facilities so that industrial and other workers and schoolchildren could supplement their rations with meals away from home. These measures, taken as a whole, may be summarised as 'fair shares for all', a phrase that implies not only special provision for those with special needs, such as energy foods for heavy manual workers and growth promoting nutrients for children and child-bearing women, but a fair distribution of foods in short supply.

Many people were involved in the development and implementation of the policies, but two of those already mentioned stand out: J. C. Drummond, who was seconded from London University to the Ministry of Food in October 1939 and was appointed Scientific Adviser on 1 February 1940, and Lord Woolton who became Minister of Food in April 1940. Both men subsequently became celebrities.

Nutrition policies

Soon after his appointment as Scientific Adviser, Drummond produced a notable document 'on certain nutritional aspects of the food position' in which he reviewed the pre-war nutritional situation in the United Kingdom and the probable effects on it of war, particularly among the poor. He stressed the need for providing bread of high nutritive value, for increasing the consumption of potatoes, oatmeal, cheese and green vegetables, for supplying not less than a pint of milk a day to expectant and nursing mothers and all children up to the age of 15 years and for fortifying margarine with vitamins A and D. Many of these proposals were subsequently put into effect. It is clear from the official documents prepared during the war by Drummond and others that Drummond set out from the start not only to maintain but to improve the nutritional value of the British diet (Hollingsworth & Wright, 1954). This aim could not have been realised, as it was, had it not been for the support of Lord Woolton, who according to Drummond (1947) 'invariably balanced evidence and arguments on the psychological side against the recommendations of the scientists'. In other words, political support is needed, and was provided in wartime Britain, if food and nutrition policies are to be put satisfactorily into effect.

The first official indication of Drummond's influence on food policy appeared in May 1940 in the Ministry of Food's import programme for the second year of war, to which was appended *A Survey of Wartime Nutrition* which set out in detailed and quantitative form his views on the type of nutritional strategy the Ministry should adopt. At that time it was novel to apply modern concepts of nutrition to the job of feeding a nation at war, and it was Drummond's unique contribution to collaborate successfully with statisticians and economists to produce a document that could form the practical basis of the national food policy (Hollingsworth, 1957).

Practical measures

The measures planned and put into effect were superimposed on a system of general rationing which provided all persons with equal domestic rations at controlled prices of bacon, fats, sugar, preserves and sweets, equal domestic rations of cheese (except for certain classes of workers who were entitled to extra cheese for sandwiches), equal domestic rations of tea (except for children under five who got none) and domestic rations of equal cash value for carcase meat (with the modifications of a half ration for children under five, an extra half ration for expectant mothers and, after the end of 1946, an extra allowance for underground coal miners). There was a 'Points' rationing scheme by which non-perishable foods, mainly canned and dried, too scarce to ration, could be bought against special coupons. This scheme was introduced to counter public criticism that these foods, previously unrationed, were being distributed unequally. Eggs and milk were allocated by special schemes of which those for milk were of great nutritional importance. Nearly half the energy value of the wartime working class diet was derived from foods rationed by weight, cash value or points or under controlled distribution (Ministry of Food, 1951).

Milk schemes

There were several schemes relating to milk.

1. Steps were taken to increase the consumption of milk and milk products: milk production was increased; milk was diverted from manufacturing to the liquid market; imports of dried skimmed milk and cheese were increased.
2. The National Milk Scheme was introduced to provide cheap milk for expectant mothers, infants and children up to the age of five years.
3. The School Milk Scheme was expanded. Since about 1927 the National Milk Publicity Council had been promoting the sale of milk in schools, and in 1934 the Milk Marketing Boards and the distributive trades, in co-operation with the Education Departments, started the Milk-in-Schools Scheme with the object of providing free milk for necessitous children and to enable other children to buy it at $\frac{1}{2}$d for $\frac{1}{3}$ pint. The scheme gradually grew in importance until in 1939 over half the pupils in grant-aided schools were taking school milk. After war broke out more school milk was taken, so that during the war about one-third of schoolchildren had $\frac{2}{3}$ pint daily and over one third had $\frac{1}{3}$ pint daily. In an effort to increase take-up school milk became free of charge in all schools in August 1946, but was restricted to $\frac{1}{3}$ pint for each child. By October of that year over 90% of schoolchildren were taking school milk. The free supply continued until the autumn term of 1968.
4. A somewhat abortive Milk Cocoa Drink Scheme was introduced for adolescents, but this never took off.

Table 29.1. *Wartime milk allowances*

Priority class	Weekly allowance of milk
Expectant mothers	7 pt cheap or free plus adult's allowance at full price
Children 0–1 year	7 pt cheap or free plus 5 pt at full price (or the equivalent as full cream dried milk – National Dried Milk)
Children 1–5 years	7 pt cheap or free
Children 5–18 years	$3\frac{1}{2}$ pt at full price
Certain groups of invalids	7–14 pt at full price

5. The Milk Supply Scheme provided for the differential rationing of milk. The concept of priority class consumers was introduced (Table 29.1).

Other people were classified as 'non-priority' consumers. The weekly allowances to priority consumers were guaranteed throughout the year. As the milk supply varied seasonally the amount left over for non-priority consumers did not remain constant: in the autumn and winter it often fell to 2 pt a head weekly and in the late spring and summer it usually rose to 3–4 pt a head weekly. At certain seasons over half the milk supply went to priority consumers. Controls came off the milk supply in January 1950, and after that date the only priority allowances were the 7 pt weekly supplied cheap or free under the Welfare Foods Service to expectant mothers and children up to the age of five years, a provision that ceased in April 1971, and school milk, arrangements for which changed in 1970.

Vitamin Welfare Scheme

Another scheme designed to improve the condition of the vulnerable groups was the Vitamin Welfare Scheme, under which blackcurrant syrup and purée, and cod liver oil were available for young children, which started at the end of 1941. About a year later, the blackcurrant products were replaced by orange juice and the scheme was extended to include expectant mothers, who later became eligible for vitamin A and D tablets on the grounds that some women disliked cod liver oil.

Schemes to improve the nutritional value of foods

There were schemes for improving the nutritional value of important foods for the whole population. In Drummond's words, good was done by stealth. Vitamins A and D were added to margarine to make it nutritionally similar to butter, to increase the intakes of vitamins A and D, and to compensate to some extent for the shortage of eggs, one of the few foods naturally rich in vitamin D.

Flour of 85 % extraction was introduced primarily in order to economise in wheat and thus save shipping for wheat imports, but it also raised the national consumption of vitamins of the B group. Calcium carbonate (*creta praeparata*) was added to flour to raise calcium consumption and to counteract any interference with absorption of calcium by the phytic acid in high extraction flour.

There was considerable effort to increase the production and consumption of carrots and leafy green vegetables, which was coupled with a sustained educational campaign to conserve the vitamin C content of green vegetables in cooking, or by serving fresh salads.

Nutrition education

Unfamiliar foods, particularly dried eggs and dried skimmed milk, were introduced and the need to teach people how to use them, together with the effort to promote good cooking methods for cabbage, led to a widespread programme of cookery instruction and, eventually, education in nutrition, by means of leaflets, posters, lectures and demonstrations. The central point of this national effort was the Food Advice Division of the Ministry of Food, which worked under Drummond's guidance, and its influence was widespread and lasting. This would not have been possible without the enthusiastic and trained support of countless teachers of domestic science, dietitians, school meals organisers, hospital caterers and public health workers who demonstrated that good nutrition could be taught and practised.

Communal feeding

Nutrition propaganda was much helped by the support of such bodies as the King Edward's Hospital Fund for London which published two important memoranda on hospital diet (King Edward's Hospital Fund for London, 1943, 1945). The Fund and the Ministry of Health both appointed advisory dietitians before the end of the war, and gradually the whole concept of hospital catering in Britain changed for the better, though there may still be room for improvement.

There was also development in the provision of school meals. Since 1906, Local Education Authorities had been empowered to provide meals free or at reduced charge for necessitous and other children who would otherwise have been unable to profit from the education provided. The Education Act of 1944 converted this power into a duty towards all schoolchildren, the object being to ensure for them an adequate diet, particularly in respect of animal protein. To make this possible, especially generous allowances of rationed foods, including double the ordinary catering meat allowance, were available for school meals.

Communal feeding of all kinds was encouraged and the principle was accepted that occasional meals eaten in catering establishments were additional to domestic rations because most of such meals were eaten by people whose employment did not permit them to return home for a meal. However, the supply of rationed foods to the catering industry was strictly controlled. Hospitals were treated as residential establishments and rationed accordingly. Factories were required to establish canteens which were entitled to greater quantities of rationed foods than were restaurants for the general public. Special British restaurants (so-called) were established to provide cheap and nourishing meals for people obliged to eat away from home and for whom no other catering facilities were available. A special cheese ration was introduced in 1941, and the Rural Pie Scheme a year later, for agricultural workers unable to get meals in a canteen. There were also schemes for feeding people who had suffered from severe air raids.

Food legislation

The war also brought advances in food legislation for the protection of the consumer. The new Food and Drugs Act of 1938 came into force after the outbreak of war. Power under the Act was assumed by the Ministry of Food in the form of Defence (Sale of Food) Regulations. The wartime orders made by the Ministry grew into a comprehensive system of control over the advertising, labelling and composition of foods with important new developments concerning claims as to the nutritive value of foods. All this was consolidated into subsequent legislation.

Effects on health of wartime policy

By all known measurements of health, the wartime policy was judged to be successful. To quote again from the Lasker Group Award citation:

'By effective employment of its great powers, the Ministry of Food, in consultation with the Ministry of Health... succeeded to a remarkable degree in providing a diet for all the workers of the country in conformity with their physiological requirements, irrespective of income.'

'Although almost all other environmental factors which might influence the public health deteriorated under the stress of war, the public health in Great Britain was maintained and in many respects improved.'

'The rates of infantile, neonatal and maternal mortality and of stillbirths all reached the lowest levels in the history of the country. The incidence of anaemia and dental caries declined, the rate of growth of school children improved, progress was made in the control of tuberculosis, and the general state of nutrition of the population as a whole was up to or an improvement upon pre-war standards.'

Conclusions

The success of the programme can be attributed to a few important facts. At all times, adequate, but not excessive, supplies of food energy were available; food rations were always honoured in the shops, which had an important effect on public morale; the Government owned nearly all available foods during at least part of the distribution chain and could impose the various schemes already described; food prices were controlled; there was full employment; people could afford to buy the foods to which they were entitled and most people did; there were advisory services to inform people about food supplies and nutritional values, and the problem of informing people was easy because the message was simple. 'Eat your rations; eat plenty of green and yellow vegetables; fill up on bread and potatoes.'

But people became bored with the diet, and after the war was over there was a widespread wish for the easing of food restrictions. 'The population was vocal in its discontent, and the importance of palatability and acceptability of food supplies became abundantly clear.' (Hollingsworth, 1957). Food rationing came quietly to an end in 1954 and all food controls were gradually removed.

A comparison of the diets of working-class families with children before the war and after the removal of food controls (Baines, Hollingsworth & Leitch, 1963) showed that food consumption by comparable groups of families at the two dates was remarkably similar, apart from milk then still available through the special schemes already described. The post-war diets of all kinds of families were of greater nutritional value than their pre-war counterparts because of the milk schemes and the food fortification schemes.

At that time we did not foresee that the belief would grow in high places that, because wartime nutritional problems were solved, the unknown problems of peace and plenty did not require new thought and new research, particularly in the social aspects of nutrition and the problems of choice when foods became abundant and more varied than ever before. In the words of the ARC/MRC Committee on Food and Nutrition Research (Agricultural Research Council/Medical Research Council, 1974) 'There is still uncertainty about the exact quantitative requirements of some nutrients but even in 1939 our knowledge was sufficiently detailed to enable the Government to evolve a most successful food policy during World War II. Indeed, this achievement created the belief that most of the problems in nutrition had been solved and that the additional national resources which became available after the war might be more effectively deployed in supporting other scientific activities'. This belief was a serious negative result of success.

References

Agricultural Research Council/Medical Research Council (1974). *Food and Nutrition Research*. London: HMSO.

Baines, A. H. J., Hollingsworth, D. F. & Leitch, I. (1963). Diets of working-class families with children, before and after the second world war. *Nutrition Abstracts and Reviews*, **33**, 653–68.

Bayliss, W. M. (1917). *The Physiology of Food and Economy in Diet*. London: Longmans Green.

Board of Trade (1938). *Report of the Food (Defence Plans) Department for the Year ended 31st December* 1937. London: HMSO.

British Medical Association (1933). *Report of the Committee on Nutrition*. London: British Medical Association.

Crawford, W. & Broadley, H. (1938). *The People's Food*. London: William Heinemann.

Drummond, Sir Jack (1947). Scientific approach to food problems during the war. *Nutrition: Dietetics: Catering*, **1**, 47–62.

Hammond, R. J. (1951). *Food Vol I: The Growth of Policy*, pp. 51–61. London: HMSO and Longmans Green.

Hollingsworth, D. (1957). The application of the newer knowledge of nutrition. In *The Englishman's Food*, 2nd edn. Chap. XXIV Drummond, J. C. & Wilbraham, A., eds. London: Jonathan Cape.

Hollingsworth, D. F. & Wright, N. C. (1954). Obituary – Sir Jack Cecil Drummond. *British Journal of Nutrition*, **8**, 319–24.

King Edward's Hospital Fund for London (1943). *Memorandum on Hospital Diet*, London.

King Edward's Hospital Fund for London (1945). *Second Memorandum on Hospital Diet*, London.

League of Nations (1937). *Final Report of the Mixed Committee on the Relation of Nutrition to Health, Agriculture and Economic Policy*. Geneva: Series of League of Nations Publications II Economic and Financial IIA 10.

Ministry of Food (1951). *The Urban Working-Class Diet 1940 to 1949 First Report of the National Food Survey Committee*. London: HMSO.

Ministry of Health (1937). *First Report of the Advisory Committee on Nutrition*. London: HMSO.

Orr, J. B. (1936). *Food, Health and Income*. London: Macmillan.

30

Translating nutrition knowledge into policy

W. P. T. JAMES and ANN RALPH

It seems appropriate at this Jubilee celebration of the Nutrition Society to consider the changing perceptions of how we should translate nutrition knowledge into policy and compare our present views with those of 50 years ago. Miss Hollingsworth (p. 329) has set out the remarkable effort which went into establishing food and nutrition policies in wartime. Decisions were taken rapidly because this was essential at a time of national crisis. If one goes back to prewar days, it is clear that there had been much debate and scientific controversy well before the development and implementation of policies were precipitated by war.

Dr Petty (1987) has analysed, from archival material obtained from the Medical Research Council, the Ministry of Health and the Board of Education, the controversies that surrounded the public health applications of nutritional science between the two World Wars. Perception of public health in relation to nutrition had been established at the turn of the century by the Committee on Physical Deterioration, which had been formed because of the high rejection rate of so many recruits to the Boer War on grounds of poor physique and health. By 1918 McCollum had already coined the term 'protective foods' for two food classes, i.e. milk and leafy vegetables, and made public health workers more receptive to the need for dietary quality as well as quantity. Then followed the excitement of the vitamin discoveries and their link to public health which heralded the first nutrition revolution of this century. In the 1920s and 1930s nutrition research received a tenth of the MRC's total research budget and Britain remained a world leader in nutrition research. This meant that there was a cadre of prestigious professionals concerned with nutritional issues linked to politically effective leaders such as Fletcher and Mellanby. Mellanby, on taking over as MRC Secretary in 1933, worked directly with Whitehall and successfully pressed for the formation of an Interdepartmental Advisory Committee on Nutrition, formed in February 1935.

Fletcher and Mellanby were, however, opposed by such eminent figures as Paton and Cathcart, both of Glasgow, who emphasised the social and environmental basis of health problems, claiming that parental effectiveness and not diet was often the key to children's health. By virtue of their dominance of key committees, they both actively opposed nutritional studies, e.g. into the dietary aetiology of rickets. They had, however, to contend with such politically active scientists as Boyd Orr who, in *Food, Health and Income* (Boyd Orr, 1936), published 5 years before the Society was founded, linked poverty rather than parental efficiency to deficient diets and poor health. The issues were brilliantly portrayed, and national policy was extrapolated from community studies which were far from perfect. Retrospective criticism of all these studies does not detract from the commitment of the investigators to provide nutrition research suitable for translating into national policy.

Policy developments based on the first revolution

By 1941 about 60% of school children in England and Wales received cheap milk and this rose by the end of the war to 75%. The National Milk Scheme was also established in 1940 to ensure that every pregnant woman, nursing mother and under-5 year-old child could receive a pint of milk. The cost was 2d but milk could be obtained free of charge if family circumstances indicated the need. Thus not only was there a population strategy of preventive nutrition but also the clear recognition of the importance of selective measures for 'the vulnerable groups'. This scheme proved so successful that 96% of those eligible received sufficient milk to overcome the major concerns about thiamin and calcium deficiency.

The policy of providing school meals was also implemented widely because in 1941 the Government stimulated action by local authorities with an offer to cover 70–95% of the cost of the food. So by the end of the war a third of all children in elementary schools were provided with a substantial lunch. Government policy was not confined to children. All factories employing more than 250 'hands' were obliged to provide a canteen for meals. Policy also involved food fortification, e.g. of bread and margarine enriched with vitamins A and D, from 1940 onwards.

Drummond, immediately after the war, gave an illuminating account of the extraordinary variety of measures taken, including not only rationing and controlled distribution, but price controls and subsidies (Drummond, 1948). Drummond noted that the food available to the population before the war was sufficient to meet all nutritional needs, but so disparate were incomes that nearly a third of the population had been considered undernourished. The rationing, price control and subsidies were therefore measures for coping with the purchasing power of the poor.

Sir Donald Acheson, in his trenchant review of nutrition policy by the British Government for the 10th Boyd Orr Memorial Lecture (Acheson, 1986), notes that the learning of a scientific lesson does not guarantee its application and there can be a long gap between a scientific discovery and its translation into effective policy. Acheson notes that 'in 1939, happily for Britain, the right people were for once in the right place at the right time. Lord Woolton, with the scientific advice of Sir Jack Drummond at the Ministry of Food, and Sir Wilson Jamieson with the help of John Boyd Orr at the Ministry of Health, together formulated a national nutrition policy'.

By the time the Nutrition Society was founded in 1941 the science of nutrition seemed well established and the issue was how to collate all the information. By 1945 Magnus Pyke had produced the first *Manual of Nutrition* (Pyke, 1945) from the Ministry of Food and a huge body of knowledge had been compiled on the nutritive value of wartime foods by the Medical Research Council (MRC, 1945). Data on food consumption levels were set out by the Combined Food Boards (1944) which compared the British experience with that of the United States and Canada. The British Ministries of Food and Health were understandably delighted to be presented with the Lasker Group award from the American Public Health Association in 1947 (see Acheson, 1986). The glow of pride in officialdom must have pervaded most discussions of nutrition research and how to translate it into policy during the first few years of our Society.

The postwar period

After the war Britain was set on establishing a universal programme of school meals and school milk. Preschool children and their pregnant or nursing mothers received cheap or free milk, orange juice and cod liver oil. When the National Health Service was introduced in 1948, the poor were given access to an effective and free medical service. These immense social programmes were accepted by both major political parties and everybody recognised the one overwhelming lesson of wartime policies: Britain was totally inadequate in its farm production.

An analysis of the postwar Reports from Ministries of Health and Agriculture suggests that the health aspects of nutrition were taken to be those of fine-tuning in relation to food compositional standards or food fortification. The declared and widely accepted top priority for the Ministry of Agriculture, Fisheries and Food (MAFF) was to support the farming and food industry. Their agenda was altruistic and clear: to produce safe, nutritious food as cheaply as possible, thereby making it available to the poorest in the land. This was a totally logical and progressive policy which solved the pre-war controversies. The milk industry, which had been on the verge of bankruptcy in the 1920s, now had a transformed image because of the combined marketing operation undertaken by both the Ministry of Health and the dairy industry. Although milk was still hazardous because of the risk of tuberculosis and brucellosis, its production clearly had to increase markedly if everybody was to have a plentiful supply of milk. This dietary item was now seen as the principal protective food.

The second nutritional revolution: agriculture

Since World War II therefore we have seen in Britain and in most of Europe a massive transformation of the agricultural and food industries nurtured by a huge investment of Government finance as subsidies and in many different ways including agricultural and food research. By the end of the 1970s there were over 30 Institutes of Agricultural Research employing over 6000 staff on issues relating to food production and processing. At least ten Institutes of the Agricultural Research Service (encompassing both the Agricultural Research Council and the Scottish Office Institutes), with between 100 and 400 staff, were directly involved in research in animal nutrition. Research would be of little value to the farmer, however, without a carefully organised extension and training service, so the Agricultural Development and Advisory Service (ADAS) and Agricultural Colleges developed and expanded, with local authorities adding their own agricultural training facilities. The milk and meat industries received sustained and massive subsidies so that farmers could build dairies, clear their land, develop new systems of rotation cropping and then, with massive industrial and Government support, intensive monoculture systems to maximise efficiency. In this agricultural context, research was translated with practical measures to help the farmer with extraordinary efficiency.

Public health and medical research in Britain after the war

Developments in British public health seemed unimportant with the onset of the National Health Service, which was seen as the effective provider of public health. The principal task of those involved in community medicine was to make the NHS more effective, thereby protecting public health.

Health services research became important and helped to maintain some academic analysis. Doctors working in community medicine still had responsibility for identifying outbreaks of food poisoning and for improving immunisation rates, but the field became a dull routine which few aspiring academic doctors would consider joining.

The bonanza in public funding during the 1960s did not encompass research in human nutrition. Waterlow and Dean ran small and cheap units in Jamaica and Uganda, McCance had a small team in Cambridge, Platt a group in Mill Hill and Harris continued with the largest research unit – the Dunn – which had a staff complement of ten scientists until 1963 when Kodicek took over and increased the work on basic biochemical research with a local scientific staff of 15.

Nutrition was no longer considered of national importance as can be seen from the COMA Reports which became concerned with the vulnerable sectors of society only. Meanwhile the Food Advisory Committee of MAFF promulgated a series of Reports concerned with curbing the excesses of the rapidly developing food industry. This Committee had one nutritional scientist as a representative, but the nutritional questions were not as pressing as those of consumer protection.

By the end of the 1960s nutritional research had effectively dissociated itself from the medical profession, which therefore took up the burden of nutrition research on the basis of obvious need. Paediatricians became interested in childhood obesity; surgeons in the rudiments of body composition and nutrient needs so that they could feed their patients intravenously; gastroenterologists developed enteral feeding and renal physicians explored diets for patients with renal failure who were embarking on dialysis. Cardiologists, diabetologists and geriatricians used dietitians for coping with any dietary problems as an adjunct to drug therapy or other management. Leading medical figures with substantial influence were also extremely disparaging about the importance of nutrition in medicine. McMichael, Booth and Mitchell were major influential figures who denied the importance of nutrition in western diseases, but rarely expressed themselves in print so that the validity of their case could be examined.

Meanwhile nutrition in that bastion of British public health, the London School of Hygiene, became increasingly involved in tropical public health. Professor Morris's MRC Unit was investigating coronary heart disease in the UK but concentrated on the importance of exercise and water softness. Other epidemiological research by Meade, Miall and Acheson was also concerned with the new features of heart disease, of high blood pressure and of environmental aspects of health, but rarely with diet. Despite the work of Keys and Dahl, nutrition was a strangely neglected topic, perhaps because Jean Marr in Morris's MRC Unit had emphasised the proper scientific point that assessing the diet accurately of large numbers of subjects for epidemiological research was extremely difficult and in her view, impossible (Marr, 1971). This view was amplified by ourselves (James, Bingham & Cole, 1981) and helped to stall research in nutritional epidemiology until Willett proceeded to obtain valuable data using dietary questionnaires (Willett *et al.*, 1985).

The beginnings of the third nutrition revolution in Britain

The Neuberger Report, published in 1973, is a landmark in thinking about post-war nutritional research. By then human nutrition research in Britain was in a desperate state. Platt's and McCance's units had closed, and the Dunn represented almost all the MRC's contribution to nutritional science. As Neuberger's team of eminent scientists noted, there was a host of complex diseases of public health importance which seemed to have a nutritional basis and therefore warranted a new approach. But nutritionists and young investigators linked to the Nutrition Society were not involved in these issues because there was almost a generation gap in the recruitment of top quality people into the field. Research on obesity, cardiovascular diseases and cancer was therefore being conducted by physicians and scientists with little or no nutritional background and with no contact with the major forces of nutritional science now harnessed to research in animal science and animal husbandry.

The approach to nutrition in Britain from the 1970s onwards depended in practice on ex-patriot scientists from the Third World. Those returning from the colonies always had a population perspective, but this meant that they might persist with their tropical interests, which in a British context meant considering only the vulnerable groups such as babies and children as worthy of interest. Thus the ex-Ugandan doctor, Sylvia Darke, in charge of the Nutrition Unit at the Department of Health, did an excellent job in promoting changes in infant formulae, in securing funds for monitoring child growth, in considering the problems of Asian immigrant children and of the elderly, but she, like Waterlow and Whitehead, had little interest in obesity or other diseases of affluence with effects on morbidity and mortality coming only late in life.

On the other hand, when Burkitt and Trowell retired to Britain from Uganda, they compared the medical problems of Britain with those of East

Africa and concluded that many of Britain's diseases were of dietary origin; Garrow had also returned from Jamaica and now embarked on his obesity research. Then Waterlow and Whitehead followed to revitalise research in Western diseases at the London School of Hygiene and Tropical Medicine and Dunn Nutrition Unit while continuing their own interest in tropical child health. Given the tropical perspectives of these nutrition leaders and their need to re-establish themselves in Britain, it is little wonder that it took a decade for them to move into prominent positions on Government committees and to the point where they felt able to influence British nutrition policies. Meanwhile, in 1974, COMA, with a substantial complement of iconoclasts, issued its unimpressive Report on dietary aspects of heart disease (COMA, 1974). This was in marked contrast to the remarkably up-to-date and refreshing Report published in 1976 by the Royal College of Physicians (Royal College of Physicians and British Cardiac Society, 1976) under the chairmanship of an ex-Ugandan cardiologist, Shaper. Shaper and then Rose were involved in a dispassionate analysis of heart disease and, whilst not great promoters of nutritional research, they recognised the importance of diet. They also displayed a feature of policy-making which had been neglected for 30 years, i.e. the ability to develop policy from an epidemiological perspective, using data which was not necessarily their own. Although the Royal College Report was well received, the doctors concerned were not part of the Whitehall power base so, on this occasion, the right people were not in the right place at the right time.

The response to the Royal College Report was so unsatisfactory that concerned members of the Committee, such as Dr Keith Ball, set up the Coronary Prevention Group which has played such an effective part in changing national perceptions of nutrition policy in Britain. Meanwhile, at the Dunn we were banned from continuing our research on dietary aspects of colon cancer since Booth and other external reviewers considered it part of the nonsensical fibre story and unworthy of support when the problem could be solved by research in molecular biology. Cummings' own research on dietary fibre was tolerated provided it was expressed in the context of colonic physiology, and our other studies on developing techniques for studying salt intake were considered irrelevant and unworthy of MRC support.

Thus the medical and nutritional establishments viewed the new world of clinical nutrition as deserving only modest support, and were allergic to the fundamental principles we were trying to establish whereby physiological studies were linked to metabolic epidemiology and thereby to public health and potential issues of policy. The medical community and other nutritionists thought that only small subsections of society could possibly need special dietary advice.

Three individuals contributed substantially to the change in perceptions of nutrition policy-making in the UK: Sir Francis Avery Jones, Geoffrey Rose and Sir Donald Acheson. Sir Francis and Professor Rose began by operating on policy-making through channels other than the Department of Health. In the mid-1970s Sir Francis pressed for scientific assessments of the role of dietary fibre in public health problems by the Royal College of Physicians. This Report (Royal College of Physicians of London, 1981), ably collated by Heaton, came out clearly in favour of changes in the types of dietary carbohydrate consumed by the majority of the population. Then the Royal College, stimulated by Sir Francis, convened another group to work on obesity. Simultaneously Geoffrey Rose was preparing, with Henry Blackburn of Minnesota, a major WHO document on cardio-vascular disease (World Health Organisation, 1982). Thus policy-makers in Government were being assailed by expert groups, all highlighting the need for changes in nutrition policy.

The saga surrounding the production of the NACNE Report has been set out by Cannon and Walker in *The Food Scandal*. This public furore was led by the media. Certain members of the Department of Health and of the British Nutrition Foundation were accused of operating secretly to suppress new initiatives in the nutritional field, particularly if these developments were a threat to particular industrial interests. However, Prime Minister Margaret Thatcher's response to the charge that Government was suppressing a Report which would help individuals choose a more appropriate lifestyle prompted the Department of Health to publish a modified NACNE Report while it convened a new COMA Panel to reconsider the issue of diet and cardiovascular disease. This Panel contained both reactionaries and reformers, but the political skills of the Chairman led to Governmental acceptance of the need for major changes in nutrition policy, with specific recommendations for actions from bodies including the Ministry of Agriculture (COMA, 1984). That almost nothing has happened in the last 7 years reflects the classic problems of inertia, bureaucratic delay and the failure of Government officials to accept the need for practical measures other than a minor tinkering with meat subsidies and poorly interpretable food labelling.

Philosophically there has also been a huge switch in emphasis on the nature of political action during the Thatcher years. Market-led consumer-based action is seen to be the only legitimate means of progress with planning, and central Government in theory playing a minor role. Thus those who object to implementing a nutrition policy consider that dietary change should depend exclusively on nutrition education. No account is taken of the huge vested interests aided by Government subsidies and Government officials' overt or covert support. Philosophically, tax changes, regulations and structural changes in society are considered part of unacceptable social engineering, illogical though these attitudes are (James, 1988).

The present position

One month before this Jubilee Meeting the Government issued a consultative document *The Health of the Nation* which now accepts all the arguments which we expected to set out as an agenda for future action. Whilst many would wish to see one or more changes in detail the broad philosophical sweep is remarkable, with a text which sets out a health strategy for Government for the first time ever. The change in thinking is as great as that involved in the establishment of the National Health Service and its breathtaking range is given added substance because this is not a covert Report but a Cabinet-agreed Governmental proposal involving a range of Government departments. Furthermore, it is evident that the Labour Party has similar views, so the challenge will be one of ensuring that the change in policy is implemented. One of its features is the acceptance of Geoffrey Rose's argument on the significance of average blood pressures, body weights, serum cholesterol, etc. and the implication that health education alone is no longer the only means for making progress. Government departments accept their responsibility too.

We can now see parallels emerging with policy-making of the 1940s, i.e. coherent integrated strategies aimed at society in general as well as at vulnerable groups. The relevant research has been accumulating for 30 years and is far more detailed and coherent than that which led to wartime policies. In the 1970s and 1980s we have had to contend with huge vested interests developed originally with Government help and subsidy. Pressures have included misinformation and the selective financial backing of academics with converse views. On this basis the issuing of *The Health of the Nation* Report is an even more remarkable event. We can, however, again discern the return to Acheson's scenario for effective change: the right people were at last again in the right place at the right time. The recent change in British Prime Minister has permitted huge swings in Government policy and we have been fortunate to have a farsighted, intelligent and discerning Secretary of State for Health in William Waldegrave. Rose's intellectual rigour, and the mobilisation of major consumer organisations to promote the latest WHO Report calling for effective nutritional policies have also created the opportunity for change. All these factors have been used by Sir Donald Acheson, who can now be seen as one of the great leaders of British public health. His contribution to changing Government action on AIDS, to re-establishing the speciality of public health in Britain and now to bringing nutrition back to the centre of public health policy is a remarkable achievement after only 8 years as Chief Medical Officer of Health.

Conclusions

With these remarkable recent changes in health policy some members of the Nutrition Society might assume that research will have little to do with policy-making from now on. However, it is believed that nutrition research is in its infancy, with fundamental work on dietary bioactive molecules, physiological biochemistry and molecular biology all contributing to new insights on policy. Implementing the evolving policies, however, will also demand an immense amount of research. The Society therefore has major new challenges as it enters a fascinating new phase.

References

Acheson, D. (1986). Food policy, nutrition and government. Tenth Boyd Orr Memorial Lecture. *Proceedings of the Nutrition Society*, **45**, 131–8.

Boyd Orr, J. (1936). *Food, Health and Income*. Macmillan.

Combined Food Boards (1944). *Food Consumption Levels in the United States, Canada and the United Kingdom*. London: HMSO.

Committee on Medical Aspects of Food Policy (1974). *Diet and Coronary Heart Disease, Report on Health and Social Subjects 7*. DHSS. London: HMSO.

Committee on Medical Aspects of Food Policy (1984). *Diet and Cardiovascular Disease. Report on Health and Social Subjects 28*. DHSS. London: HMSO.

Drummond, Sir J. (1948). Nutritional requirements of man in the light of wartime experience. Eleventh Gluckstein Memorial Lecture, Royal Institute of Chemistry.

James, P. (1988). Dietary reform: an individual or national response? *Royal Society of Arts Journal*, **136**, 373–87.

James, W. P. T., Bingham, S. & Cole, T. J. (1981). Epidemiological assessment of dietary intake. *Nutrition and Cancer*, **2**, 203–12.

Marr, J. W. (1971). Individual dietary surveys. Purposes and methods. *World Review of Nutrition and Dietetics*, **13**, 105–64.

Medical Research Council (1945). Nutritive value of wartime foods. *War Memorandum No. 14*. London: HMSO.

Petty, C. (1987). The impact of the newer knowledge of nutrition: Nutrition science and nutrition policy, 1900–1939. PhD Thesis, University of London.

Pyke, M. (1945). *Manual of Nutrition*. Ministry of Food. London: HMSO.

Royal College of Physicians and British Cardiac Society (1976). Prevention of coronary heart disease. *Journal of the Royal College of Physicians of London*, **10**, 213–75.

Royal College of Physicians of London (1981). *Report on the Medical Aspects of Dietary Fibre.*

The Neuberger Report (1974). Joint ARC–MRC Committee on Food and Nutrition Research. London: HMSO.

Willett, W. C., Sampon, L., Stamfer, M. J. *et al.* (1985). Reproducibility and validity of a semiquantitative food frequency questionnaire. *American Journal of Epidemiology*, **122**, 51–65.

World Health Organization (1982). Prevention of coronary heart disease. *Technical Report Series, 678.* Geneva.

31

The epidemiology of diet and health

GEOFFREY A. ROSE

Incidence rates: a great state of flux

In the 50 years since the foundation of the Nutrition Society the most striking features in the pattern of human disease have been instability and inequalities. There is scarcely a single major disease whose incidence is not changing, or for which there are not large regional or social inequalities. A condition which is common in one time or place will nearly always be found to be rare at some other time or place.

If the present rate of increase of osteoporotic hip fractures is maintained, then the rate in Britain will be doubled by the end of the century. In the island of Naurua, in the south Pacific Ocean, diabetes used to be rare; but independence from Australia brought sudden prosperity, and with it came overnutrition, obesity, and a 50% prevalence of diabetes. Duodenal ulcer used to be rare in Britain (as it still is in the poor countries of the world). It then became extremely common, but now in Britain it is diminishing; in contrast, it is increasing rapidly in the industrialising sectors of the developing world, such as Hong Kong. Coronary heart disease, although of great antiquity among the aristocracy, emerged earlier this century as a pandemic; then in many countries after about 40 years it began to recede. Now, however, at the same time as rates are falling in western populations they are rising catastrophically in eastern Europe.

Alongside these dramatic temporal changes we have become aware also of large regional and social class inequalities, involving most of the major causes of death and morbidity (Marmot, Shipley & Rose, 1984). Ethnic minorities have distinctive health problems, so that among Asians in Britain we see excess rates for diabetes, coronary heart disease and stroke, rickets and tuberculosis. Experience elsewhere has shown that, to the extent that they become culturally integrated, migrants tend to acquire the health characteristics of their adoptive country; thus the Japanese in America, for example, are taller and have more coronary risk factors and coronary disease than native Japanese.

The potential for prevention

These inequalities and rapid changes in incidence imply that the occurrence of most diseases depends on how people live; most diseases are due to modifiable causes, and hence they could be prevented. Old fatalistic views of causation have given way to a recognition that we ought to be able to alter the incidence rates of most major diseases.

Disease occurs when external agents penetrate the interior of the body, disturbing the vital constancy of the internal environment of cells and tissues. The largest and most vulnerable interface between the exterior and the interior is the alimentary tract, and so it is not surprising to find that diet dominates aetiology.

Aetiology has two branches, dealing respectively with the causes of cases and the determinants of the overall frequency of disease. Much research has been concentrated on the role of nutrition in explaining why some individuals within a population become sick whilst others stay well. It is, however, of much greater importance to the public health to study the relation between the diet of whole populations and their incidence rates of disease: advice to individuals can help only the individuals concerned, but changes in national nutrition may alter the health of the nation.

Knox (1977) undertook a systematic ecological study of the relation at national level between food consumption and disease. His first finding was the remarkable strength of the correlations, all the more surprising since the data were so crude: when he related 50 foods to 70 causes of death, he found that nearly 20 per cent of all the correlations were significant at the 5 per cent level, and many of the correlation coefficients were high (> 0.8).

Equally striking was the systematic nature of the pattern of these correlations, many foods showing similar correlations (positive or negative) with a whole range of diseases. This could mean either that a particular diet is just one part of a constellation of disease-related characteristics of a nation's life style, or else that a particular diet may reduce the risks of many major diseases. Recent thinking has inclined towards the latter view, with a gratifying convergence of dietary conclusions from research into a whole range of diseases. A recent recommendation from the World Health Organisation (1990) states that 'the health needs of the population are best met by a high-carbohydrate, low-fat diet, rich in starchy foods (e.g., cereals, tubers and pulses) and including a substantial intake of vegetables and fruit.' Such a diet, it is thought, should minimise the risk of many diseases.

A complex situation

The relation between diet and national health has proved more complex to study than the nutritional health of individuals: the data are poor, and different nutrients are so closely intercorrelated that it is difficult to tease out any specific effects. The situation is well illustrated by breast cancer, a condition of major public health importance (it is the commonest cancer in women, and its incidence is rising). Internationally the mortality rate is highly correlated with total fat intake ($r = 0.9$ at ages 55 to 64 years, Knox, 1977). Even more remarkable than the closeness of the association is its strength: an increase in the national average fat intake of around 40 g daily is associated with a doubling of deaths from breast cancer. In women, the intake of fat may be as important for breast cancer as it is for coronary heart disease; or on the other hand, fat may be acting only as a marker for some other nutrient with which it happens to be highly correlated. This is a pressing issue for further research: no one has yet found any way to prevent breast cancer, but nutrition might hold an answer.

Nutrition and chronic disease

At the start of this century the public health scene was dominated by the interrelated problems of infectious diseases and dietary deficiencies; now it is dominated by the problems of chronic diseases and old age – cardiovascular diseases, obesity, diabetes, cancers, dementia, and the complications of smoking and alcohol. Nutrition remains a central factor in public health; but deficiencies are now less important than the effects of the energy-dense unbalanced diet associated with affluence. The key issues of nutrition and chronic disease are exemplified by the cardiovascular diseases, which will now be considered more closely.

Coronary heart disease

The Framingham Study identified serum cholesterol as a personal risk factor (Kannel *et al.*, 1971), but it was Ancel Keys, a nutritional physiologist, who first confronted the more fundamental question of the underlying causes of the epidemic of heart disease. His famous demonstration that there is hardly any overlap between the serum cholesterol distributions of Finland and Japan taught us to investigate disease from a

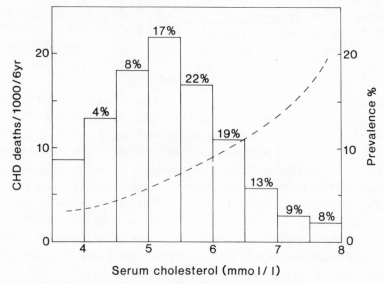

Fig. 31.1. Prevalence distribution (bars) of serum cholesterol concentration related to age-adjusted mortality from coronary heart disease (interrupted line) in men aged 40–59. The number above each bar is the percentage of the deaths, statistically attributable to the cholesterol effect, arising at that level. (Data from Martin *et al.*, 1986).

new viewpoint, that of the sick population; and it showed the need to look at whole distributions and not merely their extremities.

Widespread awareness of the preventive implications of Keys' work originated with the World Health Organisation report (1982), where we stressed that most of the excess cholesterol-associated risk did not occur among the clinically 'hypercholesterolaemic' minority, but rather among the far larger group with values around or a little above the average. This is well illustrated (Fig 31.1) by a recent American cohort study of 361 662 men (Martin et al., 1986): *many people exposed to a small risk generate more disease than a small number exposed to a conspicuous risk.* The key to the aetiology and control of coronary heart disease is not the identification and care of high-risk individuals, but rather an improvement in the national diet; the problem is not clinical hypercholesterolaemia but the average diet of the nation.

Using these arguments we advised the nation to eat less saturated fatty acids, primarily by reducing total fats but with some assistance from substitution by polyunsaturates (Committee on Medical Aspects of Food Policy, 1984). The public has responded in most western countries by maintaining its total fat intake (expressed as a proportion of energy) but making large changes in its constitution. We now have a hitherto unknown pattern of our national diet, very high in total fat and high in polyunsaturates of vegetable origin. Only time will reveal its long-term effects; but in the short term the increased consumption of polyunsaturates (with its accompanying increase in vitamin E) has proved to be the single best correlate of declining coronary mortality, first in the USA and now also in Britain and many other countries. Conversely, in eastern Europe a fall in the dietary P/S ratio has accompanied their dramatic rise in coronary mortality.

The epidemiological findings, strongly supported by laboratory work on thrombotic mechanisms, are pointing towards a new view of advice to prevent heart disease: polyunsaturates, formerly recommended simply as saturate-sparers, are now seen as strongly protective in their own right. At the same time it must be recognised that the epidemiological data do not distinguish the effects of polyunsaturates from those of vitamin E: the intakes are too closely correlated. It is more than 40 years since vitamin E was first recommended in the treatment of atherosclerosis, and the role of antioxidants remains an issue of lively debate.

Blood pressure

Blood pressure has as big an impact as serum cholesterol on cardiovascular disease (both coronary disease and stroke), but its importance at a population level was relatively neglected until quite recently. As with serum cholesterol, the problem in western populations is that the whole distribution is shifted upwards. Risk increases across the whole range (Martin *et al.*, 1986), and most of the complications arise among those whose pressures would be widely regarded as 'normal'.

The average blood pressure in children is similar everywhere: the problem is the biologically abnormal rise of pressure with age which characterises economically developed populations. This rise is substantially due to nutritional factors – salt, obesity, alcohol and (probably) nitrogen intake (Intersalt Cooperative Research Group, 1988). It has to be concluded that changes in the national diet in respect of these factors might reduce the burden of cardiovascular disease as much as changes in fat intake (Stamler *et al.*, 1989). For example, a reduction of one-third in average sodium intake in the UK would be expected to reduce the incidence of hypertension needing treatment by one-third (Rose & Day, 1990) and of total coronary heart disease by one-sixth (Law, Frost & Wald, 1991).

The Intersalt study found large differences in average sodium intake between populations, but equally striking was the wide range between individuals within the same population: the desired level for the national average is already being achieved by a third of the population. However, health education and advice to individuals is a quite insufficient response to the problem, since around 75% of the salt consumed is already present in the food when purchased. The key to most of the improvements in the national diet is in the hands of the food industry and government, but these ponderous organisations will only respond to public demands.

Nutrition in pregnancy and early childhood

The influence of nutrition on maternal and child health has long been recognised, but recent work by Barker and others has opened up a new dimension to research and, in due course no doubt, to practice. Earlier studies (Rose, 1964; Forsdahl, 1977) had suggested that sectors of the population with high infant mortality would in mid-life suffer an excess of cardiovascular disease. Barker (1991) has now shown that birthweight, and also weight at 1 year, correlate strikingly with coronary heart disease (Fig 31.2) and blood pressure 50 years later.

These are particular examples of a widely important phenomenon. During fetal and infant life it seems that there is a series of critical periods during which particular organs and tissues develop (including brain, pancreas, and the immune system) and physiological regulators are programmed (including those for blood pressure and metabolism); and what happens during these critical periods has a major influence on health throughout the rest of life. It is not yet clear what are the external factors which determine whether this organ development and programming go well or badly; but the strong correlations between adult health and growth in early life suggest the critical importance of nutrition during pregnancy and infancy.

In order to explain and perhaps control the major diseases of adult life, together with the disturbing social inequalities in health, it may be necessary to improve not only the nutrition of adults but also the nutrition of pregnant mothers and small babies. Much remains to be understood, but further exciting research can be expected.

Nutrition of individuals and populations

Clinical and laboratory research has shown the importance of nutrition to individual health, and epidemiology has emphasised the link between national diet and public health. Recently it has become clear that these are

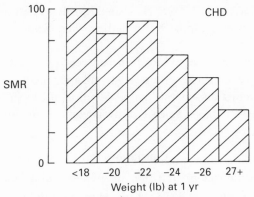

Fig. 31.2. The relation between standardised mortality ratios (SMR) for coronary heart disease (CHD) and weight at 1 year in 6500 males. (Data from Barker, 1991.)

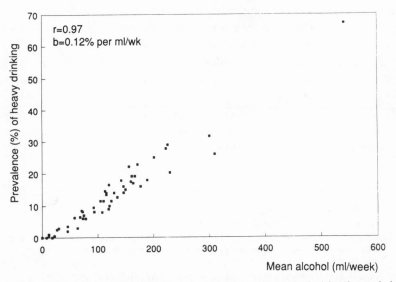

Fig. 31.3. The relation between the population's average alcohol intake and the prevalence of heavy drinking (> 300 ml/week) in 10 079 men and women aged 20–59, from 52 samples in 32 countries (Rose & Day, 1990).

not two problems but one. The Intersalt study (Intersalt Cooperative Research Group, 1988) obtained well-standardised measures of some nutritional and other health-related variables in 52 population samples from 32 countries. Using these data it was shown (Rose & Day, 1990) that the average value for the whole population predicts precisely the prevalence of deviant individuals. Figure 31.3 illustrates this for alcohol intake, where the correlation coefficient is 0.97. Currently the average alcohol intake of

English adults is about 150 ml/week. Using the Intersalt estimates it seems that if this value were reduced by 10%, then there would be 10% fewer heavy drinkers.

For body mass index the correlation between the population average and the prevalence of overweight was 0.94; and applying the slope estimate to the British population suggests that a reduction of 1 kg in average body weight would reduce the prevalence of overweight by one-third.

Conclusions

Concern for the impact of nutrition on public health arises from two sources, namely, the problems of deviant individuals (e.g. obesity, alcoholism, diabetes, hypertension, hypercholesterolaemia) and the fact that even average values are associated with excess risk (e.g. blood pressure and cholesterol). Since the prevalence of deviance is so intimately linked with the average for the nation as a whole, it follows that both public health and the prevalence of clinical cases depend on the national diet.

The national diet is partly under the control of individuals, and health education can clearly influence food preferences; but the more powerful forces are on the supply side, involving agricultural and pricing policies, manufacture, marketing, advertising and labelling. These are all major determinants of the public health, but their operation is not much influenced by any concern for health.

References

Barker, D. J. P. (1991). The foetal and infant origins of inequalities in health in Britain. *Journal of Public Health Medicine*, **13**, 64–8.

Committee on Medical Aspects of Food Policy (1984). Report of the Committee on Medical Aspects of Food Policy: *Diet and Cardiovascular Disease*, Department of Health and Social Security. London: HMSO.

Forsdahl, A. (1977). Are poor living conditions in childhood and adolescence an important risk factor for arteriosclerotic heart disease? *British Journal of Social and Preventive Medicine*, **31**, 91–5.

Intersalt Cooperative Research Group (1988). Intersalt: an international study of electrolyte excretion and blood pressure. Results for 24 hour urinary sodium and potassium excretion. *British Medical Journal*, **297**, 319–28.

Kannel, W. B., Castelli, W. P., Gordon, T. & McNamara, P. M. (1971). Serum cholesterol, lipoproteins, and the risk of coronary heart disease. The Framingham Study. *Annals of Internal Medicine*, **74**, 1–12.

Knox, E. G. (1977). Foods and diseases. *British Journal of Social and Preventive Medicine*, **31**, 71–80.

Law, M. R., Frost, C. D. & Wald, N. J. (1991). By how much does dietary salt reduction lower blood pressure? Analysis of data from trials of salt reduction. *British Medical Journal*, **302**, 819–24.

Marmot, M. G., Shipley, M. J. & Rose, G. (1984). Inequalities in death-specific explanations of a general pattern? *Lancet*, **i**, 1003–6.

Martin, M. J., Hulley, S. B., Browner, W. S., Kuller, L. H. & Wentworth, D. (1986). Serum cholesterol, blood pressure, and mortality: implications from a cohort of 361 662 men. *Lancet*, **ii**, 933–6.

Rose, G. (1964). Familial patterns in ischaemic heart disease. *British Journal of Social and Preventive Medicine*, **18**, 75–80.

Rose, G. & Day, S. (1990). The population mean predicts the number of deviant individuals. *British Medical Journal*, **301**, 1031–4.

Stamler, J., Rose, G., Stamler, R., Elliott, P., Dyer, A. & Marmot, M. (1989). Intersalt study findings. Public health and medical care implications. *Hypertension*, **14**, 570–7.

World Health Organization (1982). *Prevention of coronary heart disease*. Report of a WHO Expert Committee. World Health Organisation Technical Report Series 678. Geneva: WHO.

World Health Organization (1990). *Diet, nutrition and the prevention of chronic diseases*. Report of a WHO Study Group. World Health Organisation Technical Report Series 797. Geneva: WHO.

32

Government food and nutrition policies for the 1990s

DAVID H. BUSS

Introduction

It is already clear that there are new situations and new consumer demands which will require new food and nutrition policies in the 1990s. Many needs are, however, already addressed in current policies, and there are increasing constraints on the freedom of the United Kingdom to act independently in some areas. This chapter therefore outlines the Government's present policies and what they have achieved, and then sets out the goals, the possibilities and some of the problems for the future.

Food from 1950 to 1990

Most of the wartime food policies were no longer needed when food rationing ended in the mid-1950s, and people were at last able to buy the good things in life that they craved, including white bread, butter, sugar and sweets (Buss, 1991). That these foods became available so rapidly and could be afforded was in large measure due to improvements in agricultural efficiency, based on Government-funded research and price support mechanisms, to improvements in our developing food industry, and to freer world trade.

By the 1960s, however, housewives were increasingly going out to work and many homes had refrigerators, so frozen and other convenience foods were wanted and started to become available. It was still necessary for Government to ensure a viable British farming industry, but no Government at that time would have dared to interfere with people's increasing freedom and ability to buy the foods they wanted – even if, with our present concerns about health, we might now think that some aspects of this diet were less than ideal.

Table 32.1. *Increasing longevity in the UK population*[a]

| Year | Life expectancy (years) | | Percentage of population aged 75 and over |
	Male	Female	
1931	58.4	62.4	—
1951	66.2	71.2	3.6
1961	67.9	73.8	4.2
1971	68.8	75.0	4.8
1981	70.8	76.8	5.3
1988	72.4	78.1	6.9

[a] Central Statistical Office (1991).

In the 1970s there was a series of poor harvests around the world and rapid inflation at home which led to substantial increases in the price of food and other goods. The Government of that time responded to consumer concern with a new policy for peacetime – subsidising the retail prices of (white) bread, butter, cheese, sugar, (whole) milk and tea. These foods were important in the diets of poorer and older people, even if not (even at that time) nutritionally the most desirable. But the complexity and expense of that policy soon led to its demise.

The 1970s also saw changes in school milk and school meal provisions, freeing both from an earlier emphasis on energy and fat in particular. Who now remembers that every school meal was once required to provide a *minimum* of 29 grams of fat (Department of Education and Science, 1975), and may have put generations of British schoolchildren off vegetables? But perhaps more important for Government's freedom of action on food policies in the longer term, the 1970s were also the decade in which we joined the European Community and started to lose the freedom to make food laws which differed from those of other Community countries.

There was a steady increase in health and life expectancy during this time (Table 32.1), but an increasing proportion of deaths from coronary heart disease. So the 1980s saw more people than ever before in Britain and in other Western countries worrying about their health and that of the nation. Among the middle classes in particular, smoking decreased; joggers appeared, compensating for their otherwise sedentary lifestyle; *and* they started to change their diets to follow the variety of health advice that sprouted in books, newspapers, magazines and increasingly on television (Buss, 1991). Food safety concerns also grew, despite the generally very high quality of the British food supply. Thus health and nutrition have become, and will continue to be, a major component of British food policies in the 1990s. But what are the present policies? And how might they be changed?

Government policies in 1991

The Government's main aim, as always, is to help people to improve their lives and health, and its broad objectives in the food and nutrition area can be summarised as (i) to ensure that there is always available at a reasonable price enough of the foods that people want; (ii) that these foods are safe, wholesome and nutritious; and (iii) that people should know what healthy diets are, and be able and encouraged to choose them, so that the burden of diet-related diseases is reduced.

The policies to achieve these objectives are an amalgam of those pursued during earlier years, with some discarded as the need disappeared but with others introduced as recently as this year. They may be considered under a number of broad headings.

Policies relating to food availability

The country continues to need, and has, policies to ensure that enough food of the kind that people want is produced or imported. This requires little attention now, even though our population is larger than in 1941 and we now feed (in effect) 40 million people from our own resources compared with only about 10 million in the 1930s. The EC Common Agricultural Policy, which is important in this area now, has been criticised by the British Government, which continues to press for reforms which will help to maintain sensible supplies without wasteful overproduction of fat and other foods while bringing down the cost of food to the consumer.

These policies have resulted in a greater abundance than ever before of high-quality fruit and vegetables, white and wholemeal cereals, dairy products, meats and fats with a range of fat contents, and an enormous range of other fresh and prepared foods. Even the smallest shops and caterers now carry the foods from which as healthy (or as unhealthy) a diet as anyone wishes can be constructed. This food is also more affordable than ever before with, on average, only 12% of consumer expenditure now needed for food compared with 30% in 1940.

Policies relating to nutritional quality

The country's food must be safe, wholesome and nutritious, and Government has taken many steps to ensure this – most recently with the

Food Safety Act 1990, which has given both central Government and local authorities extensive new powers for investigation and control.

Nutritional quality can be enhanced by the fortification policies which the Government first introduced in the early years of World War II, and by the welfare policies which have been in place for many years. Most foods in Britain may be fortified with nutrients, but it is a legal requirement that all margarine be fortified with vitamins A and D, and that most flours be fortified with iron, calcium, thiamin and niacin. Compulsory fortification is, however, a potential barrier to trade which the European Community can stop unless these nutrients can be proved essential to the health of the nation. This matter is currently under discussion.

Welfare policies include the provision of free supplements of vitamins A, C and D, calcium and iodine to expectant and nursing mothers, and vitamins A, C and D are also provided to young children. Uptake is, however, low, and the formulations and use of the products are currently being reviewed – as indeed all policies are reviewed from time to time to ensure that they are the most effective means of achieving the desired ends.

Effective nutrition policies require that Government has accurate and up-to-date information on people's food and nutrient intakes and their health, and Britain continues to have more comprehensive surveillance policies than almost any other country. Since these activities were last described in detail (Ministry of Agriculture, Fisheries and Food, 1988), many new foods have been analysed for a wide range of nutrients and the results published in supplements to the UK food composition tables and now in a new 5th edition of *The Composition of Foods* (Holland *et al.*, 1991). The first of a major series of national diet and nutrition surveys has been completed (Gregory *et al.*, 1990), and will be followed by similar surveys of diet and health in preschool children, and then in schoolchildren and the elderly before the cycle is repeated. Household diets throughout Britain continue to be monitored through the National Food Survey (Ministry of Agriculture, Fisheries and Food, 1991*a*), which from 1992 will be extended to include information on sweets, alcoholic drinks and meals eaten outside the home, which were previously not included. The Department of Health is also about to start a new national health survey, concentrating on risk factors for coronary heart disease, to supplement its surveys of infant feeding practices, of children's health and growth and child dental health, as well as the General Practice Morbidity Survey and the other morbidity and mortality statistics that it collects.

This information quantifies the many improvements in diet and health in Britain, showing, for example, increases in the intakes of minerals and vitamins despite a decline in food intake by an increasingly sedentary population. Nevertheless, many people take nutrient supplements, to the point where the Government has become concerned about possible dangers from overconsumption. Recent reports from an investigative committee (Ministry of Agriculture, Fisheries and Food and Department of Health, 1991) and from a Panel on Dietary Reference Values (Department of Health, 1991*a*) are examples of recent action taken by Government to improve their policies in this area.

Nutritionists' main concern nowadays, however, is about excessive consumption of energy, fat, sugars and perhaps sodium, leading to problems with obesity, high serum cholesterol concentrations, high blood pressure and tooth decay. Since people in several other developed countries enjoy even better health than in the UK, and although their smoking, exercise and stress levels may be different, there is clearly scope for dietary improvement by many individuals. But before Government or indeed anyone else can consider setting realistic new health and dietary targets, research and expert advice are needed.

Research and advice

Most researchers, if not all educators, agree that the relationships between diet and health, and certainly the mechanisms behind them, are not fully understood. For example, despite worldwide correlations, there is little or no regional variation in serum cholesterol or dietary fat *within* Britain to correspond with the well-known regional variations in heart disease mortality (Gregory *et al.*, 1990). The Government therefore continues to support an active research programme to explore these issues, and has substantially increased its funding for food and nutrition research. From 1991/92, MAFF will be targeting new nutrition research towards the following public health issues: (i) the role of the amount and type of dietary fat in atherogenesis and heart disease; (ii) antioxidant nutrients and the prevention of disease; (iii) diet in the development of certain types of cancer; (iv) the level and type of dietary fibre for meeting health and nutrition goals; (v) the relationship between dietary calcium, peak bone mass and osteoporosis; (vi) the possibility of determining criteria for optimal nutrition status and the role of early nutrition on events in later life (including old age). There is also a substantial commitment to research on the determinants of food choice and the presentation of nutritional information to the public, for without such information any dietary advice is unlikely to be well focused (Ministry of Agriculture, Fisheries and Food, 1991*b*).

While ambiguities and uncertainties remain, the Government takes advice on public health issues from the Chief Medical Officer's respected independent Committee on Medical Aspects of Food Policy (COMA). In recent years this committee has provided advice on (besides the topics already mentioned) infant feeding, rickets, diet and heart disease, very low calorie diets, and sugars and human disease. Before new food laws are made on the labelling, advertising and composition of food, advice is taken from the influential and longstanding Food Advisory Committee, complemented by a number of other expert advisory committees on different aspects of food and nutrition. Interested parties, including consumers, enforcement authorities and industry, are also consulted to ensure that the laws are understood, effective and enforceable.

Labelling and education

Despite the ready availability of all the foods needed for a healthy diet, many of us still do not take full advantage of them. People cannot be forced to eat them, but because Government wants to encourage and help people to choose better diets, MAFF, DH and the Health Education Authority have recently issued a number of booklets for the general public and educators including *Eight Guidelines for a Healthy Diet*, together with *Food Sense* booklets on healthy eating and videos on food labelling and hygiene. Very recently, MAFF joined with the British Nutrition Foundation to launch a major new structured resource material for use in schools, called *Food – a fact of life*.

Food labelling is also an important way for consumers to learn about the nutritional value of their foods, so MAFF issued voluntary guidelines as long ago as 1987 to help to ensure a consistent approach from manufacturers and retailers. We were one of the first countries to do this, and were influential in the EC discussions which led to the Nutrition Labelling Directive which will harmonise such labelling throughout the Community. We were, however, disappointed that it was not possible to agree a second Directive which would have enabled selective compulsory nutrient labelling if there was a health need and after other measures had been tried.

A new health strategy for the 1990s

Despite the broad success of these policies, the Government has recognised the need for diet and health issues to take an even higher profile in the 1990s. A consultation document called *The Health of the Nation* (Department of Health, 1991*b*) therefore sets out a new and comprehensive strategy for health promotion and disease prevention which includes reducing deaths from coronary heart disease in the under 65s by one-third; reducing the risk of certain cancers; reducing the number of obese people and those with excessive alcohol consumption; and substantially reducing the number of decayed, missing and filled teeth in 12 year-olds. The proposed dietary targets for the year 2005 include (i) at least 60 % of the population should be deriving less than 15 % of their food energy from saturated fatty acids; (ii) at least 50 % of the population should be deriving less than 35 % of their food energy from fat; (iii) fewer than 7 % of adults should be obese; and (iv) fewer than 1 in 6 men and 1 in 18 women should be exceeding sensible alcohol limits.

These are daunting targets, given the difficulty of achieving current fat targets despite major changes in the British diet in the directions proposed by COMA (Department of Health, 1991a). The means of achieving them have yet to be agreed, but will require great efforts on the part of nutritionists, dietitians, caterers, the food and farming industries, local authorities, consumer groups and consumers themselves, as well as central Government, if these important targets are to be met.

References

Buss, D. H. (1991). The changing household diet. In *Fifty Years of the National Food Survey 1940–1990*, Slater, J. M., ed., pp. 47–54. London: HMSO.
Central Statistical Office (1991). *Social Trends 21*. London: HMSO.
Department of Education and Science (1975). *Nutrition in Schools*. London: HMSO.
Department of Health (1991a). *Dietary Reference Values for Food Energy and Nutrients for the United Kingdom*. London: HMSO.
Department of Health (1991b). *The Health of the Nation*. London: HMSO.
Gregory, J., Foster, K., Tyler, H. & Wiseman, M. (1990). *The Dietary and Nutritional Survey of British Adults*. London: HMSO.
Holland, B., Welch, A., Unwin, I. D., Buss, D. H., Paul, A. & Southgate, D. A. T. (1991). *McCance and Widdowson's The Composition of Foods*, 5th edn. Letchworth: Royal Society of Chemistry.
Ministry of Agriculture, Fisheries and Food (1988). *The British Diet: Finding the Facts*. London: HMSO.
Ministry of Agriculture, Fisheries and Food (1991a). *Household Food Consumption and Expenditure: 1990*. London: HMSO.
Ministry of Agriculture, Fisheries and Food (1991b). *MAFF Food Research Strategy and Requirements Document 1991/92*. London: Ministry of Agriculture, Fisheries and Food.
Ministry of Agriculture, Fisheries and Food and Department of Health (1991). *Dietary Supplements and Health Foods*. London: Ministry of Agriculture, Fisheries and Food.

Part seven

Food composition, food education and the
role of the food industry

33

The composition of foods

D. A. T. SOUTHGATE

A knowledge of chemical composition of foods is the first essential in the dietary treatment of disease or in any quantitative study of human nutrition

(McCance & Widdowson, 1940)

The truth of this quotation, published the year before the foundation of the Nutrition Society, has been borne out by the contributions that compilations of the composition of foods have made to a wide range of nutritional investigations and in the treatment of nutritional related diseases.

The researchers who laid the foundations of the nutritional sciences also recognised the need for a knowledge of the composition of foods in their studies, and initiated food analyses and compilation of the data from these analyses. König in Germany and Atwater in the United States were responsible for the first major series of food composition tables (König, 1878; Atwater & Woods, 1896), although it is probable that Percy and Vaquelin in France should be given the credit for making the first compilation (Somogyi, 1975). König and Atwater laid the foundations for the two most comprehensive series of data on the composition of foods that are available at the present time; the Bundeslebensmittelschussel and the US Department of Agriculture Handbook No. 8.

The development of tables on the composition of foods in the United Kingdom has been described by Widdowson (1967, 1975), and it is not necessary to discuss the early years of what we all know as 'McCance and Widdowson' except to draw attention to three important features that characterised these tables; first, they were designed to be used in the area of research of the authors so that they included values for cooked foods, because this was the level of consumption which was of most importance for individual studies, secondly, they included values for a range of inorganic nutrients because this was one of the authors' major research interests, and thirdly they included values for the different major categories of carbohydrates, based on direct analysis, again because the authors knew that these values were required by the major users of the tables at that time, the clinicians and dietitians concerned with the management of diabetes mellitus. McCance and Widdowson thus created a basic tool or, to use modern jargon, an 'information source' for nutritionists.

The first edition of *The Chemical Composition of Foods* was published in 1940 and was revised in 1946 to include some wartime foods and recipes (McCance & Widdowson, 1940, 1946). The 1930s and 1940s were marked by a rapid increase in nutritional research and knowledge of the constituents that were essential in the diet, and by the 1950s it was clear that there was a need to expand tables of food composition if they were to continue in their role in the nutritional treatment of disease and nutrition research.

Pressures for change to meet the needs of the nutritional sciences

In the 1950s two major pressures were active in all countries where food composition tables had been produced. First, the nutritional sciences had developed and it was clear that the coverage of nutrients needed to be expanded; thus it was essential to include values for the vitamins, and the development of column chromatography as an analytical tool meant that it was now possible to give data for the amino acid composition of proteins and so provide the basis for evaluating amino acid intakes and for treating disorders of amino acid metabolism. Techniques for the study of the carbohydrates had also undergone a rapid development and it was possible to analyse the components of the unavailable carbohydrate fraction.

The second major pressure was the expansion of the food industry, and processed foods were becoming increasingly important in the diet. The primary producers had also benefited by the application of agricultural research and great changes in agronomic and horticultural practices had taken place, as had also occurred in the storage and marketing of their produce. There was thus a need to increase the number of food items in the tables to accommodate the newer foods and to revise the values for foods whose method of production had changed in such a way as to alter their nutrient content. These pressures led to the preparation of the third edition, published in 1960 (McCance & Widdowson, 1960). It is important to note that several of the more perceptive nutritional researchers during the 1950s saw the benefits that would come from computerising the data in food composition tables, initially because of the radical benefits it would bring to the calculation of nutrient intakes.

Development of the present generation of food composition tables and the growth of nutritional databases

Research in the nutritional sciences in the 1960s continued to develop, and relationships between diet and the incidence of chronic diseases, especially cardiovascular disease, began to emerge (Keys, 1970). The requirements of nutritional epidemiology began to create demands for additional values in food composition compilations. In essence these were extensions of the pressures for revising the tables experienced in the 1950s; the demand for increased numbers of nutrients to be covered and the continuous development of the food industry in producing new food products, especially convenience 'ready-to-eat' foods created the need for increasing the numbers of food items. The primary production of food was also developing new methods for storage and marketing of foods which resulted in changes in nutrient content. There were, in addition, other changes taking place that also led to the requirement for more food items in the compilations. The growth of immigration and foreign travel was serving to increase the numbers of different types of food imported into, or produced in, the United Kingdom.

These twin pressures for more food items and expanded coverage of nutrients continue to exert themselves at the present time. They result in an ever-increasing size of compilations of food composition data. When we began work on the fourth edition of *The Composition of Foods* (Paul & Southgate, 1978) in the late 1960s it was clear that the revision would need to be done with preparations for computerisation forming an integral part of the revision. At that time (1968) the data in the food composition tables was seen as a large data set which would make considerable demands on computer storage capacity. The pace of development in computing capacity has meant that now one can use the nutritional database on the simplest of personal computers.

The role of analytical chemistry has been important in developing new methods and improving methods for the analysis of nutrients in the expansion of the food composition data. Instrumental techniques for the analysis of inorganic constituents have transformed the accuracy and speed of analysis for all the inorganic nutrients, especially the trace constituents. Chromatographic techniques enable fatty acid compositions to be characterised in terms of the isomeric forms, and gas-liquid chromatography (Christie, 1973) and HPLC techniques have made the measurement of the component sugars (Shaw, 1988) in foods and in non-starch polysaccharides a matter of, almost, routine in many laboratories. In the field of vitamin analysis, chromatographic techniques have provided powerful specific methods that are in the process of replacing the older microbiological assays (Brubacher, Muller-Mulot & Southgate, 1985; Finglas & Faulks, 1987) and at the same time a new generation of protein-binding and ELISA techniques are being developed which offer exquisite sensitivity and specificity and are much more rapid to perform (Finglas & Southgate, 1990).

International developments in the field of food composition tables and nutritional databases

I have focused most of my remarks on the developments in the UK and it is now necessary to consider international developments. Most countries who had food composition tables have experienced the same kinds of pressures and have developed in similar ways, and it was this common experience that led the Group of European Nutritionists to set up a working party to consider the principles involved in preparing tables of food composition. The Group knew that there was much common use of existing compositional data within Europe and elsewhere, and the patterns of food production and the developments in food trade were such at that time that we could foresee the possibility of developing a common table for Europe. We felt that it was important to address some key issues to make the development of national tables more consistent scientifically, and compatible with one another.

The outcome of this working group was a series of guidelines dealing with the principles for preparing food composition tables (Southgate, 1975), based on the principles that had evolved during the successive editions of *The Composition of Foods* (McCance & Widdowson, 1940, 1946, 1960) and the work that was in progress on the fourth edition.

The focus at that time was on the printed table and, although in principle computerised nutritional databases share much in common with printed compilations, databases lend themselves to a wider range of uses and these introduce other features that must be taken into account.

Printed tables have some attributes that give them advantages over current databases although, as will be evident later, I believe that these will rapidly disappear. The advantages of printed tables are first, their portability so that they can be used easily everywhere; as the compilations grow in size to meet the needs of the users this is no longer true for some of the most recent compilations (Cashell, English & Lewis, 1989); secondly, the numerical data is presented together with qualifying textual matter which gives the origins of the data, descriptions of the food items and the parts analysed and most importantly, textual matter that describes the limitations of the data which directly affect the ways in which the values can and cannot be used. Printed tables have the disadvantage that, as they become larger, they become more difficult to use, for example to locate a particular food. They are also greatly inferior to a computerised database when one wishes to make calculations from the data or to make nutritional comparisons on the basis of the data.

A computerised database, however, takes the form of a matrix of food items by nutrient values. Calculations can be made rapidly from this matrix without knowledge of the true identity of the food item or of the meaning or validity of the nutrient values.

The growth of nutritional epidemiological studies where nutrient intakes of large populations of individuals needed to be assessed was made possible or certainly much easier by the development of nutritional databases, but it was soon recognised that for international studies or indeed any studies that involved the use of two or more databases any comparisons that were made could be vitiated unless one was certain that the data in the different databases were compatible and that the food items were clearly and unequivocally identifiable across the databases.

Two groups of workers concerned with international nutritional studies, virtually simultaneously, began to address this issue of compatibility. Infoods (International Food Data Systems) (Rand & Young, 1983) initially thought that this might best be done by setting up a large database that would effectively include all foods on an international scale. The initial discussions around this concept showed that the most practical way to proceed was to establish a network of national and regional databases, using common principles for naming and identifying foods: using comparable standards for producing and controlling data quality and using agreed nomenclature for nutrients and agreed modes of expression and conventions (for example, for calculating energy value and vitamin activities). Infoods then set about addressing these various elements. This was accompanied by a parallel survey of user requirements.

Eurofoods was the name chosen by a group in Europe, which about the same time recognised the importance of database compatibility (West, 1985). The group included a number of users and, although the issues they identified were similar to those of Infoods, the initial approaches differed slightly and included studies of analytical methodology (Katan & Hollman, 1988). The practical matter of merging databases (Arab, 1988) involves such problems as missing values which create potential difficulties when calculating from a database (Bergstrom, 1990).

Eurofoods also tackled the issue of food identification in a different way by setting up a coding system that would give a unique code for each individual food, because it was recognised that nomenclature of foods across the different languages and cultures of Europe could not be encompassed in a textual way (Wittler & Arab, 1988).

Nutrient descriptors

Interchanging values between databases depends on having agreed nomenclature for nutrients and agreements on the modes of expression and the units to be used. The rules for the nomenclature of nutrients, which effectively define the nutrient chemically or in terms of its nutritional activity, are well established and it has been possible to assemble an agreed set of nutrient 'tags' which incorporate a definition and the units in which data should be transferred and ideally expressed in databases (Klensin *et al.*, 1989).

Interchange software

Programs for using these nutrient descriptor tags in data exchange are being developed.

Food nomenclature

This is a much more difficult problem, especially since the system adopted must be applicable to all foods, including processed foods and mixed dishes prepared domestically. Two types of system have evolved, an hierarchical code 'Eurocode' which gives a unique code for each individual food (Wittler & Arab, 1988) and a factored food vocabulary system, initially based on a system devised for animal feeds, which characterises the food accorded to a number of facets 'Langual' (Feinberg, Ireland-Ripent & Favier, 1991). This is a food description system and does not necessarily give a unique code for each different food. A multifaceted approach in which an open ended approach is advocated is described by Truswell *et al.* (1991).

Data quality

The quality of the data in a nutritional database depends on a number of factors, the sampling of the food item to provide a representative analytical sample, the handling of the sample before analysis, the choice of analytical method to measure the nutrients and the quality assurance procedures adopted during the analytical operations. These form a group of criteria which are applicable to values generated specifically for use in a nutritional database or taken from the literature in the course of making a compilation. These have been reviewed by Greenfield and Southgate (1985), and by Southgate and Greenfield (1988) and will be published in detail in a manual.

Future development of nutritional databases

In concluding this paper I should like to consider briefly how nutritional databases may evolve in the future. Some of these ideas may be considered speculative, but for others research has already established their feasibility and for others the computer software is available. All that remains is for users to consider whether they would find these new developments useful, because a food composition table or a nutritional database is a tool, and the design of that tool must be such that meets the users' requirements.

Non-nutrient substances

In addition to nutrients foods contain a wide range of other constituents; in particular plants contain a large number of biologically active substances and these, with the nutrients, will play a role in determining the responses of individuals to their diets. Clearly there would be considerable merit in expanding the nutritional databases to include these components. If this was done we should have to think of the databases as food compositional databases but I see real advantages to expanding them in this way.

Nutritional information systems

As mentioned earlier, one of the disadvantages of nutritional databases is that the data are separated from the textual matter which is available within a printed table. It is possible to use the database food-item-by-nutrient matrix as the foundation for an information system. Thus, one could address text files that are linked to all the cells in the database. For example, the 'dietary fibre' column heading would take one into definition files in terms of chemistry: analytical files that describe the alternative analytical strategies available and the interpretation of the results obtained: recommended intake files and files describing how the physiological effects are related to composition. The system could be menu driven or possibly part of a 'hypertext' system which had highlighted links to a network of layers of information. Food items would be linked to nomenclature, both systematic and colloquial and to look-up tables that provided the codes that were used for the food in other databases. It is possible to envisage including photographs to assist in identification of foods. Other files would describe the effects of husbandry and variety on nutrient composition.

Software development

One development that is certain to take place is that of increasingly sophisticated programs to manipulate the nutritional data and to make an increasing range of types of calculation possible. Nutritional databases have already demonstrated their utility in calculating nutrient intakes from food intake records, 'nutritional analysis'. Programs for the reverse 'nutritional synthesis' calculations, where diets are calculated to meet specific nutrient provisions, have been widely used in formulating animal feeds; constructing human diets is considerably more complex because of the numbers of different foods eaten and because meal patterns and food preferences have to be considered. However, these programs do exist and should be of value in the prescription of diets where their use should increase the range and variety of diets that can be eaten by, say, diabetic patients.

Nutritional databases also provide the basis for developing dietary models and descriptions of dietary patterns that properly represent the multidimensional character of our diet because of the computer's ability to analyse diets in more dimensions than we can physically envisage, and these patterns may give us new insights into the relationships between diet and disease.

Conclusions

Tables of the composition of foods have contributed greatly to the development of our nutritional knowledge during the past 50 years. They have evolved from printed tables giving nutrient values for several hundreds of foods into computerised databases containing many thousands of foods and values for possibly 60 or 70 different nutrients, and yet this still represents only a fraction of the numbers of foods actually consumed, and possibly only a few per cent of the substances present in the diet, many of which may have biological activity. Over the next 50 years I foresee these compilations expanding in size so that we can explore the relationships between diet and disease even more effectively. However, we should not be too concerned with the size of the databases and neglect the importance of the quality of the data they contain.

The most important advances will come from development of new ways of looking at, and analysing, the data on dietary intakes that will be obtained by their use in nutritional research.

References

Arab, L. (1988). Towards a merged European food composition database, *Food Sciences and Nutrition*, **44F**, 37–44.

Atwater, W. O. & Woods, C. D. (1896). The chemical composition of American food materials. *Station Experimental Report No. 28*, US Official Experimental Station Storrs Conn.

Bergstrom, L. (1990). Nutrient losses and gains. *Proceedings of the Fourth Eurofoods meeting.* pp. 95–107. Uppsala: Swedish Food Administration.

Brubacher, G., Muller-Mulot, W. & Southgate, D. A. T. (1985). *Methods for the Determination of Vitamins in Food.* London: Elsevier Applied Science.

Cashell, K., English, R. & Lewis, J. (1989). *Composition of Foods.* Australia, Canberra: Australian Government Publishing Service.

Christie, W. W. (1973). *Lipid Analysis.* Oxford: Pergamon Press.

Feinberg, M., Ireland-Ripent, J. & Favier, J. C. (1991). Langual: un langage international pour la description structure des aliments. *Sciences des Aliments*, **11**, 193–214.

Finglas, P. M. & Faulks, R. M. (1987). Critical review of HPLC methods for determination of thiamin, riboflavin and niacin in foods. *Journal of Micronutrient Analysis*, **3**, 251–83.

Finglas, P. M. & Southgate, D. A. T. (1990). Objectives and strategy for future vitamin methods. *Journal of Micronutrient Analysis*, **7**, 229–35.

Greenfield, H. & Southgate, D. A. T. (1985). A pragmatic approach to the production of good quality food composition data. *ASEAN Food Journal*, **1**, 47.

Katan, M. B. & Hollman, P. C. (1988). Summary of the Eurofoods interlaboratory trial of nutrient analyses. *Food Sciences and Nutrition*, **44F**, 35–6.

Keys, A. (1970). Coronary heart disease in seven countries. *Circulation. Suppl.* 41–5.

Klensin, J. C., Feskanich, D., Lin, V., Truswell, A. S. & Southgate, D. A. T. (1989). *Identification of Food Components for INFOODS Data Interchange.* Tokyo: United Nations University Press.

Konig, J. (1878). *Chemie der menschlichen Nahrungs-und Genussmittel.* Berlin: Springer.

McCance, R. A. & Widdowson, E. M. (1940). *The Chemical Composition of Foods.* Special Report Series of the Medical Research Council No. 235. London: HMSO.

McCance, R. A. & Widdowson, E. M. (1946). *The Chemical Composition of Foods.* 2nd edn. London: HMSO.

McCance, R. A. & Widdowson, E. M. (1960). *The Composition of Foods.* Special Report Series of the Medical Research Council No. 297. London: HMSO.

Paul, A. A. & Southgate, D. A. T. (1978). *McCance and Widdowson's The Composition of Foods.* 4th edn. London: HMSO.

Rand, W. M. & Young, V. R. (1983). International network of food data
systems (Infoods): Report of a small international planning conference.
Food and Nutrition Bulletin. **5**, 15–23.

Shaw, P. E. (1988). *Handbook of Sugar Separations in Foods by HPLC.* Boca
Raton: CRC Press.

Somogyi, J. C. (1975). National food composition tables. In *Guidelines for the
Preparation of Tables of Food Composition* Southgate, D. A. T. ed. 1–5.
Basel: Karger.

Southgate, D. A. T. (1975). *Guidelines for the Preparation of Tables of Food
Composition.* Basel: Karger.

Southgate, D. A. T. & Greenfield, H. (1988). Guidelines for the production,
management and use of food composition data: AN INFOODS project.
Food Sciences and Nutrition, **44F**, 15–23.

Truswell, A. S., Bateson, D. J., Madafiglio, K. C., Pennington, J. A. T., Rand,
W. M. & Klensin, J. C. (1991). *Journal of Food Composition and Analysis,*
in press.

West, C. E. (1985) editor. Eurofoods: Towards compatibility of nutrient data
banks in Europe. *Annals of Nutrition and Metabolism.* **29**, Suppl. 1.

Widdowson, E. M. (1967). The development of British food composition tables.
Journal of the American Dietetic Association, **50**, 363–367.

Widdowson, E. M. (1975). A brief history of British food composition tables. In
Guidelines for the Preparation of Tables of Food Composition. Southgate,
D. A. T. ed., 53–57. Basel: Karger.

Wittler, M. & Arab, L. (1988). Eurocode. *Food Sciences and Nutrition,* **44F**,
1–7.

34

Nutrition education – the key to dispelling misinformation

MARGARET ASHWELL and GILL FINE

Summary

In theory, the communication of the results from nutrition research to the general public should be straightforward. In practice, nutrition information, as published in the specialised journals, can undergo a series of partial interpretations so that the information that reaches the consumer can be totally distorted i.e. it has become misinformation. Misinformation can arise from problems with the message itself, the media and the influence of the motivators. These were all present 50 years ago and are unlikely to change in the next 50 years.

To some extent, the spread of misinformation can be rectified by the encouragement of better links between the scientists and the media, the motivators and the educators, and by better direct communication between the scientists and the consumers.

This remedial action is only second best and prevention is always better than cure. The real challenge is to establish a framework for teaching children about food and nutrition in schools and to use the opportunities presented by the National Curriculum to ensure that all children leave school with the basic ability to spot a clear message, in spite of the confounding efforts of those who generate and spread the misinformation.

The British Nutrition Foundation's Schools Programme 'Food – a fact of life' is the first comprehensive programme to attempt to do this for children, ages 5–16.

Introduction

Consumer surveys have indicated the wide range of sources from which adults receive information on food and nutrition. The media, advertisements, supermarket leaflets, friends and the GP are important sources. The

GP's advice is particularly influential and trusted (McCluney, 1988), but it is rather worrying that the GP also relies heavily on the media for updating his or her knowledge (National Dairy Council, 1989).

Sources of misinformation

Information transfer

In an ideal world there would be at least seven stages of scientific information transfer. The original research papers (first stage) should appear in scientific reviews (second stage) and scientific consensus reports and textbooks (third stage) before arriving in the media (fourth stage), being incorporated into health claims on labels and in advertisements (fifth stage) and eventually being passed by word of mouth as 'gossip' (sixth stage) and to future generations as folklore and customs (seventh stage). Distortion of the nutritional message (misinformation) arises because the message itself is complex and inconsistent and because the flow of information is rarely in this logical order.

Problems with the scientific message

One of the scientific messages to cause maximum confusion through apparent inconsistency and complexity in 1991 has been the relationship between milk consumption and heart disease (Elwood *et al.*, 1991). The data came from a longitudinal prospective study of middle aged men which was set up to investigate risk factors for coronary heart disease (CHD). The men who stated that they drank over a pint of milk a day 5 years ago had the lowest incidence of CHD. Differences in total fat and saturated fatty acid intake were small and inconsistent.

To the general public this association seemed to be inconsistent with the well-publicised, but less well-documented, notion that increased fat consumption is related to heart disease. However, other data from the survey showed that the physiological risk factors such as serum LDL, cholesterol and fibrinogen were positively associated with CHD events and were therefore entirely consistent with current hypotheses. The relationship between nutrients and foods to these physiological risk factors has always been much more complex, and nutritionists recognise that interactions between the nutrients must be considered as well as interactions between dietary factors and other behavioural and genetic factors in the causation of CHD (Halliday & Ashwell, 1991).

Problems with inaccuracy

Inaccuracy is the most obvious way that the scientific message can be distorted into misinformation. A small media inaccuracy is easily amplified so that the original meaning can be totally lost by the time the message is transferred by 'gossip'. A reasonably accurate media interpretation of the original scientific message is much more likely to lead to accurate 'gossip' than is the less accurate media interpretation of the same sentence. The 'gossip' that arises from an inaccurate media article will become misinformation.

Problems with prematurity

Some sections of the media like to pluck one scientific result from an original research paper (usually performed on experimental animals) and then announce prematurely that a particular technique will solve the world's nutritional problems at a stroke, e.g. a technique for injecting rats with antibodies against adipocyte plasma membranes which caused a temporary reduction in epididymal fat cells was blown up prematurely into a permanent cure for all human obesity in the US National Examiner under the headline 'Melt fat away forever!'.

Problems with mischievousness

Mischievousness is a fairly polite term for the way in which the media like to question the integrity of either scientists, Government or the food industry. This is very common practice when journalists write about important Government reports either before or after publication, and criticize the conclusions in the Report on the basis of vested interests, e.g.

'The publication of the NACNE report was delayed for $2\frac{1}{2}$ years. The report's message was opposed by powerful representatives of the food industry, notably those paid to protect the interests of fat and sugar, who are persuasive voices in Whitehall'

(from publisher's blurb to Walker & Cannon, 1984).

Problems with embellishment

Embellishment refers to the way in which the media and the food industry can use the nutritional message to suit their own purposes. This message can be embellished with outrage or euphoria.

The media are particularly good at adding *outrage* to any bad messages about food so that the consumer perception of the risk attributable to the food is heightened by the outrage (Sandman, 1987). Thus:

$$\frac{\text{Consumer perception of}}{\text{food related-risk}} = \frac{\text{Severity of the hazard plus}}{\text{outrage associated with it.}}$$

Detailed analysis of the components of outrage can be found elsewhere. The perceived risks about Alar (a growth promoter used for fruit) and BSE (Bovine spongiform encephalopathy) are much greater than the actual risks associated with these hazards because of their outrage component (Ashwell, 1991; Ashwell & Lambert, 1991).

The nutritional message can also be embellished with outrage, but it is particularly prone to embellishment with *euphoria*. Thus:

$$\frac{\text{Consumer perception of}}{\text{food-related benefit}} = \frac{\text{Magnitude of gain plus}}{\text{euphoria associated with it.}}$$

Some marketing departments in the food industry are good at adding euphoria to the nutritional message to 'motivate' increased sales. Accurate 'health claims' can help nutrition education, but overembellished, euphoric health claims have great potential for spreading misinformation.

Embellishment with euphoria can be particularly persuasive when the combined forces of the media and industry join together. A good example is the media coverage of the effect of vitamin and mineral supplementation on the non-verbal intelligence of schoolchildren, and the subsequent increased sale of hastily renamed micronutrient supplements, to include the term IQ (see Ashwell, 1991*a*).

Misinformation in the 1940s

From the foregoing analysis and the examples given, the reader could be forgiven for thinking that problems with the message, the media and the motivation are problems of recent years. This is not so, as the following two examples will show:

The need for calcium fortification of bread
The scientific message

In the early 1940s, McCance and Widdowson realised that people in Britain might not be getting the calcium they required if milk and cheese were severely rationed and if they had to switch from their beloved white bread, made with 69 % extraction flour, to 'The National Loaf' made with higher extraction flour (85 %).

They thought that phytic acid might account for the anticalcifying effect of cereals (Harrison & Mellanby, 1939) and therefore set up a series of calcium balance experiments involving five men and five women as volunteers. In each experiment, 40–50 % of the energy was provided by the flour under study at the time. Absorption of calcium was impaired by high extraction flours (92 %), but not by low extraction flours (69 %). This impairment could be mimicked by adding sodium phytate to low extraction flours, thus implicating phytate as the calcium binding agent. Fortifying all the flours with calcium, but not vitamin D, improved the absorption of calcium and prevented the loss of calcium from the body. Calcium fortification was particularly beneficial when the diets contained large quantities of high extraction (92 %) flour.

On the basis of these experiments, McCance and Widdowson (1942) recommended that 'to every 100 g of the finest 69 % extraction white flour, 65 mg of calcium should be added; to every 100 g of National 85 % wheatmeal flour, 120 mg calcium, to 100 g of 92 % extraction wholemeal flour, 200 mg of calcium'. Thus, the nutritional message from these experiments was simple and consistent: the higher the extraction rate of the flour used to make the bread, add more calcium to counteract the extra phytate which will be present.

The interpretation of the message

The results from McCance and Widdowson's experiments were partly responsible for the Government's decision to fortify flour with calcium carbonate. Unfortunately, the decision aroused a storm of protest and was bitterly opposed. The pure food enthusiasts still remembered the eighteenth century adulteration of bread by the non-nutritional addition of chalk and powdered bone to improve the colour of white flour. A particularly vociferous opponent of calcium fortification was Isaac Harris. In 1942, he wrote a booklet called *The Calcium Bread Scandal*, and proclaimed that calcium fortification of bread would lead to kidney stones and hardening of the arteries. Harris intended his booklet to be a criticism of the 1942 Government, even though he admitted that 'in comparison to the drama which is being played in the World War, the subject of this paper may appear tame'. He accused Sir Edward Mellanby, Secretary of the MRC, of being a dictator who was only interested in calcium:

Parliament was not consulted. Thus over 40 million human beings are compelled to swallow a substance which, in excess, is a slow-acting poison. At present there is no check whatsoever on any wild-cat scheme which may be forced on the public. Today it is one food crank who becomes the dictator; tomorrow there may be another. Today it is calcium; tomorrow, Heaven knows what else may be imposed on us.

The outcome of the debate that ensued was the legal requirement to add calcium only to white flour and the 85 % extraction flour for the National Loaf. Calcium has never been added to wholemeal flour which is, scientifically speaking, the bread that needs it most! Even in the 1940s, people with non-scientific, mischievous motives managed to promote such an outrage against calcium that a potential gain was seen as a hazard.

The comparative merits of white and brown bread for growth of children
The scientific message

The experiments of Chick (1940) had shown that weanling rats grew more quickly on wholemeal flour than on white flour supplemented with B vitamins and iron, and this led to a strong belief that brown bread contained something that made it better than white bread for the growth of children.

From 1947 to 1949, Widdowson and McCance gave five different types of bread to five groups of German children in orphanages who were under height and under weight at the outset. The breads were made with five different types of flour ranging from 100 % extraction wholemeal flour to white 'prewar' 70 % extraction flour. Vitamins and iron were added to some of the white flours and all flours were fortified with calcium.

Much to the surprise of the investigators (McCance & Widdowson, 1946), the experiment, which lasted 18 months, showed that the children all grew exceptionally well in height and weight on all five types of bread, and it was not possible to differentiate between the groups (Widdowson & McCance, 1954).

Widdowson and McCance subsequently confirmed Chick's results on the 3 week-old rats, but showed that 8 week-old rats grew just as well on white flour as they did on wholemeal flour, and thus reacted like the German children. The age-related discrepancy was eventually found to be due to lysine requirements. Weanling rats, but not older rats, grow so fast that they do not get enough lysine from white bread. Children grow much more slowly than rats so they get adequate lysine and vitamins from white bread and the rest of their diet.

The interpretation of the message

This example shows how easy it is for the nutritional message to be viewed as complex and inconsistent and illustrates the dangers of extrapolating the results from animal experiments to the human situation. It also provides a good illustration of how the nutritional message can be used to suit the purpose of the media and the motivators. Chapman Pincher, of the

Daily Express, used Widdowson and McCance's results to support his campaign of outrage against the National Loaf and to have some 'mischievous' digs at the Government at the same time:

Rats, gentlemen!

Raise your teacup this morning to Professor McCance. He has succeeded where public demand and the *Daily Express* both failed.

For years this newspaper sought to restore the white loaf. The public – or those who could still remember the delicious white bread of prewar days – longed to have it back. But the gentlemen in Whitehall thought they knew best. They said that the dreary grey National Loaf was better for us. Professor McCance is the man who exploded this nonsense. Thanks to him this grey bread may soon be ousted. It seems that the diet faddists who foisted the grey loaf on the public made a slight slip. They tried out their grey flour on baby rats.

If only they had made their tests on people, as Professor McCance did, they would have found that white bread can be made every bit as nutritious as their own cheerless fancy. And the worst of it is that when the gentlemen in Whitehall were put right by Professor McCance, they kept the truth hidden. Give officialdom power to meddle with the people's diet and always that power will be abused.

Parents are perfectly capable of choosing good food for themselves and their children. Professor McCance has shown that the gentlemen in Whitehall can only be trusted with baby rats.

It is interesting to compare this quote with the final sentence of the preface of the MRC Special Report in which the scientific results were published.

Dr Widdowson and Professor McCance emphasize that the greatest caution must be used in coming to any general conclusion on the basis of these results. The conclusions drawn must be restricted to the conditions under which the scientific evidence was obtained and cannot justifiably be applied to the needs of populations in very different states of nutrition and with widely ranging dietary habits.

The fact that scientific training emphasises the importance of the qualifiers and uncertainties, and that some journalists prefer to emphasise the importance of outrage, euphoria and mischievousness are two of the main reasons why scientists often find it so difficult to communicate with journalists (see Ashwell, 1991*b* for further analysis).

Better communication to dispel misinformation

Table 34.1 lists Ten Commandments for scientists who try to communicate the nutritional message to journalists or directly to consumers. Strangely enough, they are not too dissimilar to the two golden rules for crisis management, 'Emphasise your commitment and maintain control at all times'.

Table 34.1. *Ten commandments for communicating the nutritional message*

I	*Don't pooh-pooh the outrage or the euphoria* Pretend you understand it and have sympathy with it. Then get down to talking about the risk or the benefit in terms of the hazard or the gain.
II	*Reduce the outrage or the euphoria* Make the scientific data about the hazard or the gain into a story which is more interesting than the outrage or the euphoria.
III	*Distract from the outrage or the euphoria* Put the food risk or benefit into perspective with other non-food related risks or benefits.
IV	*Make the 'middle of the road' position more interesting* Veer as near to the 'gutters' at the edge of the road as your scientific integrity will allow.
V	*Simplify your story as much as you can* It's better that *you* do this than the person who listens to you. Don't give any opportunities for the 'Chinese Whispers' syndrome.
VI	*Make your story more consumer-friendly* Insert as many everyday analogies as you can.
VII	*Personalise your story as much as you dare* Talk about your grandmother or your kids or give personal anecdotes (even if you have to make them up sometimes!)
VIII	*Raise excitement about your qualifiers and uncertainties* Don't allow them to spoil and distract from your story.
IX	*Use your sense of humour* Slip in at least one funny. It's easier on some nutritional topics than others (e.g. 'fibre') but it always helps the memorability factor.
X	*Build consumer trust and credibility* Do this gradually, and don't ever demand it at the outset.

Better communication with the motivators should also be possible. If scientists can work within, or alongside, the marketing departments in the food industry, some of the euphoric claims made about food products might be toned down a little.

Better education to dispel misinformation

The previous sections in this chapter have examined the sources of misinformation about food and nutrition. These have existed for at least 50 years and are unlikely to disappear now.

Better communication between scientists and journalists is one way to stop the spread of misinformation, but this is just one tactic, and prevention is surely likely to be better than cure. So why do some people leave school without a basic understanding about food and nutrition, making them so susceptible to misinformation?

Historically, food and nutrition have been taught mostly within Home Economics (previously known as Domestic Science), with certain aspects covered in Biology and Health Education. Pupils chose which subjects they studied and consequently the level of tuition each pupil received varied widely.

The introduction of the National Curriculum has changed this situation. All pupils have to study ten subjects from ages 5 to 14 and to continue to study some of them, notably Science, Maths, English and Technology until the age of 16. Home economics is one of five subjects that make up Technology; Biology is one of three subjects comprising Science; and Health Education is one of five cross-curricular themes intended to provide a general framework through which the various subjects that make up the whole curriculum can be delivered. *All* pupils have to study Science and technology, and both of these subjects identify food as one of the materials that must be studied. The National Curriculum therefore provides an opportunity for all pupils to receive tuition in food and nutrition. At the same time there is a danger that they will receive this tuition in a piecemeal fashion i.e. within subject boundaries – so at the end of the day pupils will have only a fragmented knowledge about certain aspects of food and nutrition.

For the past three years the British Nutrition Foundation (BNF), with the help of its education advisory groups, has been devising a Food and Nutrition Programme for use in schools from age 5–16. It is entitled 'Food – a fact of life' and combines five main themes: food components and their function, socio-economic aspects of food, food processing and production, Food preparation and hygiene, and food preservation. The content of these themes has been structured to ensure that the requisite progression has been built into the programme to enable each theme to be studied in depth. These five themes provide a framework, therefore, for teaching food and nutrition in a cohesive fashion that integrates with various national curriculum subjects, notably Science, Technology, Maths, History, Geography and with Health Education.

To assist the teachers, the Programme identifies the relevant information for each key stage. This information, together with a comprehensive text about each of the five themes, ideas for teaching activities and their application within the National Curriculum, together with a list of resources produced by other organisations, is contained in the Teacher's Manual.

A range of resources has already been produced for Key Stage 1 pupils. These include an award winning video, flash cards, photographs, a data file, activity sheets, floor charts and a picture work book. The materials have been 'trialled' in 47 schools in 29 Local Education Authorities and have been available on a nationwide basis since Autumn 1991. Materials for Stages 2, 3 and 4 will be produced during 1992 to 1994.

The BNF believes that this programme provides a cohesive structure for teaching food and nutrition in schools that will enable pupils to acquire a good understanding about food and nutrition during their school career. As a result, they will leave school with the framework of knowledge that is necessary to put scientific research findings, media messages and marketing propaganda into context. They will also be able to choose a diet that meets their nutritional and lifestyle requirements – should they wish to do so. Most important of all they will understand what good nutrition is all about, and recognise that food should be fun, not feared!

References

Ashwell, M. (1991 *a*). Consumer perception of food-related issues. *BNF Nutrition Bulletin*, **16**, 25–35.

Ashwell, M. (1991 *b*). The media and slimming. *Proceedings of the Nutrition Society*, **50(2)**, 479–92.

Ashwell, M. and Lambert, J. (1991). Nutritional aspects and consumer perception of meat. In *The European Meat Industry in the 1990s*. Smulders, F., ed., Amsterdam: Elsevier. pp. 293–317.

Chick, H. (1940). Nutritive value of white flour with vitamin B1 and of whole flour. *Lancet*, **ii**, 511–12.

Elwood, P. C. et al (1991). Epidemiological studies of cardiovascular disease. *Progress Report VII*. Cardiff: MRC Epidemiology Unit.

Halliday, A & Ashwell, M. (1991). Diet and coronary heart disease – a round table of factors. *Proceedings of the 6th FENS Conference. European Journal of Clinical Nutrition*, **45**, 99–102.

Harris, I. (1942). *The Calcium Bread Scandal*. pp. 1–23, London: Hogarth Press.

Harrison, D. C. & Mellanby, E. (1939). Phytic acid and the rickets-producing action of cereals. *Biochemical Journal*, **33**, 1660–80.

McCance, R. A., & Widdowson, E. M. (1942). Mineral metabolism of healthy adults on white and brown bread dietaries. *Journal of Physiology*, **101**, 44–85.

McCance, R. A. & Widdowson, E. M. (1946). The composition and milling of wheat. *Proceedings of the Nutrition Society*, **4**, 2–6.

McCluney, J. (1988). *Answering back: public views on food and health information*. Food Policy Research Unit, University of Bradford, Bradford: Horton Publishing.

National Dairy Council (1989). *Healthy Eating, Beliefs and Attitudes*. London: NDC.

Sandman, P. M. (1987). Risk communication: facing public outrage. *EPA Journal*, Nov; pp. 21–22.

Walker, C. and Cannon, G. (1984). *The Food Scandal*. London: Century.

Widdowson, E. M., & McCance, R. A. (1954). *Studies on the nutritive value of bread and on the effect of variations in the extraction rate of flour on the growth of undernourished children*. Medical Research Council Special Report Series No. 287, London: HMSO.

35

The responsibility of the food industry

J. EDELMAN

There is a famous cartoon which describes the history of the world and its future in ten minutes; I find it impossible to deal properly with the subject of this paper in the limited space available. To begin with I cannot even adequately define the food industry, with products ranging from pots of mustard to meat pies, from chilled lamb curry to cake decorations – and does it include drink? Secondly the meaning of the word responsibility has always been fertile ground for philosophers. All I can do is to give some idiosyncratic views I have come to since joining a food company from academic life just under twenty years ago.

For a start I am going arbitrarily to decide that what is commonly understood by the food industry does not include agriculture or primary processing, even though we are seeing a progressive disappearance of the farm gate as farmers and manufacturers get closer together. I will consider only what is often called secondary processing – what is commonly understood by the public as food manufacture: the conversion of primary agricultural products to items of food bought by the consumer in supermarkets, grocers' shops, canteens and restaurants. Finally, I am going to restrict myself to the United Kingdom. I am not going to be at all original in that I do not think the food industry can do anything about responsibility which is basically different from what it is doing now. However, it can, and will, do more of what it is doing now about providing a wide spectrum of products from which good diets can be chosen that people can afford, and it will continue to encourage nutrition education. Using my definition, the modern food industry has only been able to radically influence consumer choice, and to become a significant factor in the national diet since the 1960s, that is, since food became so abundant, and affluence for the majority of the population so great that a wide choice of elaborate food items could become part of everyday life. Some may say that this happened earlier, but it did not happen much earlier.

I was asked to touch on the history of industry's responsibilities. Until two or three generations ago, housewives, apart from the very poor, bought primary ingredients such as meat, vegetables, milk, flour and condiments and cooked them in the kitchen for the family. It is true that commodities like butter and bread which sit somewhere between primary products and secondary manufacture have been commonly available almost from time immemorial, but these were, and still are, considered to be basic ingredients by most people.

Since the growth of large cities in the nineteenth century and until quite recently, the factors in the diet that have had the greatest impact on health were its inadequacy both in quantity and nutritional quality, and ignorance about that inadequacy. Secondary factors such as contamination of food and water by microbes and poisons were important, and quite often of overriding importance. Many people were concerned with getting enough to eat, and most were interested in enjoying it when they got it: neither of these concerns ensured good nutrition. Generals were concerned about their 'pygmy armies' recruited from the proletariat, and these had certainly gone hungry, but Drummond (Drummond & Wilbraham, 1957) has pointed out that the diets of most public schools, not noted for catering for the children of impoverished families, may have been substantial but were stodgy and poor, containing no milk, fruit or salads as these were considered to be 'namby-pamby' foods and did not confer 'manly qualities'. Adequate nutrition until quite recently was considered in terms of growth and bodyweight and not a healthy longevity. It seems to me that there was little real interest at all in nutrition nationally, apart from a few heroic individuals, except during the last two World Wars, and even then nutrition was considered an immediate problem, to be solved in the short term.

There were no university departments of nutrition when the Nutrition Society was founded. Medical schools taught little or no nutrition to their students. The public was unconcerned, and it was a byword in the industry that, apart from some special products like breakfast foods or patent breads, a nutritional image hindered rather than helped sales. So it is difficult to see how food companies in general could have developed any conscious view about nutrition and health until the recent past. The first major responsibilities of the industry were concerned with adulteration and safety, and were established by the Food & Drink Act of 1875 which decreed that food and drink could not be sold if it was prejudicial to the purchaser, and this was followed in this century by a number of statutes concerning public health aspects of food. It is no coincidence that scientific developments in chemistry and microbiology at that time began to make us understand how food can become contaminated and how we could avoid this happening.

As bacteriology gained strength and grew later into general microbiology, all the multitude of previous views about the incidence and spread of disease, ranging from the phase of the moon, noxious vapours, the evil eye, to sin, fell away. Although some experts maintained that prayers, magic remedies, specifics and the burning of witches worked, they did not work every time. But there had been no alternatives. Francis Galton, that extraordinary nineteenth century polymath, carried out an interesting study on families of clergymen (Galton, 1883). His basic thesis was that if prayer was efficacious then the incidence of 'deaths at the time of birth' among clergymen's children would be expected to be lower than that of similar professional groups. The precise recording of deaths and the premise that death is a fact and not a medical opinion, led to a clear result; no significant difference from the controls was found. Sophisticated statistical analysis was not used in this study, but the efficacy of prayer at that time was, I am sure, considered to be beyond such fine tuning.

Early this century it became possible to prevent the spread of many serious illnesses by using microbiological knowledge. An important principle emerges here. There was, and is, no argument about this. There are no self-styled experts with different theories about microbiological safety. There is no confusion among the thinking public. There is no conflict with the food and water industries. We understand the principles of proper hygiene. If things go wrong by accident or malpractice or individual ignorance we know how to tackle them. I am labouring this point because we can draw an analogy with the present problems of nutrition, and I will come back to this.

Turning back to affluence and the superabundance of food which the population has enjoyed recently, it is not surprising that these have led to an insatiable public demand for a wide choice of products. This has happened for all other consumer goods so it was to be expected for what can be considered the ultimate consumer commodities, food and drink. Given our political and economic system, food manufacturing businesses inexorably evolved to give this ever wider choice, but this had to be within the legal and consumer demand that food must be safe and within the marketing constraint that it must be cheap enough to buy. Today, the normal large supermarket carries some 5000 different types of product among 20 000 lines, a wide choice indeed. It is also not surprising that the responsibility of choosing what to buy lies with the consumer; how could it be otherwise? But we can choose whether to have a personal computer or a bunch of flowers or most other classes of consumer goods. We are compelled to have two basics of life, food and shelter, and it is not surprising that both of these elicit acute social and political, and indeed ethical debate. Food is a captive market and it can be argued that the food industry has a wide responsibility to help the consumer to choose, not only widely, but wisely.

It is sometimes said that people are in some way trapped by advertising into buying what the food industry wants them to buy. It is not often realised that most products which are advertised, fail. Each of the failures is obviously given the same promotional treatment as the others. The lament, 'I know that I am wasting at least half of my advertising budget, but I don't know which half', is well known in industry. When we come to research and development, I would say from my experience that it is more like only one in 10 or 20 products which even gets to the marketing stage. Influencing the public to buy your product, accept your viewpoint or change its behaviour, is a very difficult business. And independent experts, educators and commentators have so much greater opportunities than advertisers. We are bombarded with television and radio programmes on food, nutrition and health, and with columns in newspapers and magazines; nutritional advice comes through doctors' surgeries and clinics; and what an opportunity is offered by a captive school population accounting for at least eleven years of everybody's lifetime! But the educators, like the advertisers, know how difficult it is to get a message across.

So far I have dealt with the consumer, but of course there is no such archetype, there are only consumers, and each one's choice is influenced by a host of factors: need, availability, cost, preference, custom, perceptions of safety, labelling, convenience, lifestyle and, increasingly both informed and uninformed, even devious, public comment about nutrition. Food retailers and therefore manufacturers have to balance these in some way or other when competing in the marketplace.

Industry discharges its responsibilities to all its consumers first by legal requirements: products are microbiologically safe and wholesome, and descriptions are not misleading; secondly by demands of the marketplace: that there is a wide variety of choice which people can afford Should the industry go further than this? There is good argument to say it should not. For instance, should it only make and sell products which are healthy? The pitfalls here are obvious. Goethe said 'there is nothing more terrible than to see ignorance in action'. In the 1930s starch-reduced foods were considered to be healthier than starchy foods. 'Eat less bread and potatoes' was the advice given until quite recently by many experts, and brand names were established on this principle. It is even arguable that meat and fat intake increased because of this. It is difficult to imagine a more clear cut U-turn in expert opinion. And then there is food and drink which is nutritionally unnecessary or worse, but which exists entirely for pleasure or some other basic human need such as generosity or comfort or hospitality or sheer cultural tradition. There are valid and highly ethical arguments both for and against such foods and drinks. Nevertheless, there is a growing conviction that people in industry should take greater responsi-bility for the nutritional effect of commercial products on the wellbeing of the community of which they are part. The food companies themselves are increasingly acting upon this view, and it is no accident that substantial impetus exists now. Why is that? As I see it there are two reasons. First, it is a truism that it is diets, not foods, that can be unhealthy, and the explosion in sales of ready meals or recipe dishes which has occurred in the last few years provides an opportunity to balance whole meals for the major and minor nutrients in a way that was quite impossible in the past. Manufacturers of these dishes are responding strongly to this opportunity. I will give one example. I know from my experience with the development of Quorn products that detailed attention is being paid to different segments of the market. The needs of children, teenagers, young couples, young families, older families, older couples, the retired and the aged have been researched both for nutritional benefit and food choice, and possible nutritional effects of replacing present foods by various levels of the new products are being calculated. Secondly, an insatiable thirst has emerged amongst the population for nutritional understanding. Whatever the competitive position may be, it is in everybody's interest, including Government's, to promote nutrition education. This must be the best of all possible ways to ensure the best nutritional background at the current state of knowledge.

Although we are told that all analogies are false, I will still make one and return to my comments about the prebacteriology days and the myriad of half-baked or worse theories about disease and the host of experts each exhorting his audience that his way to good health was the true way. This great chorus was silenced by science. At present, we hear a similar chorus about nutrition and health. Once again, the food manufacturers and the public need clear scientific facts to silence the less respectable experts, populists and plain quacks. But even respectable nutritionists sometimes change their views to the confusion of the public and the delight of their detractors. I have no quarrel with this. There is no science which has not drastically changed course as new problems come to light and new facts are established, and nutritional science will continue to do so. But the pace and changing direction of research inevitably puts a brake on practical application.

I have a personal example of the difficulties in applying nutrition to product development. Some few years ago I invited eminent nutritionists to meet with my marketing people to help design products which would be nutritionally 'right'. I had noticed that food companies had sometimes been reproached, and we wanted to do the right thing. There were several such meetings, but the outcome was disappointing. One of the principles we had to work to was that a food which is not eaten, which is not bought, has no nutritional value, however well designed it may be nutritionally. The nutritionists had one more or less agreed view, reduce calories, but little else. I had high hopes for my novel approach to product development; in the event my credibility with the marketing departments suffered. I was unrealistic of course. Unlike microbiology, and some may be tempted to say that this was a much simpler field (I am reminded here of Sam Goldwyn's famous aphorism, 'with hindsight I could have predicted that'), we just do not know enough about nutrition. Why is the incidence of CHD falling so sharply? Why are some cancers doing likewise? What about vitamins and IQ? Is antioxidant in the blood a better risk indicator than cholesterol? And why do some dietary sinners evade punishment and live to an active and quick witted old age? But real people have always known that real people show real differences. Epidemiology can give rise to very blunt instruments.

We have come to realise, and this is now even 'official', that individuality in all human activities must be catered for. We do it, or try to do it, or pay lip service to doing it for artistic ability, for musical ability, for mathematics, for athletics, and sport, and in medical practice. We are going to have to do it increasingly for nutrition. This is by no means an original comment. I see that at another fiftieth anniversary celebration this year, that of the Food & Nutrition Board of the American Institute of Medicine, Sandford Miller made a similar prediction. The interests of consumers, government and industry all coincide here. We must have a full spectrum of choice to enable people to buy food as they see fit in the light of present expert opinion. But as discussed above, real knowledge which we can act upon is limited by the pace of scientific research, and I will take this opportunity to congratulate the Nutrition Society on promoting this for the past 50 years. Research will continue to establish more facts about long-term nutrition and how to apply these to people. I have been uncomfortably conscious during my fifties and now sixties, that I am one of that generation which was led to believe in earlier life that a diet including liberal helpings of milk, butter, cheese, eggs and meat was a good one, recommended by doctors and dietitians and supported by Government. We now discover that we are the at risk generation! It is a brave man who embarks upon social engineering without impeccable evidence. From my experience with regulating agencies I doubt that the present evidence would be sufficient if submitted by a food company, even for minor dietary changes.

It seems sensible to me that until facts about the effects of foods upon people have been suitably codified like other aspects of food safety and quality, the responsibility of industry as a whole, whatever individual companies may choose to do, is to be adventurous and imaginative in its products and services, but conservative, even beady-eyed, before it adopts the latest theory, whatever it may be, about improving the nation's health.

References

Drummond, J. C. & Wilbraham, A. (1957). *The Englishman's Food*. London: Jonathan Cape.
Galton, F. (1883). *Inquiries into Human Faculty and its Development*. London: Macmillan and Co. p. 285.

Index